WEIGHT IN AMERICA
OBESITY, EATING DISORDERS, AND OTHER HEALTH RISKS

ISSN 1551-2118

WEIGHT IN AMERICA

OBESITY, EATING DISORDERS, AND OTHER HEALTH RISKS

Barbara Wexler

INFORMATION PLUS® REFERENCE SERIES
Formerly Published by Information Plus, Wylie, Texas

GALE
CENGAGE Learning·

Farmington Hills, Mich • San Francisco • New York • Waterville, Maine
Meriden, Conn • Mason, Ohio • Chicago

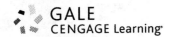

Weight in America: Obesity, Eating Disorders, and Other Health Risks

Barbara Wexler

Kepos Media, Inc.: Steven Long and Janice Jorgensen, Series Editors

Project Editors: Laura Avery, Tracie Moy

Rights Acquisition and Management: Lynn Vagg

Composition: Evi Abou-El-Seoud, Mary Beth Trimper

Manufacturing: Rita Wimberley

For product information and technology assistance, contact us at
Gale Customer Support, 1-800-877-4253.
For permission to use material from this text or product,
submit all requests online at **www.cengage.com/permissions.**
Further permissions questions can be e-mailed to
permissionrequest@cengage.com

Cover photograph: © Marques/Shutterstock.com.

While every effort has been made to ensure the reliability of the information presented in this publication, Gale, a part of Cengage Learning, does not guarantee the accuracy of the data contained herein. Gale accepts no payment for listing; and inclusion in the publication of any organization, agency, institution, publication, service, or individual does not imply endorsement of the editors or publisher. Errors brought to the attention of the publisher and verified to the satisfaction of the publisher will be corrected in future editions.

Gale
27500 Drake Rd.
Farmington Hills, MI 48331-3535

ISBN-13: 978-0-7876-5103-9 (set)
ISBN-13: 978-1-57302-705-2

ISSN 1551-2118

This title is also available as an e-book.
ISBN-13: 978-1-57302-674-1 (set)
Contact your Gale sales representative for ordering information.

TABLE OF CONTENTS

PREFACE

Weight in America: Obesity, Eating Disorders, and Other Health Risks is part of the *Information Plus Reference Series*. The purpose of each volume of the series is to present the latest facts on a topic of pressing concern in modern American life. These topics include the most controversial and studied social issues of the 21st century: abortion, capital punishment, care for the elderly, crime, the environment, health care, immigration, race and ethnicity, social welfare, women, youth, and many more. Although this series is written especially for high school and undergraduate students, it is an excellent resource for anyone in need of factual information on current affairs.

By presenting the facts, it is the intention of Gale, Cengage Learning to provide its readers with everything they need to reach an informed opinion on current issues. To that end, there is a particular emphasis in this series on the presentation of scientific studies, surveys, and statistics. These data are generally presented in the form of tables, charts, and other graphics placed within the text of each book. Every graphic is directly referred to and carefully explained in the text. The source of each graphic is presented within the graphic itself. The data used in these graphics are drawn from the most reputable and reliable sources such as from the various branches of the U.S. government and from private organizations and associations. Every effort has been made to secure the most recent information available. Readers should bear in mind that many major studies take years to conduct and that additional years often pass before the data from these studies are made available to the public. Therefore, in many cases the most recent information available in 2014 is from 2011 or 2012. Older statistics are sometimes presented as well, if they are landmark studies or of particular interest and no more-recent information exists.

Although statistics are a major focus of the *Information Plus Reference Series*, they are by no means its only content. Each book also presents the widely held positions and important ideas that shape how the book's subject is discussed in the United States. These positions are explained in detail and, where possible, in the words of their proponents. Some of the other material to be found in these books includes historical background, descriptions of major events related to the subject, relevant laws and court cases, and examples of how these issues play out in American life. Some books also feature primary documents or have pro and con debate sections that provide the words and opinions of prominent Americans on both sides of a controversial topic. All material is presented in an evenhanded and unbiased manner; readers will never be encouraged to accept one view of an issue over another.

HOW TO USE THIS BOOK

The United States has a serious weight problem. The majority of Americans weigh more than they should, and roughly one-third are considered obese. Overweight and obesity have serious health consequences, and their epidemic levels in the United States have had a major impact on society. When it comes to food, however, overweight and obesity are not the only problems that Americans face. Some suffer from eating disorders, such as anorexia nervosa and bulimia nervosa, disorders that also have a devastating effect on health. This book brings together information from academic and governmental sources on myriad aspects of overweight, obesity, and eating disorders, including their prevalence in the United States, their consequences, public opinion about them, and preventive measures.

Weight in America: Obesity, Eating Disorders, and Other Health Risks consists of 11 chapters and three appendixes. Each chapter is devoted to a particular aspect of weight in the United States. For a summary of the information that is covered in each chapter, please see the synopses that are provided in the Table of Contents. Chapters generally begin with an overview of the basic facts and background information on the chapter's topic, then proceed to examine subtopics of particular interest. For example, Chapter 8: Political, Legal, and Social Issues of Overweight and Obesity begins by considering the global politics of obesity and the World Health Organization strategy to combat overweight and obesity throughout the world. This is followed by a discussion of the U.S. war on obesity, including federal, state, and local policies to prevent and reduce obesity. The chapter then discusses how junk food fuels the obesity epidemic, describes lawsuits filed against the food industry, and questions whether nutrition labeling will help consumers make healthier food choices. It also includes a discussion of food industry initiatives to help Americans achieve healthy weights. It concludes with a discussion of weight-based discrimination, stigma, and bias. Readers can find their way through a chapter by looking for the section and subsection headings, which are clearly set off from the text. They can also refer to the book's extensive Index if they already know what they are looking for.

Statistical Information

The tables and figures featured throughout *Weight in America: Obesity, Eating Disorders, and Other Health Risks* will be of particular use to readers in learning about this issue. These tables and figures represent an extensive collection of the most recent and important statistics on weight and related issues. For example, graphics cover the percentage of obese adults by state, race, and ethnicity; the prevalence of obesity among adults; the names found on ingredient labels for added sugars; dubious diet claims; and fruit and vegetable consumption rates of adults and teens. Gale, Cengage Learning believes that making this information available to readers is the most important way to fulfill the goal of this book: to help readers understand the issues and controversies surrounding overweight and obesity in the United States and reach their own conclusions about them.

Each table or figure has a unique identifier appearing above it, for ease of identification and reference. Titles for the tables and figures explain their purpose. At the end of each table or figure, the original source of the data is provided.

To help readers understand these often complicated statistics, all tables and figures are explained in the text. References in the text direct readers to the relevant statistics. Furthermore, the contents of all tables and figures are fully indexed. Please see the opening section of the Index at the back of this volume for a description of how to find tables and figures within it.

Appendixes

Besides the main body text and images, *Weight in America: Obesity, Eating Disorders, and Other Health Risks* has three appendixes. The first is the Important Names and Addresses directory. Here, readers will find contact information for a number of government and private organizations that can provide further information on aspects of overweight and obesity and weight and eating disorders. The second appendix is the Resources section, which can also assist readers in conducting their own research. In this section, the author and editors of *Weight in America: Obesity, Eating Disorders, and Other Health Risks* describe some of the sources that were most useful during the compilation of this book. The final appendix is the detailed Index. It has been greatly expanded from previous editions and should make it even easier to find specific topics in this book.

COMMENTS AND SUGGESTIONS

The editors of the *Information Plus Reference Series* welcome your feedback on *Weight in America: Obesity, Eating Disorders, and Other Health Risks*. Please direct all correspondence to:

Editors
Information Plus Reference Series
27500 Drake Rd.
Farmington Hills, MI 48331-3535

CHAPTER 1
AMERICANS WEIGH IN OVER TIME

More die in the United States of too much food than of too little.

—John Kenneth Galbraith, *The Affluent Society* (1998)

In 2013 more Americans were fatter than ever before—in fact, they remain the heaviest since the U.S. government started tracking patterns of body weight of the U.S. adult population during the first half of the 20th century. The Centers for Disease Control and Prevention (CDC) reports in "Adult Obesity Facts" (August 16, 2013, http://www .cdc.gov/obesity/data/adult.html) that roughly 36% of adults in the United States—about 78 million—are considered obese. In "Prevalence of Obesity, in the United States, 2009–2010" (January 2012, http:// www.cdc.gov/nchs/data/databriefs/db82.pdf), Cynthia L. Ogden et al. analyze data from the CDC's 2009–10 National Health and Nutrition Examination Survey. The researchers reveal that in 2009–10, 35.7% of American adults and 16.9% of youth aged 2 to 19 years were obese. Despite billions of dollars spent on diet programs, overweight and obesity are widespread and increasingly prevalent throughout the United States.

Although Americans' body weight had been increasing incrementally during the last century, obesity skyrocketed between 1976–80 and 2009–10, from 15% to 35.7%. In *F as in Fat: How Obesity Threatens America's Future 2013* (August 16, 2013, http://www .rwjf.org/content/dam/farm/reports/reports/2013/rwjf40 7528), Jeffrey Levi et al. report that while more than two-thirds (68.7%) of American adults are either overweight or obese, after three decades of steady increases, obesity rates in nearly every state appear to have leveled off. Nonetheless, every state reports obesity rates greater than 20%, and in 13 states adult obesity rates are greater than 30%. Levi et al. observe, "It's hard to believe that—just 30 years ago—the highest adult obesity rate for any state was still lower than the lowest obesity rates today."

An analysis of data from the CDC's 2012 Behavioral Risk Factor Surveillance System reveals that the prevalence of self-reported obesity was greater than 30% in 12 states and from 25% to 29% in approximately half the states. (See Figure 1.1.) (The prevalence rate is the number of cases of a disease or condition present during a specified interval, usually a year, divided by the population.)

In "Prevalence of Obesity and Trends in the Distribution of Body Mass Index Among US Adults, 1999–2010" (*JAMA*, vol. 307, no. 5, February 1, 2012), Katherine M. Flegal et al. compare the prevalence of adult obesity from the 2009–10 National Health and Nutrition Examination Survey (NHANES) and compare it with data from 1999–2008. Although the overall prevalence of obesity for women was unchanged from 1999 to 2010, there was a noticeable change for men. Flegal et al. report that non-Hispanic African Americans had the highest rates of obesity (49.5%), compared with Mexican Americans (40.4%), Hispanics (39.1%), and non-Hispanic whites (34.3%).

In the United States many researchers believe that obesity is the second-leading cause of preventable death after smoking. There is conclusive scientific evidence that mortality (death) risk increases with increasing weight and that even slightly overweight adults—people of average height who are 10 to 20 pounds (4.5 to 9.1 kg) above their ideal weight—are at increased risk of premature death. The rising prevalence of overweight and obesity not only foretells increasing adverse effects on health and longevity but also guarantees increased costs for medical care. Overweight and obesity increase the risk of developing a range of ailments including heart disease, stroke, selected cancers, sleep apnea (interrupted breathing while sleeping), respiratory problems, osteoarthritis (loss of joint bone and cartilage), gallbladder disease, fatty liver disease (the deposition of fats, such as triglycerides in the liver, which may lead to an enlarged liver and elevated liver enzymes), and diabetes

FIGURE 1.1

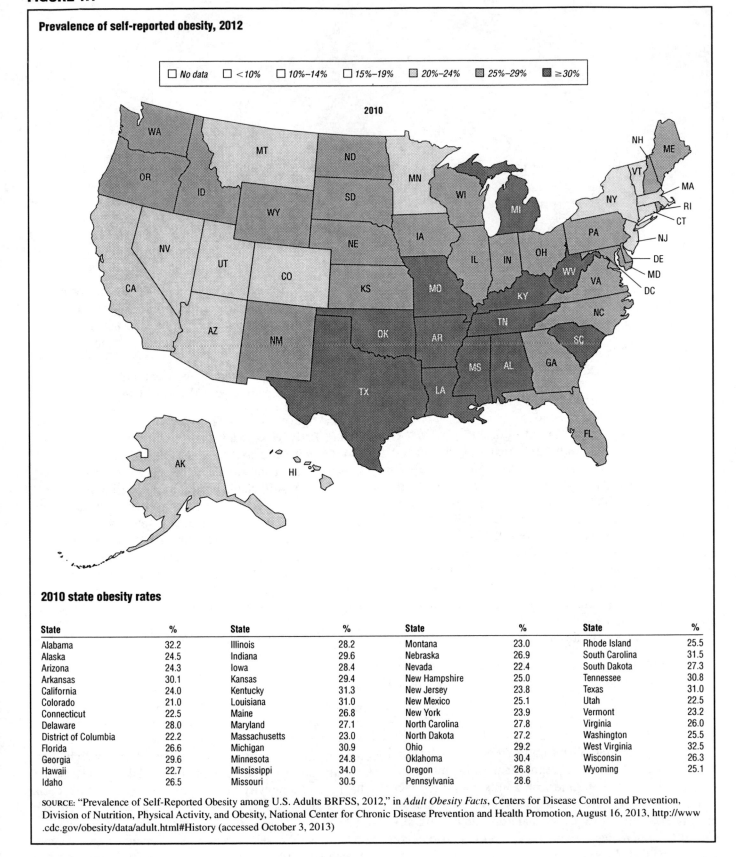

Prevalence of self-reported obesity, 2012

Legend: ☐ No data ☐ <10% ☐ 10%–14% ☐ 15%–19% ☐ 20%–24% ▨ 25%–29% ▨ ≥30%

2010

2010 state obesity rates

State	%	State	%	State	%	State	%
Alabama	32.2	Illinois	28.2	Montana	23.0	Rhode Island	25.5
Alaska	24.5	Indiana	29.6	Nebraska	26.9	South Carolina	31.5
Arizona	24.3	Iowa	28.4	Nevada	22.4	South Dakota	27.3
Arkansas	30.1	Kansas	29.4	New Hampshire	25.0	Tennessee	30.8
California	24.0	Kentucky	31.3	New Jersey	23.8	Texas	31.0
Colorado	21.0	Louisiana	31.0	New Mexico	25.1	Utah	22.5
Connecticut	22.5	Maine	26.8	New York	23.9	Vermont	23.2
Delaware	28.0	Maryland	27.1	North Carolina	27.8	Virginia	26.0
District of Columbia	22.2	Massachusetts	23.0	North Dakota	27.2	Washington	25.5
Florida	26.6	Michigan	30.9	Ohio	29.2	West Virginia	32.5
Georgia	29.6	Minnesota	24.8	Oklahoma	30.4	Wisconsin	26.3
Hawaii	22.7	Mississippi	34.0	Oregon	26.8	Wyoming	25.1
Idaho	26.5	Missouri	30.5	Pennsylvania	28.6		

SOURCE: "Prevalence of Self-Reported Obesity among U.S. Adults BRFSS, 2012," in *Adult Obesity Facts*, Centers for Disease Control and Prevention, Division of Nutrition, Physical Activity, and Obesity, National Center for Chronic Disease Prevention and Health Promotion, August 16, 2013, http://www .cdc.gov/obesity/data/adult.html#History (accessed October 3, 2013)

mellitus (abnormally high blood glucose resulting from the body's inability to use blood glucose for energy). Levi et al. observe that 10% of annual U.S. health care spending—between $147 billion and $210 billion—is related to obesity and that people who are obese spend 42% more on health care than do healthy-weight people.

Overweight and obesity also exact a personal toll, with affected individuals at increased risk for emotional, psychological, and social problems. Overweight children, teens, and adults suffer from depression, low self-esteem, and other mental health and emotional problems more than their normal-weight counterparts. Along with a physical inability to participate in many activities, people who are overweight or obese may encounter weight-based stigmatization, bias, and discrimination in school and at the workplace and may be excluded from social opportunities.

TRENDS IN U.S. BIRTH WEIGHTS

Although the ideal birth weight varies based on the expectant mother's ethnicity, for women in the United States the average ideal birth weight is approximately 7 pounds, 8 ounces (3,402 g). In the United States the percentage of babies born with low birth weight (LBW)—less than 5 pounds, 8 ounces (2,500 g)—rose between 1990 and 2010. (See Table 1.1.) According to Joyce A. Martin et al., in "Births: Final Data for 2011" (*National Vital Statistics Reports*, vol. 62, no. 1, June 28, 2013), the LBW rate declined slightly from 8.2% in 2010 to 8.1% in 2011. The percentage of infants with very low birth weight (VLBW)—less than 3 pounds, 4 ounces (1,500 g)—remained steady between 1990 (1.3%) and 2011 (1.4%). In 2011 more than twice as many non-Hispanic African American mothers gave birth to LBW and VLBW infants, 13.3% and 3%, respectively, as did non-Hispanic white mothers (7% LBW and 1.1% VLBW).

TABLE 1.1

Percentage of low birth weights and very low birth weights by race and Hispanic origin, selected years, 1981–2011

Year	All races[a]	Very low birthweight[g] Non-Hispanic White[b]	Black[b]	Hispanic[c]	All races[a]	Low birthweight[h] Non-Hispanic White[b]	Black[b]	Hispanic[c]
				Percent				
2011	1.44	1.14	2.99	1.20	8.10	7.09	13.33	7.02
2010	1.45	1.16	2.98	1.20	8.15	7.14	13.53	6.97
2009	1.45	1.16	3.06	1.19	8.16	7.19	13.61	6.94
2008	1.46	1.18	3.01	1.20	8.18	7.22	13.71	6.96
2007	1.49	1.19	3.20	1.21	8.22	7.28	13.90	6.93
2006	1.49	1.20	3.15	1.19	8.26	7.32	13.97	6.99
2005	1.49	1.21	3.27	1.20	8.19	7.29	14.02	6.88
2004	1.48	1.20	3.15	1.20	8.08	7.20	13.74	6.79
2003	1.45	1.18	3.12	1.16	7.93	7.04	13.55	6.69
2002	1.46	1.17	3.15	1.17	7.82	6.91	13.39	6.55
2001	1.44	1.17	3.08	1.14	7.68	6.76	13.07	6.47
2000	1.43	1.14	3.10	1.14	7.57	6.60	13.13	6.41
1999	1.45	1.15	3.18	1.14	7.62	6.64	13.23	6.38
1998	1.45	1.15	3.11	1.15	7.57	6.55	13.17	6.44
1997	1.42	1.12	3.05	1.13	7.51	6.47	13.11	6.42
1996	1.37	1.08	3.02	1.12	7.39	6.36	13.12	6.28
1995	1.35	1.04	2.98	1.11	7.32	6.20	13.21	6.29
1994	1.33	1.01	2.99	1.08	7.28	6.06	13.34	6.25
1993	1.33	1.00	2.99	1.06	7.22	5.92	13.43	6.24
1992[d]	1.29	0.94	2.97	1.04	7.08	5.73	13.40	6.10
1991[d]	1.29	0.94	2.97	1.02	7.12	5.72	13.62	6.15
1990[e]	1.27	0.93	2.93	1.03	6.97	5.61	13.32	6.06
1989[f]	1.28	0.93	2.97	1.05	7.05	5.62	13.61	6.18
1988	1.24	—	—	—	6.93	—	—	—
1987	1.24	—	—	—	6.90	—	—	—
1986	1.21	—	—	—	6.81	—	—	—
1985	1.21	—	—	—	6.75	—	—	—
1984	1.19	—	—	—	6.72	—	—	—
1983	1.19	—	—	—	6.82	—	—	—
1982	1.18	—	—	—	6.75	—	—	—
1981	1.16	—	—	—	6.81	—	—	—

—Data not available.
[a]Includes races other than white and black and origin not stated.
[b]Race and Hispanic origin are reported separately on birth certificates. Persons of Hispanic origin may be of any race. Race categories are consistent with 1977 Office of Management and Budget standards. Forty states and the District of Columbia reported multiple-race data for 2011 that were bridged to single-race categories for comparability with other states. Multiple-race reporting areas vary for 2003–2011.
[c]Includes all persons of Hispanic origin of any race.
[d]Data by Hispanic origin exclude New Hampshire, which did not report Hispanic origin.
[e]Data by Hispanic origin exclude New Hampshire and Oklahoma, which did not report Hispanic origin.
[f]Data by Hispanic origin exclude New Hampshire, Oklahoma, and Louisiana, which did not report Hispanic origin.
[g]Less than 1,500 grams (3 lb. 4 oz.).
[h]Less than 2,500 grams (5 lb. 8 oz.).

SOURCE: Adapted from Joyce A. Martin et al., "Table 24. Very Preterm and Preterm and Very Low Birthweight and Low Birthweight Births, by Race and Hispanic Origin of Mother: United States, 1981–2011," in "Births: Final Data for 2011," *National Vital Statistics Reports*, vol. 62, no.1, June 28, 2013, http://www.cdc.gov/nchs/data/nvsr/nvsr62/nvsr62_01.pdf#table25 (accessed October 4, 2013)

LBW and VLBW are major predictors of infant morbidity (illness or disease) and mortality. According to Martin et al., less than 2% of LBW infants in 2009 died during the first year of life, compared with 0.2% of infants born at normal weight. The risk for VLBW infants is much higher with 2009 numbers, indicating that 23% failed to survive their first year. The risk of delivering an LBW infant is greatest among the youngest and oldest mothers; however, many of the LBW births among older mothers are attributable to their higher rates of multiple births.

Birth Weight Influences Risk of Disease

Although the relationship between birth weight and development of disease in adulthood is an emerging field of research, and scientists cannot yet fully explain how and why birth weight is a predictor of health and illness in later life, mounting evidence indicates that both LBW and higher-than-average birth weight are linked to future health problems. Research reveals that LBW infants are more likely than normal-weight infants to develop disease in later life. Male infants with LBW who gain weight rapidly before their first birthday appear to be at the highest risk. Researchers hypothesize that LBW infants have fewer muscle cells at birth and that rapid weight gain during the first year of life may lead to disproportionate amounts of fat to muscle and above-average body mass. Infants with LBW who later develop above-average body mass have an increased risk for developing diseases such as type 2 diabetes (an inability to produce sufficient insulin, the hormone that regulates blood glucose), hypertension (high blood pressure), and cardiovascular disease (diseases of the heart and blood vessels).

Keith M. Godfrey, Hazel M. Inskip, and Mark A. Hanson find in "The Long-Term Effects of Prenatal Development on Growth and Metabolism" (*Seminars in Reproductive Medicine*, vol. 29, no. 3, May 2011) that LBW and poor rates of infant growth and development are associated with an increased risk for cardiovascular disease, type 2 diabetes, and osteoporosis (thinning of the bones that makes them more likely to fracture). The risk of developing these diseases increases when restricted early growth and development are followed by increased weight gain during childhood. The researchers also note that abnormally high birth weights are associated with an increased risk for obesity and type 2 diabetes.

LBW has also been linked to the development of asthma. In "Is the Association between Low Birth Weight and Asthma Independent of Genetic and Shared Environmental Factors?" (*American Journal of Epidemiology*, vol. 169, no. 11, June 1, 2009), a study of 21,588 twins, Eduardo Villamor, Anastasia Iliadou, and Sven Cnattingius find that LBW is associated with asthma during childhood and adult life.

Evidence also indicates that birth weight is related to a risk of developing breast cancer. Xiaohui Xu et al. consider 18 epidemiological (population) studies that detail 16,424 cases of breast cancer to determine whether birth weight influenced the risk of developing breast cancer in adulthood. The results of the study were published in "Birth Weight as a Risk Factor for Breast Cancer: A Meta-analysis of 18 Epidemiological Studies" (*Journal of Women's Health*, vol. 18, no. 8, August 2009). The researchers find that women who weighed more than 8 pounds, 13 ounces (4,000 g) when they were born were at greater risk for breast cancer than women who had birth weights of less than 5 pounds, 8 ounces to 6 pounds, 10 ounces (2,500 to 3,000 g) and that this risk followed a classic dose-response pattern—each incremental increase in birth weight increased the risk of developing the disease.

Athanasios Michos, Fei Xue, and Karin B. Michels indicate in "Birth Weight and the Risk of Testicular Cancer: A Meta-Analysis" (*International Journal of Cancer*, vol. 121, no. 5, September 1, 2007) that both LBW and high birth weight (HBW), or weight greater than 8 pounds, 13 ounces, increase the risk of testicular cancer in men. Men with LBW were 18% more likely and men with HBW were 12% more likely to develop testicular cancer than men of average birth weight.

HBW is also associated with an increased risk for childhood cancer. Michael R. Sprehe et al. observe in "Comparison of Birth Weight Corrected for Gestational Age and Birth Weight Alone in Prediction of Development of Childhood Leukemia and Central Nervous System Tumors" (*Pediatric Blood Cancers*, vol. 54, no. 2, February 2010) that HBW is most closely linked to an increased risk of developing acute lymphoblastic leukemia (a cancer of the blood and bone marrow and one of the most common cancers in children).

In "Birth Size, Infant Weight Gain, and Motor Development Influence Adult Physical Performance" (*Medicine and Science in Sports and Exercise*, vol. 41, no. 6, June 2009), Charlotte L. Ridgway et al. look at birth weight as an influence on adult physical performance measures, including muscle strength, endurance, and aerobic fitness. The researchers find that LBW is associated with impaired aerobic fitness and a higher resting pulse rate in adulthood, independent of adult body size. Higher birth weight is associated with earlier motor development, as evidenced in standing unaided and walking at younger ages. It is also associated with increased handgrip strength in adolescents, young adults, and even in older adults, which suggests that the effects of birth weight on physical performance may be lifelong. Higher birth weight, greater infant weight gain, and earlier motor development were independently associated with muscle strength and endurance, whereas higher birth weight and lower infant weight gain were associated with higher levels of aerobic fitness. Ridgway et al. explain that the link between higher birth weight and greater muscle strength and endurance may in part reflect the relationship between birth weight and lean muscle in adults— people with higher birth weights are likely to have increased muscle mass. Similarly, the relationship between lower infant weight gain and improved aerobic fitness may be attributable to the fact that rapid weight gain during infancy may preferentially produce fat rather than lean muscle tissue.

The only action that can alter the birth weight of an infant is if the mother modifies her weight gain during the pregnancy. In 2013 most health professionals concurred that for normal-weight women the optimal weight gain during pregnancy ranged between 15 and 25 pounds (6.8 and 11.3 kg) of fat and lean mass. Furthermore, the landmark study "Composition of Gestational Weight Gain Impacts Maternal Fat Retention and Infant Birth Weight" (*American Journal of Obstetrics and Gynecology*, vol. 189, no. 5, November 2003) conducted by Nancy F. Butte et al. of the Children's Nutrition Research Center in Houston, Texas, reveals that a newborn's birth weight and the mother's postpregnancy weight are influenced not only by how much weight is gained during the pregnancy but also by the source of the excess weight. The researchers conducted body scans of 63 women before, during, and after their pregnancies and recorded changes in the women's weight from water, protein, fat, and potassium—a marker for changes in muscle tissue, which is one component of lean mass. Butte et al. find that increases in lean mass, and not fat mass, appeared to influence infant size. Independent of how much fat the women gained during pregnancy, only lean body mass increased the birth weight of the infant, with women who gained more lean body mass giving birth to larger infants.

In "Birth Weight and Long-Term Overweight Risk: Systematic Review and a Meta-analysis Including 643,902 Persons from 66 Studies and 26 Countries Globally" (*PLoS One*, vol. 7, no. 10, October 17, 2012), Karen Schellong et al. reviewed 66 studies to analyze the relationship between birth weight and later risk of overweight. The researchers find that LBW is associated with lower long-term risk of overweight, while HBW predisposes for later overweight. Schellong et al. suggest that managing expectant mothers' nutrition and weight gain may be "a promising strategy to lower overweight risk for the long term, globally."

EARLY NUTRITION INCREASES RISK OF OBESITY. Research demonstrates that LBW and low weight gain during infancy are associated with coronary heart disease. Similarly, research indicates that rapid weight gain in infancy is shown to predict obesity in childhood.

In 2004 a landmark study funded by the National Institutes of Health and conducted at the Children's Hospital of Philadelphia, the University of Pennsylvania School of Medicine, and the University of Iowa Fomon Infant Nutrition Unit sought to determine which periods of weight gain in infancy might be associated with adult obesity.

In "Weight Gain in the First Week of Life and Overweight in Adulthood: A Cohort Study of European American Subjects Fed Infant Formula" (*Circulation*, vol. 111, no. 15, April 19, 2005), Nicolas Stettler et al. review the data for 653 subjects who had been weighed on seven occasions during infancy and were contacted when they were young adults, aged 20 to 32 years, when they again reported their height and weight. The researchers pinpointed the period between birth and age eight days as potentially critical because weight gain during the first week of life was associated with adulthood overweight status. The formula-fed babies who gained weight rapidly during their first week of life were significantly more likely to be overweight decades later. Stettler et al. conclude that "in formula-fed infants, weight gain during the first week of life may be a critical determinant for the development of obesity several decades later." The researchers also observe that their findings reinforce the recommendation by the American Academy of Pediatrics that infants should be exclusively breast-fed for the first six months of life. Among the many health benefits associated with breast-feeding is the fact that breast-fed babies are much less likely than formula-fed babies to become obese adults.

A high-calorie diet in infancy predicts not only faster early weight gain but also greater fat mass in childhood, which in turn increases the risk of obesity in adulthood. In "Nutrition in Infancy and Long-Term Risk of Obesity: Evidence from 2 Randomized Controlled Trials" (*American Journal of Nutrition*, vol. 92, no. 5, November 2010), Atul Singhal et al. report the results of a rigorous long-term study that followed infants randomly assigned to receive either a control formula or a formula containing more protein and calories than the control formula. When the children were examined at ages five and eight, those who had received the nutrient-rich formula had increased fat mass.

L. G. Andersen et al. confirm in "Weight and Weight Gain during Early Infancy Predict Childhood Obesity: A Case-Cohort Study" (*International Journal of Obesity*, vol. 36, no. 10, October 2012) that infant weight gain during the first months of life is associated with childhood obesity. This finding suggests that monitoring and controlling weight gain shortly after birth may help to prevent future obesity.

DEFINING AND ASSESSING IDEAL WEIGHT, OVERWEIGHT, AND OBESITY

Historically, the determination of desirable, healthy, or ideal weights have been derived from demographic and actuarial statistics (data compiled to assess insurance

TABLE 1.2

Defining overweight and obesity

Body weight status can be categorized as underweight, healthy weight, overweight, or obese. Body mass index (BMI) is a useful tool that can be used to estimate an individual's body weight status. BMI is a measure of weight in kilograms (kg) relative to height in meters (m) squared. The terms overweight and obese describe ranges of weight that are greater than what is considered healthy for a given height, while underweight describes a weight that is lower than what is considered healthy for a given height. These categories are a guide, and some people at a healthy weight also may have weight-responsive health conditions. Because children and adolescents are growing, their BMI is plotted on growth charts for sex and age. The percentile indicates the relative position of the child's BMI among children of the same sex and age.

Category	Children and adolescents (BMI for age percentile range)	Adults (BMI)
Underweight	Less than the 5th percentile	Less than 18.5 kg/m^2
Healthy weight	5th percentile to less than the 85th percentile	18.5 to 24.9 kg/m^2
Overweight	85th percentile to less than the 95th percentile	25.0 to 29.9 kg/m^2
Obese	Equal to or greater than the 95th percentile	30.0 kg/m^2 or greater

SOURCE: "Overweight and Obese: What Do They Mean?" in *Dietary Guidelines for Americans, 2010*, 7th ed., U.S. Department of Health and Human Services and U.S. Department of Agriculture, December 2010, http://health.gov/dietaryguidelines/dga2010/DietaryGuidelines2010.pdf (accessed October 7, 2013)

risk and formulate insurance premiums). The National Center for Health Statistics (NCHS) compiles and analyzes demographic data (the heights and weights of a representative sample of the U.S. population) to develop standards for desirable weight. In 1943 the Metropolitan Life Insurance Company (MetLife) introduced standard weight-for-height tables for men and women based on an analysis of actuarial data. The MetLife weight-for-height tables assisted adults in determining if their weight was within an appropriate range for height and frame size. Revised in 1959 and 1983, the tables were based on actuarial data, in which desirable or ideal weight was defined as the weight for height that was associated with the lowest mortality rate, or longest life span, among the client population of adults (policyholders) insured by MetLife.

Even though the MetLife and other weight-for-height tables remained in use in 2014, many health professionals and medical researchers believe these tables have limited utility. Nearly every weight-for-height table shows different acceptable weight ranges for men and women, and there continues to be considerable debate among health professionals over which table to use. The tables also lack information about body composition, such as the ratio of fat to lean muscle mass; their data are derived primarily from white populations and do not represent the entire U.S. population; they generally do not take age into consideration; and it is often unclear how frame size is determined. Furthermore, it is now known that ideal, healthy, or low-risk weight varies for different populations and varies for the same population at different times and in relation to different causes of morbidity and mortality.

The limitations of weight-for-height tables have prompted health care practitioners and researchers to adopt other measures that allow comparison of weight independent of height and frame across populations to define desirable or healthy weight as well as overweight and obesity. For example, the *Dietary Guidelines for Americans, 2010* (December 2010, http://health.gov/dietaryguidelines/dga 2010/DietaryGuidelines2010.pdf), which is published jointly

by the U.S. Department of Health and Human Services and the U.S. Department of Agriculture (USDA), uses the body mass index (BMI), a measure that incorporates height and weight to categorize adult body weight as underweight, healthy weight, overweight, or obese. Because children and adolescents are growing, their BMIs are plotted on a curve that compares them to children of the same age and sex. (See Table 1.2.) A child's relative position on this curve indicates whether he or she is underweight, healthy weight, overweight, or obese.

Overweight is generally defined as excess body weight in relation to height, when compared with a predetermined standard of acceptable, desirable, or ideal weight. One definition characterizes individuals as overweight if they are between 10 and 30 pounds (4.5 and 13.6 kg) heavier than the desirable weight for height. Overweight does not necessarily result from excessive body fat; people may become overweight as the result of an increase in lean muscle. For example, even though muscular bodybuilders with minimal body fat frequently weigh more than nonathletes of the same height, they are overweight because of their increased muscle mass rather than increased fat.

Rather than viewing overweight and obesity as distinct conditions, many researchers prefer to consider weight as a curve or continuum with obesity at the far end of the curve. People who are obese constitute a subset of the overweight population. In this definition, only some overweight people are obese, but all obese people are overweight.

Similarly, there is still no uniform definition of obesity. Some health professionals describe anyone who is more than 30 pounds (13.6 kg) above his or her desirable weight for height as obese. Others assert that body weight 20% or more above desirable or ideal body weight constitutes obesity. Extreme or clinically severe obesity is often defined as weight twice the desirable weight or 100 pounds (45.4 kg) more than the desirable weight. Obesity is also defined as an excessively high amount of adipose tissue (body fat) in relation to lean body mass such as muscle and bone. The amount of body fat (also known as adiposity), the distribution of fat throughout the body, and the size of the adipose tissue deposits are also used to assess obesity because the location and distribution of body fat are considered to be important predictors of the health risks that are associated with obesity. The location and distribution of body fat may be measured by the ratio of waist-to-hip circumference. High ratios have been associated with higher risks of morbidity and mortality.

Historically, overweight and obese body types have been characterized as apple- or pear-shaped, depending on the anatomical site where fat is more prominent. In the apple or android type of obesity, fat is mainly located in the trunk (upper body, nape of the neck, shoulder, and abdomen). Gynoid obesity, or the pear-shape, features rounded hips and more fat located in the buttocks, thighs, and lower abdomen. Fat cells around the waist, flank, and abdomen are more active metabolically than those in the thighs, hips, and buttocks. This increased metabolic activity is thought to produce the increased health risks that are associated with android obesity. In general, women are more likely to have gynoid obesity.

Research reported in the March 26, 2011, issue of the *Lancet* disputes the relationship between abdominal obesity (android obesity) and the increased risk for cardiovascular disease. In "Separate and Combined Associations of Body-Mass Index and Abdominal Adiposity with Cardiovascular Disease: Collaborative Analysis of 58 Prospective Studies" (vol. 377, no. 9771), investigators in the Emerging Risk Factors Collaboration who tracked 221,934 adults for nearly a decade find that even though obesity (BMI greater than 30) significantly increases the risk for cardiovascular disease, the distribution of the excess fat does not appear to influence this risk. The investigators deemed all distributions of body fat equally harmful in terms of heart health and suggest that in addition to obesity, high blood pressure and cholesterol and a history of diabetes are important predictors of future risk of developing cardiovascular disease.

In an effort to more accurately characterize the relationship between weight, the distribution of body fat, and risk for cardiovascular disease, A. C. Carlsson et al. compared a variety of measures including weight, height, waist circumference (WC), waist-hip ratio (WHR), waist-hip-height ratio (WHHR), WC-to-height ratio (WCHR), and BMI. In "Novel and Established Anthropometric Measures and the Prediction of Incident Cardiovascular Disease: A Cohort Study" (*International Journal of Obesity*, vol. 37, no. 12, March 28, 2013), Carlsson et al. report that that WHHR is the most accurate predictor of cardiovascular risk.

There are many ways to measure body fat. Weighing an individual underwater in a laboratory with specialized equipment provides a highly accurate assessment of body fat. By performing hydrostatic or underwater weighing, an examiner obtains an estimate of whole-body density and uses this to calculate the percentage of the body that is fat. First, the subject is weighed on a land scale. The subject then puts on a diver's belt with weights to prevent floating during the weighing procedure, sits on a chair that is suspended from a precision scale, and is completely submerged. When maximum expiration of breath is achieved, the subject remains in this submerged position for about 10 seconds while the investigator reads the scale. This procedure is repeated as many as 10 times to obtain reliable, consistent values. The weight of the diver's belt and chair are subtracted from this weight to obtain the true value of the subject's mass in water.

Simpler, but potentially less accurate assessments of body fat include skinfold thickness measurements, which involve measuring subcutaneous (immediately below the skin) fat deposits using an instrument called a caliper in locations such as the upper arm. Skinfold thickness measurements rely on the fact that a certain fraction of total body fat is subcutaneous and by using a representative sample of that fat, overall body fatness (density) may be predicted. Several skinfold measurements are obtained, and the values are used in equations to calculate body density. Using a caliper, the examiner grasps a fold of skin and subcutaneous fat firmly, pulling it away from the underlying muscle tissue that follows the natural contour of the skin. The caliper jaws exert a relatively constant tension at the point of contact and measure skinfold thickness in millimeters. Most obesity researchers believe there is an acceptable correlation between skinfold thickness and body fat—that it is possible to estimate body fatness from the use of skinfold calipers. Skinfold thickness measurements are considered more subjective than underwater weights because the accuracy of measurements of skinfold thickness depends on the skill and technique of the examiner, and there may be variations in readings from one examiner to another.

Another technique used to evaluate body fat is bioelectric impedance analysis (BIA). BIA offers an indirect estimate of body fat and lean body mass. It entails passing an electrical current through the body and assessing the body's ability to conduct the current. It is based on the principle that resistance is inversely proportional to total body water when an electrical current (with a frequency of 70 megahertz) is applied through several electrodes that are placed on body extremities. Because greater conductivity occurs when there is a higher percentage of body water and because a higher percentage of body water indicates larger amounts of muscle and other lean tissue (fat cells contain less water than muscle cells), people with less fat are better able to conduct electrical current. BIA has been shown to correlate well with total body fat that has been assessed by other methods.

TABLE 1.3

Classification of overweight and obesity by body mass index (BMI), waist circumference, and associated disease risk

	BMI (kg/m²)	Obesity class	Disease risk[a] relative to normal weight and waist circumference	
			Men ≤ 102 cm (≤ 40 in) Women ≤ 88 cm (≤ 35 in)	> 102 cm (> 40 in) > 88 cm (> 35 in)
Underweight	<18.5		—	—
Normal[b]	18.5–24.9		—	—
Overweight	25.0–29.9		Increased	High
Obesity	30.0–34.9	I	High	Very high
	35.0–39.9	II	Very high	Very high
Extreme obesity	≥40	III	Extremely high	Extremely high

[a]Disease risk for type 2 diabetes, hypertension, and cardiovascular disease.
[b]Increased waist circumference can also be a marker for increased risk even in persons of normal weight.

SOURCE: "Table ES-4. Classification of Overweight and Obesity by BMI, Waist Circumference, and Associated Disease Risk," in *Clinical Guidelines on the Identification, Evaluation, and Treatment of Overweight and Obesity in Adults: The Evidence Report*, National Institutes of Health, National Heart, Lung, and Blood Institute in cooperation with The National Institute of Diabetes and Digestive and Kidney Diseases, September 1998, http://www.ncbi.nlm.nih.gov/books/NBK2003/pdf/TOC.pdf (accessed October 7, 2013)

Other means of estimating the location and distribution of body fat include waist-to-hip circumference ratios and imaging techniques such as ultrasound, computed tomography, or magnetic resonance imaging.

Waist Circumference and Waist-to-Hip Ratio

Along with height and weight, waist circumference is a common measure used to assess abdominal fat content. An excess of body fat in the abdomen or upper body is considered to increase the risk of developing heart disease, high blood pressure, diabetes, stroke, and certain cancers. Like body fat, health risks increase as the waist circumference increases. For men, a waist circumference greater than 40 inches (101.6 cm) is considered to confer increased health risks. Women are considered at increased risk when a waist measurement is 35 inches (88.9 cm) or greater. Waist-circumference measures lose their incremental predictive value in people with a BMI greater than or equal to 35 because these individuals generally exceed the cutoff points for increased risk. Table 1.3 shows the relationship between BMI, waist circumference, and disease risk for people who are underweight, normal weight, overweight, obese, and extremely obese.

In fact, research demonstrates that clothing size, which serves as a surrogate for waist circumference, can help predict disease risk. Laura A. E. Hughes et al. find that skirt and trouser sizes correlate well with waist-circumference measurements and that bigger skirt and trouser sizes are associated with a greater risk of developing selected cancers. In "Self-Reported Clothing Size as a Proxy Measure for Body Size" (*Epidemiology*, vol. 20, no. 5, September 2009), Hughes et al. indicate that skirt size predicts the risk for endometrial cancer (cancer of the lining of the uterus) and trouser size predicts the risk for renal cell carcinoma (kidney cancer).

The waist-to-hip ratio is the ratio of waist circumference to hip circumference, which is calculated by dividing waist circumference by hip circumference. For men and women, a waist-to-hip ratio of one or more is considered to place them at greater risk. Most people store body fat at the waist and abdomen (android body fat distribution) or at the hips (gynoid body fat distribution).

Body Mass Index

BMI is a single number that evaluates an individual's weight status in relation to height. It does not directly measure the percent of body fat; however, it offers a more accurate assessment of overweight and obesity than weight alone. It is a direct calculation based on height and weight, and it is not gender specific. BMI is the preferred measurement of health care professionals and obesity researchers to assess body fat and is the most common method of tracking overweight and obesity among adults. BMI, which is calculated by dividing weight in kilograms by the square of height in meters, classifies people as underweight, normal weight, overweight, or obese. Table 1.4 shows the formula used to calculate BMI when height is measured in either inches or centimeters and weight is measured in either pounds or kilograms.

The World Health Organization and the National Institutes of Health consider individuals overweight when their BMI is between 25 and 29.9, and they are classified as obese when their BMI exceeds 30. Table 1.5 shows the relationship between height, weight, and BMI. Table 1.3 shows the classification of overweight and obesity by BMI and distinguishes between three levels of obesity. Table 1.6 shows weights in pounds and kilograms that represent the three levels of obesity at two different heights: 5 feet, 4 inches (162.6 cm) and 5 feet, 9 inches (175.3 cm).

BMI is a simple, inexpensive tool for assessing weight, but it has several limitations. BMI may deem

TABLE 1.4

How to calculate body mass index (BMI)

You can calculate BMI as follows

$$BMI = \frac{Weight\ (kg)}{Height\ squared\ (m^2)}$$

If pounds and inches are used

$$BMI = \frac{Weight\ (pounds) \times 703}{Height\ squared\ (inches^2)}$$

Calculation directions and sample

Here is a shortcut method for calculating BMI. (Example: for a person who is 5 feet 5 inches tall weighing 180 lbs.)

1. Multiply weight (in pounds) by 703

$$180 \times 703 = 126,540$$

2. Multiply height (in inches) by height (in inches)

$$65 \times 65 = 4,225$$

3. Divide the answer in step 1 by the answer in step 2 to get the BMI.

$$126,540/4,225 = 29.9$$

$$BMI = 29.9$$

SOURCE: "You Can Calculate BMI As Follows," in *The Practical Guide: Identification, Evaluation, and Treatment of Overweight and Obesity in Adults*, National Institutes of Health, National Heart, Lung, and Blood Institute, North American Association for the Study of Obesity, October 2000, http://www.nhlbi.nih.gov/guidelines/obesity/prctgd_b.pdf (accessed October 7, 2013)

muscular athletes overweight when they are extremely fit and excess weight is the result of a larger amount of lean muscle. It may similarly misrepresent the health of older adults who as the result of muscle wasting (loss of muscle mass) may be considered to have a normal or healthy weight when they may actually be nutritionally depleted or overweight in terms of body fat composition. Even though it is an imperfect method for assessing individuals, BMI is useful for tracking weight trends in the population.

Definitions and Estimates of Prevalence Vary

Historically, varying definitions of, and criteria for, overweight and obesity have affected prevalence statistics and made it difficult to compare data. Some overweight- and obesity-related prevalence rates are crude or unadjusted estimates; others are age-adjusted estimates that offer different values. Early efforts to track overweight and obesity in the U.S. population relied on the 1943, 1959, and 1983 MetLife tables of desirable weight-for-height as the reference standard for overweight. During the last three decades, most government agencies and public health organizations have estimated overweight using data from a series of surveys conducted by the NCHS. These surveys include the National Health Examination Surveys, the National Health and Nutrition Examination Surveys (NHANES), and the Behavioral Risk Factor Surveillance System.

Despite changing definitions of overweight and obesity and various methods to track changes in the U.S. population, there is irrefutable evidence that the prevalence of overweight and obesity has steadily increased among people of both sexes, all ages, all racial and ethnic groups, and all educational levels. The prevalence of obesity in the United States was first reported in the 1960 National Health Examination Survey. Most obesity data referenced in the medical literature in 2013 were drawn from the 2009–10 NHANES study and the 2013 National Health Interview Studies, along with several other national studies. Data from the 1960 National Health Examination Survey and prior NHANES studies indicated that the prevalence of obesity was relatively constant between 1960 and 1980 and sharply increased between the late 1980s and 2010.

Overweight and obesity have steadily progressed at an alarming rate since the 1980s. Cheryl D. Fryar, Margaret D. Carroll, and Cynthia L. Ogden observe in "Prevalence of Overweight, Obesity, and Extreme Obesity among Adults: United States, Trends 1960–1962 through 2009–2010" (*NCHS Health E-Stat*, September 13, 2012) that in the United States the prevalence of obesity doubled between 1976–80 and 2009–10. During the same period the prevalence of overweight remained relatively stable. Figure 1.2 and Figure 1.3 show trends in overweight, obesity, and extreme obesity among men and women aged 20 to 74 years from 1960 through 2010.

Data from the National Health Interview Study reveal that the prevalence of obesity among adults aged 20 years and older has increased over time, from 19.4% in 1997 to 28.1% in March 2013. (See Figure 1.4.) The prevalence of overweight and obesity generally increases with advancing age, then starts to decline among people over the age of 60 years. In January through March 2013 for men and women combined, the prevalence of obesity was highest among adults aged 40 to 59 years (33.6%) and lowest among adults aged 20 to 39 years (24.1%). (See Figure 1.5.) There was no significant difference in the prevalence of obesity between men and women in all four age groups.

The age-adjusted prevalence of obesity in racial and ethnic minorities, especially minority women, is generally higher than in whites in the United States. According to Brian W. Ward, Jeannine S. Schiller, and Gulnur Freeman of the NCHS, in *Early Release of Selected Estimates Based on Data from the January–March 2013 National Health Interview Survey* (September 2013, http://www.cdc.gov/nchs/data/nhis/earlyrelease/earlyrelease201309_06.pdf), in 2013 for both sexes, non-Hispanic African Americans were more likely than Hispanics and non-Hispanic whites to be obese. The age-adjusted prevalence of obesity was highest among non-Hispanic African American women (38%) and lowest among non-Hispanic white women (24.7%). (See Figure 1.6.)

TABLE 1.5

Adult BMI (body mass index) chart

BMI	19	20	21	22	23	24	25	26	27	28	29	30	31	32	33	34	35
Height	Healthy weight						Overweight					Obese					
									Weight in pounds								
4'10"	91	96	100	105	110	115	119	124	129	134	138	143	148	153	158	162	167
4'11"	94	99	104	109	114	119	124	128	133	138	143	148	153	158	163	168	173
5'	97	102	107	112	118	123	128	133	138	143	148	153	158	163	158	174	179
5'1"	100	106	111	116	122	127	132	137	143	148	153	158	164	169	174	180	185
5'2"	104	109	115	120	126	131	136	142	147	153	158	164	169	175	180	186	191
5'3"	107	113	118	124	130	135	141	146	152	158	163	169	175	180	186	191	197
5'4"	110	116	122	128	134	140	145	151	157	163	169	174	180	186	192	197	204
5'5"	114	120	126	132	138	144	150	156	162	168	174	180	186	192	198	204	210
5'6"	118	124	130	136	142	148	155	161	167	173	179	186	192	198	204	210	216
5'7"	121	127	134	140	146	153	159	166	172	178	185	191	198	204	211	217	223
5'8"	125	131	138	144	151	158	164	171	177	184	190	197	203	210	216	223	230
5'9"	128	135	142	149	155	162	169	176	182	189	196	203	209	216	223	230	236
5'10"	132	139	146	153	160	167	174	181	188	195	202	209	216	222	229	236	243
5'11"	136	143	150	157	165	172	179	186	193	200	208	215	222	229	236	243	250
6'	140	147	154	162	169	177	184	191	199	206	213	221	228	235	242	250	258
6'1"	144	151	159	166	174	182	189	197	204	212	219	227	235	242	250	257	265
6'2"	148	155	163	171	179	186	194	202	210	218	225	233	241	249	256	264	272
6'3"	152	160	168	176	184	192	200	208	216	224	232	240	248	256	264	272	279

Notes: Locate the height of interest in the left-most column and read across the row for that height to the weight of interest. Follow the column of the weight up to the top row that lists the BMI. BMI of 18.5–24.9 is the healthy range, BMI of 25–29.9 is the overweight range, and BMI of 30 and above is the obese range.

SOURCE: "Figure 2. Adult BMI Chart," in *Dietary Guidelines for Americans, 2005,* 6th ed., U.S. Department of Health and Human Services and U.S. Department of Agriculture, January 2005. http://www.health.gov/dietaryguidelines/dga2005/document/pdf/DGA2005.pdf (accessed October 7, 2013)

TABLE 1.6

Obesity cut points for adults 5'4" and 5'9"

Height	Obesity class I	Obesity class II	Obesity class III
5'4"	174 pounds	204 pounds	232 pounds
5'4"	79 kilograms	93 kilograms	105 kilograms
5'9"	203 pounds	236 pounds	270 pounds
5'9"	92 kilograms	107 kilograms	123 kilograms

SOURCE: Margot Shields, Margaret D. Carroll, and Cynthia L. Ogden, "Table. Obesity Cut Points for Adults 5'4" and 5'9"," in "Adult Obesity Prevalence in Canada and the United States," *NCHS Data Brief*, no. 56, National Center for Health Statistics, March 2011, http://www.cdc.gov/nchs/data/databriefs/db56.pdf (accessed October 7, 2013)

FIGURE 1.2

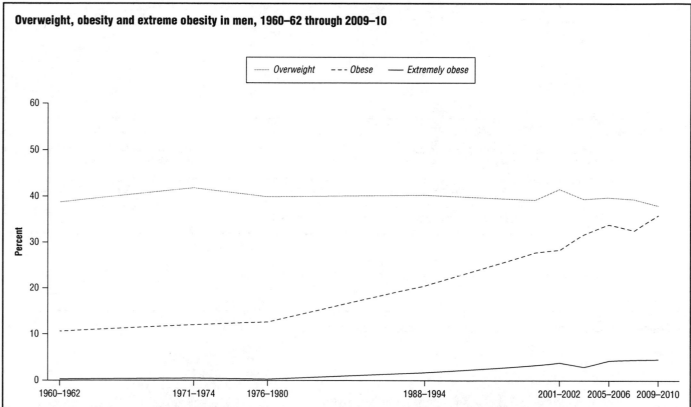

Overweight, obesity and extreme obesity in men, 1960–62 through 2009–10

Notes: Age adjusted by the direct method to the 2000 U.S. Census population using age groups 20–39, 40–59, and 60–74. Overweight is a body mass index (BMI) of 25 kg/m² or greater but less than 30 kg/m²; obesity is a BMI greater than or equal to 30 kg/m²; and extreme obesity is a BMI greater than or equal to 40 kg/m².

SOURCE: Cheryl D. Fryar, Margaret D. Carroll, and Cynthia L. Ogden, "Figure 1. Trends in Overweight, Obesity, and Extreme Obesity among Men Aged 20–74 Years: United States, 1960–1962 through 2009–2010," in "Prevalence of Overweight, Obesity, and Extreme Obesity among Adults: United States, Trends 1960–1962 through 2009–2010," *NCHS Health E-Stats*, Centers for Disease Control and Prevention, National Center for Health Statistics, September 2012, http://www.cdc.gov/nchs/data/hestat/obesity_adult_09_10/obesity_adult_09_10.pdf (accessed October 7, 2013)

WHY ARE SO MANY AMERICANS OVERWEIGHT?

Historically, overweight and obesity were largely attributed to gluttony—solely the result of inappropriate eating. The scientific study of obesity has identified genetic, biochemical, viral, and metabolic alterations in humans and experimental animals, as well as the complex interactions of psychosocial and cultural factors that create susceptibility to overweight and obesity. Even though overweight and obesity are thought to result from

multiple causes, for the overwhelming majority of Americans overweight and obesity result from excessive consumption of calories and inadequate physical activity—eating too much and exercising too little.

Some observers maintain that Americans were destined to become overweight when their diets remained unchanged even as the inventions of the industrial revolution such as cars, automation, and a variety of laborsaving devices sharply reduced levels of physical activity. The widespread availability of high-calorie foods and less physically

FIGURE 1.3

Overweight, obesity and extreme obesity in women, 1960–62 through 2009–10

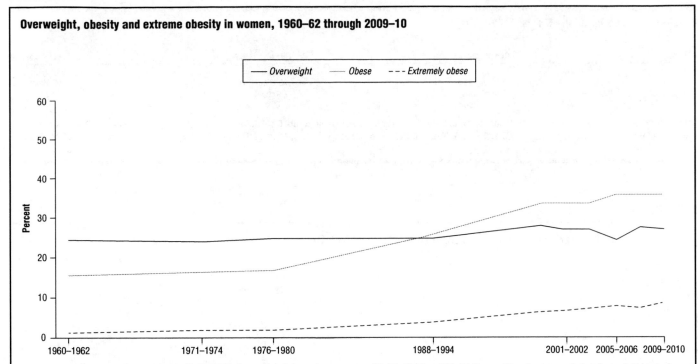

Notes: Age adjusted by the direct method to the 2000 U.S. Census population using age groups 20–39, 40–59, and 60–74. Pregnant females were excluded. Overweight is a body mass index (BMI) of 25 kg/m² or greater but less than 30 kg/m²; obesity is a BMI greater than or equal to 30 kg/m²; and extreme obesity is a BMI greater than or equal to 40 kg/m².

SOURCE: Cheryl D. Fryar, Margaret D. Carroll, and Cynthia L. Ogden, "Figure 2. Trends in Overweight, Obesity, and Extreme Obesity among Women Aged 20–74 Years: United States, 1960–1962 through 2009–2010," in "Prevalence of Overweight, Obesity, and Extreme Obesity among Adults: United States, Trends 1960–1962 through 2009–2010," *NCHS Health E-Stats*, Centers for Disease Control and Prevention, National Center for Health Statistics, September 2012, http://www.cdc.gov/nchs/data/hestat/obesity_adult_09_10/obesity_adult_09_10.pdf (accessed October 7, 2013)

FIGURE 1.4

Prevalence of obesity among adults aged 20 years and older, 1997–March 2013

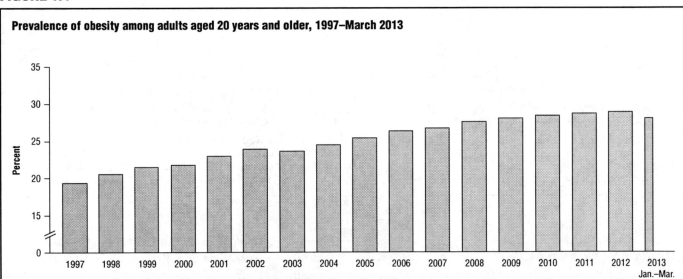

Notes: Data are based on household interviews of a sample of the civilian noninstitutionalized population. Obesity is defined as a body mass index (BMI) of 30 kg/m² or more. The measure is based on self-reported height (m) and weight (kg). Estimates of obesity are restricted to adults aged 20 and over for consistency with the Healthy People 2020 (3) initiative. The analyses excluded people with unknown height or weight (about 6% of respondents each year).

SOURCE: Brian W. Ward, Jeannine S. Schiller, and Gulnur Freeman, "Figure 6.1. Prevalence of Obesity among Adults Aged 20 Years and over: United States, 1997–March 2013," in *Early Release of Selected Estimates Based on Data from the January–March 2013 National Health Interview Survey*, Centers for Disease Control and Prevention, National Center for Health Statistics, September 2013, http://www.cdc.gov/nchs/data/nhis/earlyrelease/earlyrelease201309_06.pdf (accessed October 7, 2013)

FIGURE 1.5

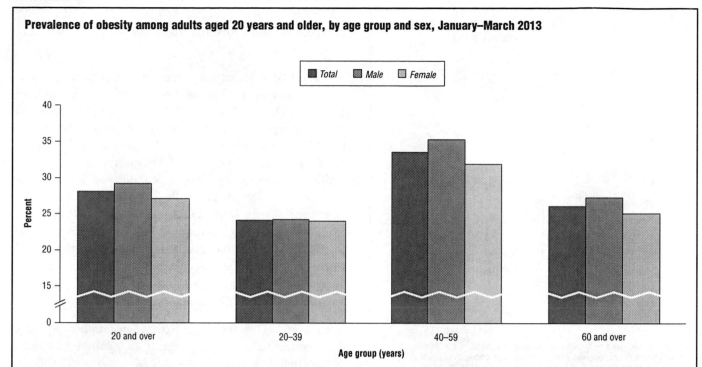

Prevalence of obesity among adults aged 20 years and older, by age group and sex, January–March 2013

Notes: Data are based on household interviews of a sample of the civilian noninstitutionalized population. Obesity is defined as a body mass index (BMI) of 30 kg/m² or more. The measure is based on self-reported height (m) and weight (kg). Estimates of obesity are restricted to adults aged 20 and over for consistency with the Healthy People 2020 (3) initiative. The analyses excluded the 3.6% of persons with unknown height or weight.

SOURCE: Brian W. Ward, Jeannine S. Schiller, and Gulnur Freeman, "Figure 6.2. Prevalence of Obesity among Adults Aged 20 Years and over, by Age Group and Sex: United States, January–March 2013," in *Early Release of Selected Estimates Based on Data from the January–March 2013 National Health Interview Survey*, Centers for Disease Control and Prevention, National Center for Health Statistics, September 2013, http://www.cdc.gov/nchs/data/nhis/earlyrelease/earlyrelease201309_06.pdf (accessed October 7, 2013)

demanding jobs conspired to make Americans fatter. Others contend that the rise in overweight and obesity began during the 1970s, when Americans came to rely on processed, convenient, and calorie-dense, saturated-fat-laden fast foods. In "The Epidemic of Childhood Obesity: A Case for Primary Prevention and Action" (*Bariatric Nursing and Surgical Patient Care*, vol. 4, no. 3, September 2009), Renee Ellen Fox and Deborah E. Trautman cite the interaction of myriad biological and social factors including "dramatic decreases in the amount of calories expended daily, increases in calorie intake and portion sizes, societal changes such as women entering the workforce in large numbers, more meals eaten in restaurants, and changes in television and video game viewing patterns."

Recent research also implicates a viral cause of obesity. Mary Miu and Yee Waye note in "New Insights into How Adenovirus Might Lead to Obesity: An Oxidative Stress Theory" (*Free Radical Research*, vol. 45, no. 8, August 2011) that the human adenovirus-36 (Ad-36) is capable of inducing adiposity in experimentally infected animals and is known to increase the replication, differentiation, lipid accumulation, and insulin sensitivity in fat cells. (Adenoviruses typically produce respiratory infections.) In the United States antibodies to Ad-36 are more prevalent in obese subjects than in nonobese subjects.

Research also confirms genetic origins of obesity. In "Genes and Obesity: A Cause and Effect Relationship" (*Endocrinology Nutrition*, vol. 58, no. 9, November 2011), Emilio González Jiménez asserts that although obesity usually results from an interaction of specific gene polymorphisms and environmental triggers, about 5% of obesity is attributable to mutations in specific genes. More than 100 genes linked to obesity have been reported. Some of these genes govern hunger and satiety signals, some are involved in the development and growth of fat cells, and some are involved in energy expenditure.

Qianghua Xia and Struan F. A. Grant observe in "The Genetics of Human Obesity" (*Annals of the New York Academy of Science*, vol. 1281, April 2013) that while obesity due to single gene disorders has been well described and genome-wide searches have identified specific sites, called loci, where genetic variants associated with polygenic (caused by more than one gene) obesity are located, the genes within these many loci have not yet been identified. Xia and Grant opine that new technologies will help identify the obesity-associated gene

FIGURE 1.6

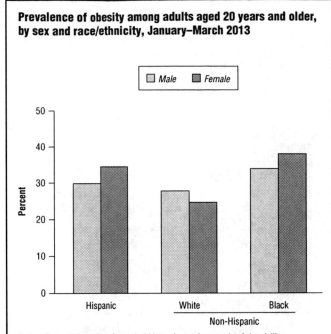

Prevalence of obesity among adults aged 20 years and older, by sex and race/ethnicity, January–March 2013

Notes: Data are based on household interviews of a sample of the civilian noninstitutionalized population. Obesity is defined as a body mass index (BMI) of 30 kg/m² or more. The measure is based on self-reported height (m) and weight (kg). Estimates of obesity are restricted to adults aged 20 and over for consistency with the Healthy People 2020 (3) initiative. The analyses excluded the 3.6% of persons with unknown height or weight. Estimates are age adjusted using the projected 2000 U.S. population as the standard population and using five age groups: 20–24, 25–34, 35–44, 45–64, and 65 and over.

SOURCE: Brian W. Ward, Jeannine S. Schiller, and Gulnur Freeman, "Figure 6.3. Age-Adjusted Prevalence of Obesity among Adults Aged 20 Years and over, by Sex and Race/Ethnicity: United States, January–March 2013," in *Early Release of Selected Estimates Based on Data from the January–March 2013 National Health Interview Survey*, Centers for Disease Control and Prevention, National Center for Health Statistics, September 2013, http://www.cdc.gov/nchs/data/nhis/earlyrelease/earlyrelease201309_06.pdf (accessed October 7, 2013)

variants, which in turn will help investigators develop more effective therapies.

The American Diet Has Changed

The American diet has changed dramatically since the mid-20th century. According to the USDA, in *Agriculture Fact Book, 2001–2002* (March 2003, http://www.usda.gov/factbook/2002factbook.pdf), during the 1950s food production in the United States provided about 800 fewer calories per person per day than in 2000. Of the 3,800 calories produced per person per day in 2000, the USDA estimates that about 1,100 calories were wasted, either through spoilage, plate waste, or cooking, leaving an average of about 2,700 calories per person per day. The USDA data reveal that between 1970 and 2000 the average number of calories consumed daily rose by 530 calories, an increase of 24.5%. This 24.5% increase consisted of 9.5 percentage points of grains (primarily refined grain products), 9 percentage points of added fats and oils, 4.7 percentage points of added sugars,

1.5 percentage points of fruits and vegetables, and 1 percentage point of meats and nuts. There was a 1.5 percentage point decline in dairy product and egg consumption.

The USDA states that Americans consumed an average of 4 pounds (1.8 kg) more fish and shellfish, 7 pounds (3.2 kg) more red meat, and 46 pounds (20.9 kg) more poultry per person per year in 2000 than they did during the 1950s. Americans consumed more meat—57 pounds (25.9 kg) more per year in 2000 than they did during the 1950s. Despite record-high per capita (per person) consumption of meat in 2000, the proportion of fat in the U.S. food supply from meat, poultry, and fish declined from one-third (33%) during the 1950s to a quarter (24%) in 2000. This decline resulted from the marketing of lower-fat ground and processed meat products, a shift away from red meat to poultry, and closer trimming of outside fat on meat, which commenced in 1986.

According to the USDA, the consumption of milk dropped from an annual average of 36.4 gallons (137.8 L) per person during the 1950s to 22.6 gallons (85.6 L) in 2000, a decrease of 38%. The USDA posits a link between the trend toward dining out and the reduction in beverage milk consumption. According to the USDA, soft drinks, fruit drinks, and flavored teas appear to be displacing milk as the beverages of choice for Americans. By contrast, Americans ate more cheese, from 7.7 pounds (3.5 kg) during the 1950s to 29.8 pounds (13.5 kg) in 2000.

The average use of added fats and oils increased 67%, from 44.6 pounds (20.2 kg) during the 1950s to 74.5 pounds (33.8 kg) in 2000. Added fats include butter, shortenings, and oils used in commercially prepared foods. All fats that naturally occur in foods, such as those in milk and meat, were excluded from the USDA analysis. Americans consumed an average of 23% more salad and cooking oil in 2000 than they did during the 1950s, and more than twice as much shortening. During the same period the consumption of butter and margarine declined by about the same proportion—25%. During the 1950s added fats and oils accounted for the largest proportion of fat in the food supply (41%), followed by animal proteins—meat, poultry, and fish (32%). By 2000 added fats and oils accounted for 53% of total fat consumption, most likely because Americans' appetites for fried foods in fast-food outlets and high-fat snack foods grew, as did the use of salad dressings. USDA food consumption surveys, which assess the prevalence of discretionary fats in the American diet, continue to find that margarine, salad dressing, and mayonnaise, along with cakes and other sweet baked goods, are among the top-10 food sources of fat in the American diet.

The USDA indicates that the consumption of fruit and vegetables increased 20%, from 587.5 pounds (266.5 kg) during the 1970s to 707.7 pounds (321 kg) in 2000. The USDA attributes some of the increase to the introduction of convenient, ready-to-eat, precut, and packaged fruit and vegetables and to increasing consumer health awareness. Despite these gains, the CDC explains in *State Indicator Report on Fruits and Vegetables, 2013* (2013, http://www.cdc.gov/nutrition/downloads/State-Indicator-Report-Fruits-Vegetables-2013.pdf), a state-by-state study of fruit and vegetable consumption, that 37.7% of adults report consuming fruit less than one time daily and 22.6% consumed less than one serving of vegetables in 2013. (See Table 1.7.) Vegetable consumption by adolescents was even worse—37.7% said they ate vegetables less than once a day and 36% said they ate less than one serving of fruit per day. Among adults the median (half are higher and half are lower) vegetable intake was higher in California, Oregon, and New Hampshire and lower in North Dakota, South Dakota, Iowa, Louisiana, and Mississippi. (See Table 1.7 and Figure 1.7.)

According to the USDA, the per capita use of flour and cereal products reached 199.9 pounds (90.7 kg) in 2000, up from an annual average of 155.4 pounds (70.5 kg) during the 1950s and 138.2 pounds (62.7 kg) during the 1970s, when grain consumption was at a record low. This increase reflects plentiful grain stocks, robust consumer demand for store-bought bakery items and grain-based snack foods, and increased consumption of fast-food products such as buns, pizza dough, and tortillas. Despite the overall increase in grain consumption, the average American's diet contained mostly refined grain products and fell short of the recommended minimum three daily servings of whole-grain products.

The NHANES conducted by the CDC (August 29, 2013, http:www.ars.usda.gov/ba/bhnrc/fsrg) reports that Americans' consumption of whole grains increased 23.4% between 2008 and 2010. In 2007–08 Americans ate an average of 0.6 servings per person and by 2009–10, they consumed 0.8 servings per day. Despite this increase, American adults still consumed far less than the recommended three to five servings per day.

The USDA cites a variety of factors that have contributed to the changes in the American diet over the past 50 years, including fluctuations in food prices and availability, increases in real (adjusted for inflation) disposable income, and more food assistance for the poor. New products, particularly the expanding array of convenience foods, also alter patterns of consumption, as do more imports, growth in the away-from-home food market, intensified advertising campaigns, and increases in nutrient-enrichment standards and food fortification. Social and demographic trends driving changes in food choices include smaller households, more two-wage earner households, more single-parent households, an aging population, and increased ethnic diversity.

Americans Enjoy Eating Out

A variety of societal trends are thought to contribute to Americans' propensity to overeat, including eating outside the home, as well as ready access to, and preference for, sugar- and fat-laden foods. Table 1.8 shows how expenditures for eating away from home have steadily increased and more than doubled from $307.6 billion in 1995 to $641.2 billion in 2011. Purchases of food away from home rose between 2003 and 2008; however, the economic recession that lasted from late 2007 to mid-2009 prompted Americans to limit their eating out. Aylin Kumcu and Phil Kaufman of the Economic Research Service note in "Food Spending Adjustments during Recessionary Times" (*Amber Waves*, September 2011) that there was a 5% decline in inflation-adjusted food spending during the recession—the largest decrease in 25 years. They indicate that this decline was largely attributable to reductions in food-away-from-home spending, such as at fast-food and sit-down restaurants. Table 1.8 shows that after a drop in 2009, expenditures at eating and drinking places rose in 2010 and 2011.

Many nutritionists and obesity researchers assert that controlling portion size, which is key to controlling calorie consumption, is more difficult in restaurants, where portions are frequently quite large. Increasingly, restaurants have translated consumer demand for value into more food for less money. Because humans are genetically programmed to eat when food is abundant, larger portions trigger the natural impulse to eat more.

Besides portion size, large containers also appear to increase intake. In "Container Size Influences Snack Food Intake Independently of Portion Size" (*Appetite*, vol. 58, 2012), David Marchiori, Olivier Corneille, and Olivier Klein report that larger containers stimulate food intake independent of portion size. They gave study participants a medium portion of M&M's in a small container, a medium portion in a large container, or a large portion in a large container. Marchiori, Corneille, and Klein explain that the larger container increased intake by 129% despite the portion size remaining constant.

BIGGER PORTIONS IN RESTAURANTS. Samara Joy Nielsen and Barry M. Popkin of the University of North Carolina, Chapel Hill, looked at portion sizes consumed in the United States to determine whether average portion sizes had increased over time and reported their findings in "Patterns and Trends in Food Portion Sizes, 1977–1998" (*JAMA*, vol. 289, no. 4, January 22, 2003). In this landmark study, Nielsen and Popkin analyze data collected by national nutrition surveys (the Nationwide Food Consumption Survey and the Continuing Survey of Food

TABLE 1.7

Fruit and vegetable consumption by adults and adolescents, by state, 2013

State	Adults				Adolescents			
	Percentage who report consuming fruits and vegetables less than one time daily		Median intake of fruits and vegetables (times per day)		Percentage who report consuming fruits and vegetables less than one time daily		Median intake of fruits and vegetables (times per day)	
	Fruits	Vegetables	Fruits	Vegetables	Fruits	Vegetables	Fruits	Vegetables
U.S. national	37.7	22.6	1.1	1.6	36.0	37.7	1.0	1.3
Alabama	43.8	24.3	1.0	1.6	44.4	45.7	1.0	1.0
Alaska	38.7	19.7	1.1	1.7	39.1	34.1	1.0	1.3
Arizona	38.0	20.6	1.1	1.7				
Arkansas	47.5	28.6	1.0	1.5	49.4	43.2	1.0	1.0
California	30.4	16.5	1.3	1.8				
Colorado	35.7	19.1	1.1	1.7				
Connecticut	32.0	20.6	1.3	1.7	34.6	35.3	1.3	1.3
Delaware	39.2	23.8	1.0	1.6	46.0		1.0	
Dist of Columbia	31.7	20.1	1.3	1.8				
Florida	37.7	22.6	1.1	1.6	37.2	42.1	1.0	1.1
Georgia	41.9	23.2	1.0	1.6	42.9	43.1	1.0	1.0
Hawaii	39.5	22.6	1.0	1.7	45.1	40.8	1.0	1.1
Idaho	38.1	20.1	1.1	1.6	33.9	32.2	1.0	1.3
Illinois	36.0	25.2	1.1	1.6	38.7	42.3	1.0	1.1
Indiana	41.6	27.3	1.0	1.5	44.7	42.0	1.0	1.1
Iowa	39.8	26.9	1.0	1.4	36.1	35.1	1.0	1.3
Kansas	41.4	22.2	1.0	1.6	40.4	35.7	1.0	1.3
Kentucky	45.9	25.2	1.0	1.5	49.7	43.2	1.0	1.1
Louisiana	46.7	32.5	1.0	1.4	47.8	50.1	1.0	0.9
Maine	33.2	18.9	1.2	1.7	37.5		1.0	
Maryland	36.4	22.8	1.1	1.6	38.7	38.9	1.0	1.3
Massachusetts	31.6	20.7	1.2	1.7				
Michigan	37.3	23.2	1.1	1.6	37.8	36.8	1.0	1.3
Minnesota	36.2	23.6	1.1	1.5				
Mississippi	50.8	32.3	0.9	1.4	39.8	42.4	1.0	1.1
Missouri	43.9	25.2	1.0	1.5				
Montana	39.2	21.7	1.0	1.6	38.4	33.5	1.0	1.3
Nebraska	40.1	26.2	1.0	1.5	41.0	38.0	1.0	1.3
Nevada	36.9	24.4	1.1	1.6				
New Hampshire	30.3	17.6	1.3	1.8	36.8	31.8	1.0	1.3
New Jersey	33.9	22.2	1.1	1.6	39.1	34.9	1.0	1.3
New Mexico	38.0	21.9	1.1	1.7	40.8	37.1	1.0	1.3
New York	33.9	23.0	1.2	1.6	34.7		1.3	
North Carolina	40.8	21.9	1.0	1.6	44.5	39.6	1.0	1.1
North Dakota	39.1	27.1	1.1	1.4	36.4	39.4	1.0	1.1
Ohio	40.5	26.0	1.0	1.5	42.4	42.2	1.0	1.1
Oklahoma	50.2	26.8	0.9	1.5	44.3	40.4	1.0	1.1
Oregon	32.0	15.3	1.1	1.9				
Pennsylvania	36.1	23.9	1.1	1.5				
Rhode Island	32.9	20.7	1.2	1.6	36.5	35.3	1.0	1.3
South Carolina	44.4	27.3	1.0	1.5	50.6	47.8	0.7	1.0
South Dakota	39.6	26.3	1.0	1.4	41.2	38.8	1.0	1.1
Tennessee	46.3	25.4	1.0	1.6	44.9	41.4	1.0	1.1
Texas	40.3	21.8	1.0	1.6	42.1	47.5	1.0	1.0
Utah	34.9	19.8	1.1	1.7	32.5	31.8	1.0	1.3
Vermont	31.4	18.1	1.3	1.7	30.7	26.4	1.3	1.6
Virginia	38.4	22.2	1.1	1.7	39.8	41.7	1.0	1.1
Washington	35.0	18.8	1.1	1.7				
West Virginia	47.2	26.2	1.0	1.5	37.8	34.9	1.0	1.3
Wisconsin	35.6	26.0	1.1	1.5	34.1	35.7	1.0	1.3
Wyoming	38.2	22.4	1.1	1.6	37.9	31.4	1.0	1.3

Note: Some states may not have estimates for F&V intake among adolescents which may be due to either not collecting survey data, not achieving a high enough overall response rate to receive weighted results, or omitting 1 or more questionnaire items during administration of the survey.

SOURCE: "Table 1. State Indicator Report on Fruits and Vegetables, 2013: Behavioral Indicators," in State Indicator Report on Fruits and Vegetables 2013, Centers for Disease Control and Prevention, National Center for Chronic Disease Prevention and Health Promotion, Division of Nutrition, Physical Activity, and Obesity, 2013, http://www.cdc.gov/nutrition/downloads/State-Indicator-Report-Fruits-Vegetables-2013.pdf (accessed October 7, 2013)

Intakes by Individuals) that were conducted in the United States in 1977–78, 1989–91, 1994–96, and 1998, detailing the consumption habits of more than 63,000 people. For each survey year, the researchers analyze the average portion sizes that were consumed of specific food items (salty snacks, desserts, soft drinks, fruit drinks, french fries, hamburgers, cheeseburgers, pizza, and Mexican food) by eating location (home, restaurant, and fast-food outlet). Nielsen and Popkin report that between 1977 and 1996 the average portions of salty snacks such as chips

FIGURE 1.7

Median daily vegetable intake among adults, 2013

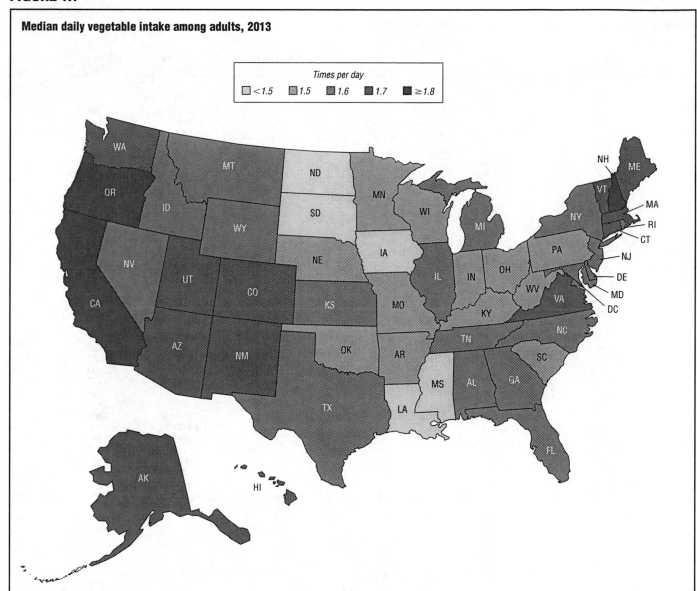

SOURCE: "Median Daily Vegetable Intake among Adults in the United States," in *State Indicator Report on Fruits and Vegetables 2013*, Centers for Disease Control and Prevention, National Center for Chronic Disease Prevention and Health Promotion, Division of Nutrition, Physical Activity, and Obesity, 2013, http://www.cdc.gov/nutrition/downloads/State-Indicator-Report-Fruits-Vegetables-2013.pdf (accessed October 7, 2013)

increased by 60% and soft drinks grew by 50%. The average bag of chips grew from 1 ounce (28.4 g) in 1977 to 1.6 ounces (45.4 g) in 1996. During this same period an average dispensed soft drink increased from 13.1 ounces (387.4 mL) to 19.9 ounces (588.5 mL). As a result, the average chips-and-soda snack in 1996 contained 150 more calories than it did in 1977.

The portion-size changes were also observed with many fast-food offerings. During the 20 years studied, the size of the average hamburger grew by 23%, to 7 ounces (198.4 g), and the servings of fries grew by 16%, to 3.5 ounces (99.2 g). In 1996 a regular-sized burger-and-fries meal contained 155 more calories than it did in 1977. Worse still, Nielsen and Popkin found that portion

size had also expanded in Americans' homes, indicating widespread ignorance about appropriate portion size. Interestingly, portion sizes were smallest in restaurants, although they, too, had increased during the study period. For example, the average restaurant portion of spaghetti with tomato sauce and meatballs doubled in size from 500 to 1,025 calories.

In "Reducing Portion Sizes to Prevent Obesity: A Call to Action" (*American Journal of Preventive Medicine*, vol. 43, no. 5, November 2012), Lisa R. Young and Marion Nestle observe that portion sizes of many foods continued to increase throughout the first decade of the 21st century. Furthermore, nearly 150 new large-size portions, including burgers, pizza, candy bars, and

TABLE 1.8

Food away from home, total expenditures, selected years 1929–2011

Year	Eating and drinking places[a]	Hotels and motels[a]	Retail stores, direct selling[b]	Recreational places[c]	Schools and colleges[d]	All other[e]	Total[f]
			Million dollars				
1929	2,101	362	—	—	175	1,483	4,121
1933	1,235	250	—	—	105	869	2,459
1935	1,257	271	—	—	161	1,145	2,834
1936	1,430	320	—	—	175	1,236	3,161
1937	1,696	351	—	—	194	1,375	3,616
1938	1,626	312	—	—	191	1,260	3,389
1939	1,782	321	—	—	203	1,307	3,613
1940	1,938	353	—	—	219	1,385	3,895
1941	2,369	386	—	—	263	1,781	4,799
1942	2,992	453	—	—	310	2,539	6,294
1943	3,837	604	—	—	332	3,572	8,345
1944	4,471	681	—	—	326	4,415	9,893
1945	5,218	736	—	—	373	4,908	11,235
1946	5,859	846	—	—	525	3,802	11,032
1947	6,243	854	—	—	842	3,864	11,803
1948	6,338	846	—	—	983	4,069	12,236
1949	6,294	786	—	—	979	3,943	12,002
1950	6,472	774	—	—	1,051	4,172	12,469
1951	7,172	783	—	—	1,124	5,167	14,246
1952	7,549	805	—	—	1,138	5,435	14,927
1953	7,834	790	—	—	1,215	5,392	15,231
1954	8,008	752	1,416	274	1,311	3,676	15,437
1955	8,490	809	1,408	313	1,390	3,539	16,009
1956	8,992	875	1,534	354	1,530	3,506	16,791
1957	9,409	932	1,592	342	1,661	3,609	17,545
1958	9,447	922	1,599	356	1,809	3,756	17,889
1959	10,102	982	1,677	385	1,949	3,739	18,834
1960	10,505	1,028	1,716	421	2,082	3,855	19,607
1961	10,907	1,061	1,740	452	2,264	3,961	20,385
1962	11,624	1,134	1,812	472	2,463	4,090	21,595
1963	12,247	1,200	1,854	484	2,624	4,148	22,557
1964	13,156	1,289	1,988	496	2,814	4,279	24,022
1965	14,444	1,409	2,162	522	3,062	4,598	26,197
1966	15,768	1,541	2,346	544	3,329	5,173	28,701
1967	16,595	1,623	2,436	563	3,632	5,570	30,419
1968	18,695	1,703	2,713	616	3,903	5,830	33,460
1969	20,207	1,716	2,984	661	4,256	6,291	36,115
1970	22,617	1,894	3,325	721	4,475	6,551	39,583
1971	24,166	2,086	3,626	762	4,990	6,621	42,251
1972	27,167	2,390	3,811	832	5,370	7,017	46,587
1973	31,265	2,639	4,218	963	5,605	7,960	52,650
1974	34,029	2,864	4,520	1,167	6,287	9,178	58,045
1975	41,384	3,199	4,952	1,369	7,060	10,145	68,109
1976	47,536	3,769	5,341	1,511	7,854	10,822	76,833
1977	52,491	4,115	5,663	2,606	8,413	11,547	84,835
1978	60,042	4,863	6,323	2,810	9,034	13,012	96,084
1979	68,872	5,551	7,157	2,921	9,914	14,756	109,171
1980	75,883	5,906	8,158	3,040	11,115	16,194	120,296
1981	83,358	6,639	8,830	2,979	11,357	17,751	130,914
1982	90,390	6,888	9,256	2,887	11,692	18,663	139,776
1983	98,710	7,660	9,827	3,271	12,338	19,077	150,883
1984	105,836	8,409	10,315	3,489	12,950	20,047	161,046
1985	111,760	9,168	10,499	3,737	13,534	20,133	168,831
1986	121,699	9,665	11,116	4,059	14,401	20,755	181,695
1987	137,190	11,117	9,302	4,396	13,470	21,119	196,594
1988	150,724	11,905	10,359	5,082	13,889	22,474	214,433
1989	160,226	12,179	11,369	6,089	14,609	24,016	228,488
1990	171,616	12,508	12,786	7,206	15,299	25,605	245,020
1991	180,062	12,460	13,515	7,936	16,186	26,226	256,385
1992	184,697	13,204	11,817	8,509	17,666	27,596	263,489
1993	197,865	13,362	11,790	9,361	18,330	27,864	278,572
1994	207,464	13,880	12,015	10,103	19,271	28,460	291,193
1995	221,205	14,211	11,848	11,110	20,064	29,158	307,596
1996	223,406	14,553	11,959	11,512	20,867	29,696	311,993
1997	242,362	15,381	10,680	12,126	21,901	32,022	334,472
1998	255,376	16,069	11,335	12,790	23,053	32,528	351,151
1999	266,451	16,710	12,463	13,493	23,920	34,148	367,185
2000	287,332	18,003	13,608	14,224	24,468	36,212	393,847
2001	293,911	20,813	14,597	14,780	25,394	36,810	406,305
2002	295,341	21,513	17,319	15,873	26,735	37,602	414,382

TABLE 1.8

Food away from home, total expenditures, selected years 1929–2011 [CONTINUED]

Year	Eating and drinking places[a]	Hotels and motels[a]	Retail stores, direct selling[b]	Recreational places[c]	Schools and colleges[d]	All other[e]	Total[f]
	Million dollars						
2003	324,995	21,914	18,272	17,327	28,077	39,215	449,800
2004	338,105	23,462	19,430	18,265	30,185	40,507	469,954
2005	372,094	24,570	20,677	20,225	31,521	42,625	511,712
2006	397,682	25,328	21,616	22,665	34,581	45,215	547,087
2007	419,891	25,588	22,297	24,288	35,548	47,490	575,102
2008	431,391	26,085	22,942	24,639	37,797	48,803	591,657
2009	429,739	25,257	22,085	24,142	39,894	49,667	590,784
2010	446,442	25,541	22,785	24,673	42,450	50,114	612,005
2011	468,687	25,828	24,392	25,679	44,292	52,364	641,242

— = Not available.

[a]Includes tips.

[b]Includes vending machine operators but not vending machines operated by organizations.

[c]Motion picture theaters, bowling alleys, pool parlors, sports arenas, camps, amusement parks, golf and country clubs (includes concessions beginning in 1977).

[d]Includes school food subsidies.

[e]Military exchanges and clubs; railroad dining cars; airlines; food service in manufacturing plants, institutions, hospitals, boarding houses, fraternities and sororities, and civic and social organizations; and food supplied to military forces, civilian employees and child day care centers.

[f]Computed from unrounded data.

SOURCE: "Table 3. Food away from Home: Total Expenditures," in *Food Expenditures*, U.S. Department of Agriculture, Economic Research Service, October 1, 2012, http://www.ers.usda.gov/briefing/cpifoodandexpenditures/Data/Expenditures_tables/table3.htm (accessed October 25, 2013)

beverages, were introduced during the same period. For example, Hardee's Monster Thickburger contains a whopping 1,420 calories. Young and Nestle observe that while European portion sizes have also grown, they are not as big as U.S. portions. For example, the largest portion of french fries offered by British Burger King has 200 fewer calories than the largest U.S. portion.

ECONOMIC RECESSION AFFECTS FOOD CONSUMPTION AND WEIGHT. In "The Effects of the Financial Crisis on Actual and Anticipated Consumption" (University of Michigan Retirement Research Center Working Paper WP 2011-255, http://www.mrrc.isr.umich.edu/publications/papers/pdf/wp255.pdf), Michael D. Hurd and Susann Rohwedder compare consumption changes during the economic recession (2007 through 2009) with consumption changes during previous years. They posit that spending on necessities such as food consumed at home is likely to be reduced less than spending on dining out, which is optional. As anticipated, purchases of food to be consumed at home showed a much smaller decline than did meals eaten away from home.

Some studies report that like smoking, excess weight tends to decrease during temporary economic downturns, while leisure-time and physical activity increase. This trend presumably occurs because people have less money to spend on dining out and tobacco and, if they are unemployed or underemployed, they have more time to engage in physical activity. Other research, such as "Does a Slump Really Make You Thinner? Finnish Micro-level Evidence 1978–2002" (*Health Economics*, vol. 16, no. 1, 2007) suggests that economic improvement results in a decrease in BMI.

In "Do Economic Constraints on Food Choice Make People Fat? A Critical Review of Two Hypotheses for the Poverty-Obesity Paradox" (*American Journal of Human Biology*, vol. 24, no. 3, May–June 2012), Daniel J. Hruschka observes that in wealthy countries, poorer and less educated people are more likely to be overweight than their more prosperous countrymen. Hruschka questions the conventional thinking that "economic deprivation leads people to choose cheaper foods which in turn fosters overconsumption of energy," and notes that during the recent U.S. recession, obesity among women slowed across income groups.

BIGGER PORTIONS AT HOME. Increased portion sizes at home are reflected in recipes and cookbooks. Lisa R. Young notes in *The Portion Teller: Smartsize Your Way to Permanent Weight Loss* (2005) that recipes call for bigger portions using the same ingredients than they did in past decades. For example, a brownie recipe from Irma S. Rombauer and Marion Rombauer Becker's *Joy of Cooking* (1964) recommended dividing it into 30 servings, whereas the same recipe in the 1997 edition of the book was divided into only 16 servings. Similarly, a 1987 recipe for Toll House cookies yielded 60 servings, whereas in earlier decades the same recipe yielded 100 servings. Other popular food items have increased in size and caloric content. In "Portion Distortion" (February 2013, http://www.nhlbi.nih.gov/health/public/heart/obesity/wecan/portion/index.htm), the National Heart, Lung, and Blood Institute compares portion sizes and the corresponding calories of several popular foods between 1983 and 2003. Researchers find that in 1983 a bagel measured 3 inches (7.6 cm) in diameter and contained 140 calories. In 2003 a 6-inch (15.2 cm) bagel contained 350 calories.

Nielsen and Popkin also note other changes in eating behavior. For example, they find that in 1996 Americans obtained 19% of their total calories from snacks—double the amount of 1977—and 81% from meals. They conclude that "control of portion size must be systematically addressed both in general and as it relates to fast food pricing and marketing. The best way to encourage people to eat smaller portions is if food portions served inside and outside the home are smaller."

Even though the Nationwide Food Consumption Survey and the Continuing Survey of Food Intakes by Individuals have not been repeated since 1996, there is no evidence that portion sizes have returned to their previous sizes or have even decreased in size. In a review of research about portion size, Ingrid H. M. Steenhuis and Willemijn M. Vermeer of Vrije Universiteit Amsterdam observe in "Portion Size: Review and Framework for Interventions" (*International Journal of Behavioral Nutrition and Physical Activity*, vol. 6, no. 58, August 21, 2009) that since the 1970s portion sizes, especially of high energy dense (high caloric) foods eaten at home and in restaurants, have increased. The researchers confirm that "portion distortion," a term that is used to describe the phenomenon of people becoming acclimated to larger portions so that they not only do not view them as excessive but also have more difficulty selecting appropriate amounts of food, definitely increases consumption by at least 30%.

The contribution of increased portion size to increased daily intake of energy from food and drink was confirmed by research conducted by Kiyah J. Duffey and Barry M. Popkin and reported in "Energy Density, Portion Size, and Eating Occasions: Contributions to Increased Energy Intake in the United States, 1977–2006" (*PLoS Medicine*, vol. 8, no. 6, June 2011). The researchers analyze data from the Nationwide Food Consumption Survey (1977–78), the Continuing Survey of Food Intakes by Individuals (1989–91), and the NHANES (1994–98 and 2003–06) to determine the contribution of changes in the energy density of foods consumed, the portion size, and the number of meals and snacks per day. They find that the daily total energy intake increased by 570 calories between 1977 and 2006. Duffey and Popkin indicate that even though all three factors contributed to changes in the average daily total energy intake over the past 30 years, increases in the number of eating occasions and portion size accounted for most of the change. In fact, the consumption of food and beverage portions increased across all eating and drinking occasions (meals and snacks).

Is the Food Industry the Culprit?

In "The Perils of Ignoring History: Big Tobacco Played Dirty and Millions Died. How Similar Is BigFood?" (March 2009, http://vancouver.ca/parks/active community/pdf/FoodTobacco_YaleUni.pdf), Kelly D. Brownell and Kenneth E. Warner implicate marketing strategies employed by the food industry as a significant factor in the rise of obesity. Furthermore, they liken food industry practices to those of the tobacco industry, concluding that:

> The tobacco industry had a playbook, a script, that emphasized personal responsibility, paying scientists who delivered research that instilled doubt, criticizing the "junk" science that found harms associated with smoking, making self-regulatory pledges, lobbying with massive resources to stifle government action, introducing "safer" products, and simultaneously manipulating and denying both the addictive nature of their products and their marketing to children. The script of the food industry is both similar to and different from the tobacco industry script.... Because obesity is now a major global problem, the world cannot afford a repeat of the tobacco history, in which industry talks about the moral high ground but does not occupy it.

Kelly D. Brownell et al. explain in "Personal Responsibility and Obesity: A Constructive Approach to a Controversial Issue" (*Health Affairs*, vol. 29, no. 3, March–April 2010) that people gain weight when their environment promotes highly palatable food and cite research suggesting that some foods can trigger symptoms of addiction. The researchers aver that the traditional approach to diet and obesity has been one of rugged individualism—educating individuals and exhorting them to alter their behavior, often without regard to environmental influences. Instead of focusing solely on personal responsibility, Brownell et al. propose efforts on the part of government and the food industry to create conditions that encourage responsible choices. Furthermore, they call on the food industry to limit its "relentless" and often "stealth" marketing techniques such as food marketing that is incorporated into video games.

David A. Kessler also implicates the food industry in *The End of Overeating: Taking Control of the Insatiable American Appetite* (2009). He asserts that conditioned overeating is not a personal character flaw; rather, it is a biological response to the widespread availability of foods that are high in salt, fat, and sugar. Kessler blames the food industry for engineering highly processed industrial foods that use salt, fat, and added sugar to trigger cravings in some people and addiction in other people who are susceptible.

Some industry observers believe that one ingredient in particular triggers cravings: high-fructose corn syrup (HFCS). In "Brain Functional Magnetic Resonance Imaging Response to Glucose and Fructose Infusions in Humans" (*Diabetes, Obesity, and Metabolism*, vol. 13, no. 3, March 2011), Jonathan Q. Purnell et al. explain that the brain responds differently to glucose (sugar) than it does to fructose. Consuming glucose increases responses in the reward- and executive-function parts of the brain, whereas fructose inhibits these responses. This action may explain why fructose consumption appears to promote obesity—it actually stimulates hunger, which in turn increases consumption and weight gain.

Fructose also appears to trigger fat storage more efficiently than other sugars do. Even though all sugars are stored in the body as fat, some researchers think that fructose is more readily converted into fat than other sugars. Fructose encourages the liver to promote fat by activating enzymes that create higher levels of cholesterol and triglycerides (fatty substances that are normally present in the bloodstream and all the cells of the body) and make muscles more insulin resistant. Elevated levels of cholesterol and triglycerides increase the risk of coronary heart disease, and insulin resistance can lead to diabetes.

HFCS does more than sweeten; it also acts as a preservative, giving sweet foods a longer shelf life. Since the 1970s high-fructose corn syrup has been used to sweeten nearly every product on supermarket shelves. Some researchers feel that because it is so ubiquitous, many Americans are unknowingly consuming excessive amounts of fructose. Table 1.9 shows the per capita consumption of HFCS, which peaked in 1999 and has since slowly declined.

During the first decade of the 21st century HFCS received negative publicity, and as a result consumption continued to decline. In response, the Corn Refiners Association launched a controversial advertising campaign in 2009 that was intended to rebrand high-fructose corn syrup as "corn sugar." In a letter dated May 30, 2012 (http://www.fda.gov/aboutFDA/CentersOffices/OfficeofFoods/CFSAN/CFSANFOIAElectronicReadingRoom/ucm305226.htm) the Food and Drug Administration (FDA) rejected the Corn Refiners Association's request to rename its sweetener. The FDA explained that the use of the term *corn sugar* for HFCS would suggest that HFCS is a solid, dried, and crystallized sweetener obtained from corn rather than a syrup. The agency also stated that because the term *corn sugar* is commonly used to describe dextrose, a different sugar, using it to describe HCFS could cause needless confusion.

In *The Fattening of America: How the Economy Makes Us Fat, if It Matters, and What to Do about It* (2008), Eric A. Finkelstein and Laurie Zuckerman observe that Americans consumed 1,000 calories more per week in 2008 than they did in 1985. Finkelstein and Zuckerman describe how declining food costs, especially for high-calorie, low-nutrient foods, and modern technology combined to reduce the cost of producing higher-calorie processed food products. They note that when the staples used to produce fast foods became cheaper, the food industry intensified marketing efforts to induce consumers to buy and eat more. Table 1.10 shows that food expenditures decreased as a percentage of disposable personal income from 10.5% in 1996 to 9.8% in 2011.

TABLE 1.9

Estimated number of per capita calories of high-fructose corn syrup consumed daily, 1970–2012

Year	Primary weight (market level)[a] lb/yr	Loss from primary to retail weight percent	Weight at retail level lb/yr	Loss from retail/institutional to consumer level percent	Weight at consumer level lb/yr	Loss at consumer level: Nonedible share percent	Loss at consumer level: Other (uneaten food, spoilage, etc.) percent	Per capita consumption (adjusted for loss) lbs/yr	oz/daily	g/daily	Calories per serving number	Serving weight grams	Calories consumed daily[b] number	Servings (teaspoons) consumed daily[c] teaspoons
1970	0.5	0.0	0.5	11.0	0.5	0.0	34.0	0.3	0.0	0.4	16.0	4.2	2	0.1
1971	0.8	0.0	0.8	11.0	0.7	0.0	34.0	0.5	0.0	0.6	16.0	4.2	2	0.1
1972	1.2	0.0	1.2	11.0	1.0	0.0	34.0	0.7	0.0	0.8	16.0	4.2	3	0.2
1973	2.1	0.0	2.1	11.0	1.8	0.0	34.0	1.2	0.1	1.5	16.0	4.2	6	0.4
1974	2.8	0.0	2.8	11.0	2.5	0.0	34.0	1.6	0.1	2.0	16.0	4.2	8	0.5
1975	4.9	0.0	4.9	11.0	4.3	0.0	34.0	2.9	0.1	3.6	16.0	4.2	14	0.8
1976	7.2	0.0	7.2	11.0	6.4	0.0	34.0	4.2	0.2	5.2	16.0	4.2	20	1.2
1977	9.6	0.0	9.6	11.0	8.5	0.0	34.0	5.6	0.2	7.0	16.0	4.2	27	1.7
1978	10.8	0.0	10.8	11.0	9.6	0.0	34.0	6.3	0.3	7.9	16.0	4.2	30	1.9
1979	14.8	0.0	14.8	11.0	13.1	0.0	34.0	8.7	0.4	10.8	16.0	4.2	41	2.6
1980	19.0	0.0	19.0	11.0	16.9	0.0	34.0	11.1	0.5	13.8	16.0	4.2	53	3.3
1981	22.8	0.0	22.8	11.0	20.3	0.0	34.0	13.4	0.6	16.7	16.0	4.2	63	4.0
1982	26.6	0.0	26.6	11.0	23.7	0.0	34.0	15.6	0.7	19.4	16.0	4.2	74	4.6
1983	31.2	0.0	31.2	11.0	27.8	0.0	34.0	18.3	0.8	22.8	16.0	4.2	87	5.4
1984	37.2	0.0	37.2	11.0	33.1	0.0	34.0	21.9	1.0	27.2	16.0	4.2	104	6.5
1985	45.2	0.0	45.2	11.0	40.2	0.0	34.0	26.5	1.2	33.0	16.0	4.2	126	7.9
1986	45.7	0.0	45.7	11.0	40.7	0.0	34.0	26.8	1.2	33.4	16.0	4.2	127	7.9
1987	47.7	0.0	47.7	11.0	42.5	0.0	34.0	28.0	1.2	34.8	16.0	4.2	133	8.3
1988	49.0	0.0	49.0	11.0	43.6	0.0	34.0	28.8	1.3	35.7	16.0	4.2	136	8.5
1989	48.2	0.0	48.2	11.0	42.9	0.0	34.0	28.3	1.2	35.2	16.0	4.2	134	8.4
1990	49.6	0.0	49.6	11.0	44.1	0.0	34.0	29.1	1.3	36.2	16.0	4.2	138	8.6
1991	50.3	0.0	50.3	11.0	44.8	0.0	34.0	29.5	1.3	36.7	16.0	4.2	140	8.7
1992	51.9	0.0	51.9	11.0	46.2	0.0	34.0	30.5	1.3	37.9	16.0	4.2	144	9.0
1993	54.5	0.0	54.5	11.0	48.5	0.0	34.0	32.0	1.4	39.8	16.0	4.2	152	9.5
1994	56.2	0.0	56.2	11.0	50.0	0.0	34.0	33.0	1.4	41.0	16.0	4.2	156	9.8
1995	57.7	0.0	57.7	11.0	51.3	0.0	34.0	33.9	1.5	42.1	16.0	4.2	160	10.0
1996	57.8	0.0	57.8	11.0	51.5	0.0	34.0	34.0	1.5	42.2	16.0	4.2	161	10.0
1997	60.4	0.0	60.4	11.0	53.8	0.0	34.0	35.5	1.6	44.1	16.0	4.2	168	10.5
1998	62.0	0.0	62.0	11.0	55.2	0.0	34.0	36.4	1.6	45.3	16.0	4.2	172	10.8
1999	63.8	0.0	63.8	11.0	56.8	0.0	34.0	37.5	1.6	46.5	16.0	4.2	177	11.1
2000	62.7	0.0	62.7	11.0	55.8	0.0	34.0	36.8	1.6	45.8	16.0	4.2	174	10.9
2001	62.6	0.0	62.6	11.0	55.7	0.0	34.0	36.8	1.6	45.7	16.0	4.2	174	10.9
2002	62.9	0.0	62.9	11.0	55.9	0.0	34.0	36.9	1.6	45.9	16.0	4.2	175	10.9
2003	61.0	0.0	61.0	11.0	54.3	0.0	34.0	35.8	1.6	44.5	16.0	4.2	170	10.6
2004	59.9	0.0	59.9	11.0	53.3	0.0	34.0	35.2	1.5	43.7	16.0	4.2	167	10.4
2005	58.8	0.0	58.8	11.0	52.3	0.0	34.0	34.5	1.5	42.9	16.0	4.2	163	10.2
2006	57.8	0.0	57.8	11.0	51.4	0.0	34.0	34.0	1.5	42.2	16.0	4.2	161	10.0
2007	55.8	0.0	55.8	11.0	49.7	0.0	34.0	32.8	1.4	40.7	16.0	4.2	155	9.7
2008	52.6	0.0	52.6	11.0	46.8	0.0	34.0	30.9	1.4	38.4	16.0	4.2	146	9.1
2009	49.7	0.0	49.7	11.0	44.2	0.0	34.0	29.2	1.3	36.3	16.0	4.2	138	8.6
2010	48.3	0.0	48.3	11.0	43.0	0.0	34.0	28.4	1.2	35.3	16.0	4.2	134	8.4
2011	46.6	0.0	46.6	11.0	41.5	0.0	34.0	27.4	1.2	34.0	16.0	4.2	130	8.1
2012	46.2	0.0	46.2	11.0	41.1	0.0	34.0	27.1	1.2	33.7	16.0	4.2	129	8.0

Note: Estimated number of daily per capita calories calculated by adjusting high high fructose corn syrup (HFCS) deliveries for domestic food and beverage use for food losses.

[a]U.S. per capita HFCS estimated deliveries for domestic food and beverage use, calendar year.

[b]Number of daily teaspoons multiplied by calories per serving.

[c]Grams per day divided by serving weight.

SOURCE: "Table 52. High Fructose Corn Syrup: Estimated Number of per Capita Calories Consumed Daily, by Calendar Year," in *Sugar and Sweeteners Yearbook Tables*, U.S. Department of Agriculture, Economic Research Service, May 28, 2012, http://www.ers.usda.gov/data-products/sugar-and-sweeteners-yearbook-tables.aspx#.UseHQrS4reo (accessed October 25, 2013)

TABLE 1.10

Food expenditures by families and individuals as a share of disposable personal income, 1929–2011

Year	Disposable personal income	Expenditures for food					
		At home[a]		Away from home[b]		Total[c]	
	Billion dollars	Billion dollars	Percent	Billion dollars	Percent	Billion dollars	Percent
1929	83.4	16.9	20.3	2.6	3.1	19.5	23.4
1930	74.7	15.8	21.2	2.3	3.1	18.1	24.2
1931	64.3	12.7	19.8	2.1	3.3	14.8	23.0
1932	49.2	9.6	19.5	1.7	3.5	11.3	23.0
1933	46.1	10.1	21.9	1.5	3.3	11.6	25.2
1934	52.8	11.1	21.0	1.7	3.2	12.8	24.2
1935	59.3	12.1	20.4	1.8	3.0	13.9	23.4
1936	67.4	12.7	18.8	2.0	3.0	14.7	21.8
1937	72.2	13.3	18.4	2.2	3.0	15.5	21.5
1938	66.6	12.6	18.9	2.1	3.2	14.7	22.1
1939	71.4	13.0	18.1	2.3	3.2	15.2	21.3
1940	76.8	13.5	17.6	2.4	3.1	15.9	20.7
1941	93.8	15.3	16.3	2.9	3.1	18.2	19.4
1942	118.6	18.5	15.6	3.6	3.0	22.1	18.6
1943	135.4	20.7	15.3	4.5	3.3	25.2	18.6
1944	148.3	22.1	14.9	5.1	3.4	27.2	18.4
1945	152.2	23.6	15.5	5.7	3.7	29.3	19.2
1946	161.4	28.4	17.6	6.5	4.0	34.9	21.6
1947	171.2	32.8	19.2	7.4	4.3	40.2	23.5
1948	190.6	34.9	18.3	7.5	3.9	42.4	22.3
1949	190.4	34.3	18.0	7.8	4.1	42.0	22.1
1950	210.1	35.7	17.0	7.6	3.6	43.3	20.6
1951	231.0	40.0	17.3	8.4	3.6	48.4	20.9
1952	243.4	41.8	17.2	8.8	3.6	50.6	20.8
1953	258.6	42.3	16.4	9.0	3.5	51.3	19.9
1954	264.3	42.4	16.0	9.3	3.5	51.7	19.6
1955	283.3	42.9	15.1	9.8	3.5	52.7	18.6
1956	303.0	44.4	14.7	10.4	3.4	54.8	18.1
1957	319.8	48.1	15.0	10.9	3.4	59.0	18.4
1958	330.5	49.8	15.1	11.1	3.4	60.9	18.4
1959	350.5	50.1	14.3	12.1	3.5	62.3	17.8
1960	365.4	51.5	14.1	12.6	3.4	64.0	17.5
1961	381.8	52.0	13.6	13.1	3.4	65.1	17.1
1962	405.1	52.9	13.1	13.9	3.4	66.8	16.5
1963	425.1	53.3	12.5	14.5	3.4	67.9	16.0
1964	462.5	55.5	12.0	15.7	3.4	71.2	15.4
1965	498.1	58.4	11.7	16.9	3.4	75.4	15.1
1966	537.5	61.0	11.3	18.6	3.5	79.6	14.8
1967	575.3	61.4	10.7	19.8	3.4	81.1	14.1
1968	625.0	64.5	10.3	21.7	3.5	86.2	13.8
1969	674.0	69.0	10.2	23.4	3.5	92.3	13.7
1970	735.7	75.5	10.3	26.4	3.6	102.0	13.9
1971	801.8	79.5	9.9	28.1	3.5	107.6	13.4
1972	869.1	86.0	9.9	31.3	3.6	117.3	13.5
1973	978.3	94.9	9.7	34.9	3.6	129.8	13.3
1974	1,071.6	107.3	10.0	38.5	3.6	145.8	13.6
1975	1,187.4	117.4	9.9	45.9	3.9	163.3	13.8
1976	1,302.5	125.1	9.6	52.6	4.0	177.7	13.6
1977	1,435.7	133.8	9.3	58.5	4.1	192.3	13.4
1978	1,608.3	147.3	9.2	67.5	4.2	214.8	13.4
1979	1,793.5	164.0	9.1	76.9	4.3	240.9	13.4
1980	2,009.0	180.8	9.0	85.2	4.2	266.0	13.2
1981	2,246.1	195.5	8.7	95.8	4.3	291.3	13.0
1982	2,421.2	201.0	8.3	104.5	4.3	305.5	12.6
1983	2,608.4	211.4	8.1	113.7	4.4	325.1	12.5
1984	2,912.0	224.0	7.7	121.9	4.2	345.8	11.9
1985	3,109.3	234.0	7.5	128.6	4.1	362.6	11.7
1986	3,285.1	242.7	7.4	137.9	4.2	380.6	11.6
1987	3,435.3	252.7	7.4	144.4	4.2	397.1	11.6
1988	3,726.3	271.7	7.3	155.5	4.2	427.2	11.5
1989	3,991.4	290.1	7.3	163.3	4.1	453.4	11.4
1990	4,254.0	314.5	7.4	175.2	4.1	489.6	11.5
1991	4,444.8	328.6	7.4	184.0	4.1	512.6	11.5
1992	4,736.7	332.1	7.0	190.8	4.0	522.9	11.0
1993	4,921.6	340.0	6.9	204.8	4.2	544.8	11.1
1994	5,184.3	352.9	6.8	215.4	4.2	568.2	11.0
1995	5,457.0	359.4	6.6	229.2	4.2	588.6	10.8
1996	5,759.6	374.2	6.5	232.1	4.0	606.3	10.5
1997	6,074.6	387.4	6.4	248.3	4.1	635.6	10.5
1998	6,498.9	396.1	6.1	260.9	4.0	657.0	10.1
1999	6,803.3	414.0	6.1	272.9	4.0	686.8	10.1

TABLE 1.10

Food expenditures by families and individuals as a share of disposable personal income, 1929–2011 [CONTINUED]

| Year | Disposable personal income | Expenditures for food | | | | | | |
| | | At home[a] | | Away from home[b] | | Total[c] | |
	Billion dollars	Billion dollars	Percent	Billion dollars	Percent	Billion dollars	Percent
2000	7,327.2	431.6	5.9	292.9	4.0	724.5	9.9
2001	7,648.5	453.6	5.9	302.0	3.9	755.6	9.9
2002	8,009.7	474.7	5.9	307.7	3.8	782.4	9.8
2003	8,377.8	489.9	5.8	335.3	4.0	825.2	9.9
2004	8,889.4	509.1	5.7	350.4	3.9	859.4	9.7
2005	9,277.3	533.7	5.8	383.0	4.1	916.7	9.9
2006	9,915.7	552.0	5.6	410.9	4.1	962.9	9.7
2007	10,423.6	579.2	5.6	432.0	4.1	1,011.1	9.7
2008	11,024.5	607.5	5.5	443.8	4.0	1,051.4	9.5
2009	10,788.8	605.0	5.6	442.6	4.1	1,047.7	9.7
2010	11,179.7	622.0	5.6	458.1	4.1	1,080.2	9.7
2011	11,593.5	659.4	5.7	479.9	4.1	1,139.3	9.8

[a]Food-at-home includes cash purchases from grocery stores and other retail outlets, including purchases with food stamps and WIC (women, infants, and children) vouchers and food produced and consumed on farms (valued at farm prices), but excludes government-donated foods.
[b]Food-away-from-home includes meals and snacks purchased by families and individuals and food furnished to employees, but excludes food paid for by government and business, such as donated foods to schools, meals in prisons and other institutions, and expense-account meals.
[c]Total may not add due to rounding.

SOURCE: "Table 7. Food Expenditures by Families and Individuals As a Share of Disposable Personal Income," in *Food Expenditures*, U.S. Department of Agriculture, Economic Research Service, October 1, 2012, http://www.ers.usda.gov/briefing/cpifoodandexpenditures/data/Expenditures_tables/table7.htm (accessed October 25, 2013)

CHAPTER 2
WEIGHT AND PHYSICAL HEALTH

If we could give every individual the right amount of nourishment and exercise, not too little and not too much, we would have found the safest way to health.

—Hippocrates

During the 20th century and the first decade of the 21st century, advances in public health and medical care helped Americans lead longer, healthier lives. Two important measures of the health of the population are infant mortality (death) rates and life expectancy at birth rates. By the end of the 20th century, infant mortality rates had significantly decreased and life expectancy had increased by 29.4 years. Table 2.1 shows the long-term upward trend in life expectancy as well as recent gains. In 2010 life expectancy at birth for the total population reached a record high of 78.7 years, up from 75.4 years in 1990.

As deaths from infectious diseases declined during the second half of the 20th century, mortality from chronic diseases, such as heart disease and cancer, increased. Table 2.2 displays the 10 leading causes of death in the United States in 1980 and 2010. Overweight and obesity are considered contributing factors to at least four of the 10 leading causes of death in 2010: diseases of the heart, malignant neoplasms (tumors), cerebrovascular diseases (diseases affecting the supply of blood to the brain), and diabetes mellitus. Obesity may also be implicated in some deaths attributable to another leading cause of death: nephritis, nephrotic syndrome, and nephrosis (kidney disease or chronic renal failure). Table 2.2 also reveals the rise of diabetes as a cause of death. In 1980 it was the seventh-leading cause of death, claiming 34,851 lives. By 2010 it was the underlying cause of 69,071 deaths. Epidemiologists (scientists who study the occurrence and distribution of diseases and the factors that govern their spread) and medical researchers believe the increasing prevalence of diabetes in the U.S. population and the resultant rise in deaths attributable to diabetes are

direct consequences of the obesity epidemic in the United States.

Overweight and obesity increase not only the risk of morbidity (illness or disease) and mortality but also the severity of diseases such as hypertension (high blood pressure), arthritis, and other musculoskeletal problems. Table 2.3 lists the health consequences that may result from overweight and obesity among adults and children. It also estimates the likelihood of these health consequences. For example, adults who are obese are twice as likely to suffer from high blood pressure than adults who have a healthy weight.

In "Obesity and Mortality Risk: New Findings from Body Mass Index Trajectories" (*American Journal of Epidemiology*, vol. 178, no. 11, September 7, 2013), Hui Zheng, Dmitry Tumin, and Zhenchao Qian examine the relationship between body mass index (BMI) and life expectancy in the United States. The researchers find that BMI trajectories (trends of increasing or decreasing BMI) were better predictors of mortality risk than just BMI at a single time point. The researchers note that people in the overweight stable trajectory had the highest survival rate, followed by those in the overweight obesity, normal weight upward, class I obese upward, normal weight downward, and class II/III obese upward trajectories. Zheng, Tumin, and Qian also report that approximately 7.2% of deaths after the age of 51 years were in the class I and class II/III obese upward trajectories and caution that "trajectories of increasing obesity past 51 years of age pose a substantive threat to future gains in life expectancy."

IS OBESITY A DISEASE?

Researchers now recognize that obesity does not simply result from willful overeating and laziness, but from a complex combination of genetic, metabolic, behavioral, and environmental factors. Rather than viewing it as a lifestyle choice or personal failing, several groups favor declaring

TABLE 2.1

Life expectancy at birth, at 65 years of age, and at 75 years of age, according to race and sex, selected years 1900–2010

[Data are based on death certificates]

Specified age and year	All races			White			Black or African American[a]		
	Both sexes	Male	Female	Both sexes	Male	Female	Both sexes	Male	Female
At birth				Life expectancy, in years					
1900[b, c]	47.3	46.3	48.3	47.6	46.6	48.7	33.0	32.5	33.5
1950[c]	68.2	65.6	71.1	69.1	66.5	72.2	60.8	59.1	62.9
1960[c]	69.7	66.6	73.1	70.6	67.4	74.1	63.6	61.1	66.3
1970	70.8	67.1	74.7	71.7	68.0	75.6	64.1	60.0	68.3
1980	73.7	70.0	77.4	74.4	70.7	78.1	68.1	63.8	72.5
1990	75.4	71.8	78.8	76.1	72.7	79.4	69.1	64.5	73.6
1995	75.8	72.5	78.9	76.5	73.4	79.6	69.6	65.2	73.9
2000	76.8	74.1	79.3	77.3	74.7	79.9	71.8	68.2	75.1
2001	77.0	74.3	79.5	77.5	74.9	80.0	72.0	68.5	75.3
2002	77.0	74.4	79.6	77.5	74.9	80.1	72.2	68.7	75.4
2003	77.2	74.5	79.7	77.7	75.1	80.2	72.4	68.9	75.7
2004	77.6	75.0	80.1	78.1	75.5	80.5	72.9	69.4	76.1
2005	77.6	75.0	80.1	78.0	75.5	80.5	73.0	69.5	76.2
2006	77.8	75.2	80.3	78.3	75.8	80.7	73.4	69.9	76.7
2007	78.1	75.5	80.6	78.5	76.0	80.9	73.8	70.3	77.0
2008	78.2	75.6	80.6	78.5	76.1	80.9	74.3	70.9	77.3
2009	78.5	76.0	80.9	78.8	76.4	81.2	74.7	71.4	77.7
2010	78.7	76.2	81.0	78.9	76.5	81.3	75.1	71.8	78.0
At 65 years									
1950[c]	13.9	12.8	15.0	14.1	12.8	15.1	13.9	12.0	14.0
1960[c]	14.3	12.8	15.8	14.4	12.9	15.9	13.9	12.7	15.1
1970	15.2	13.1	17.0	15.2	13.1	17.1	14.2	12.5	15.7
1980	16.4	14.1	18.3	16.5	14.2	18.4	15.1	13.0	16.8
1990	17.2	15.1	18.9	17.3	15.2	19.1	15.4	13.2	17.2
1995	17.4	15.6	18.9	17.6	15.7	19.1	15.6	13.6	17.1
2000	17.6	16.0	19.0	17.7	16.1	19.1	16.1	14.1	17.5
2001	17.9	16.2	19.2	18.0	16.3	19.3	16.2	14.2	17.7
2002	17.9	16.3	19.2	18.0	16.4	19.3	16.3	14.4	17.8
2003	18.1	16.5	19.3	18.2	16.6	19.4	16.5	14.5	18.0
2004	18.4	16.9	19.6	18.5	17.0	19.7	16.8	14.9	18.3
2005	18.4	16.9	19.6	18.5	17.0	19.7	16.9	15.0	18.3
2006	18.7	17.2	19.9	18.7	17.3	19.9	17.2	15.2	18.6
2007	18.8	17.4	20.0	18.9	17.4	20.1	17.3	15.4	18.8
2008	18.8	17.4	20.0	18.9	17.5	20.0	17.5	15.5	18.9
2009	19.1	17.7	20.3	19.2	17.7	20.3	17.8	15.9	19.2
2010	19.1	17.7	20.3	19.2	17.8	20.3	17.8	15.9	19.3
At 75 years									
1980	10.4	8.8	11.5	10.4	8.8	11.5	9.7	8.3	10.7
1990	10.9	9.4	12.0	11.0	9.4	12.0	10.2	8.6	11.2
1995	11.0	9.7	11.9	11.1	9.7	12.0	10.2	8.8	11.1
2000	11.0	9.8	11.8	11.0	9.8	11.9	10.4	9.0	11.3
2001	11.2	9.9	12.0	11.2	10.0	12.1	10.5	9.0	11.5
2002	11.2	10.0	12.0	11.2	10.0	12.1	10.5	9.1	11.5
2003	11.3	10.1	12.1	11.3	10.2	12.1	10.7	8.7	11.6
2004	11.5	10.4	12.4	11.6	10.4	12.4	10.9	9.4	11.2
2005	11.5	10.4	12.3	11.5	10.4	12.3	10.9	9.4	11.2
2006	11.7	10.6	12.5	11.1	10.6	12.5	11.1	9.1	12.0
2007	11.9	10.7	12.6	11.9	10.8	12.6	11.2	9.8	12.1
2008	11.8	10.7	12.6	11.8	10.7	12.6	11.3	9.8	12.2
2009	12.1	11.0	12.9	12.1	10.4	12.9	11.6	10.2	12.5
2010	12.1	11.0	12.9	12.1	11.0	12.8	11.6	10.2	12.5

obesity a disease. Proponents assert that many public health benefits would result from designating obesity as a disease, including:

- Reducing the social stigma and prejudice that are associated with obesity, and promoting attitudinal changes to reduce weight-based discrimination

- Enabling more people to seek treatment for obesity by providing health insurance coverage for treatment

- Increasing public awareness of the severity of obesity as a threat to health and longevity

- Stimulating scientific and medical research on the prevention and treatment of the condition and speeding approval of new antiobesity drugs

Advocates of classifying obesity as a disease, including the World Health Organization, the National Institutes of Health, the National Academy of Sciences, the Federal Trade Commission, the Maternal and Child Health Bureau, the American Heart Association, the American Academy of Family Physicians, the American Society for Bariatric Surgery, the American Society of Bariatric Physicians, and the American

TABLE 2.1

Life expectancy at birth, at 65 years of age, and at 75 years of age, according to race and sex, selected years 1900–2010 [CONTINUED]

[Data are based on death certificates]

Specified age and year	White, not Hispanic			Black, not Hispanic			Hispanic[d]		
	Both sexes	Male	Female	Both sexes	Male	Female	Both sexes	Male	Female
At birth					Life expectancy, in years				
2006	78.2	75.7	80.6	73.1	69.5	76.4	80.3	77.5	82.9
2007	78.4	75.9	80.8	73.5	69.9	76.7	80.7	77.8	83.2
2008	78.4	76.0	80.7	73.9	70.5	77.0	80.8	78.0	83.3
2009	78.7	76.3	81.1	74.3	70.9	77.4	81.1	78.4	83.5
2010	78.8	76.4	81.1	74.7	71.4	77.7	81.2	78.5	83.8
At 65 years									
2006	18.7	17.2	19.9	17.1	15.1	18.5	20.2	18.5	21.5
2007	18.8	17.4	20.0	17.2	15.3	18.7	20.5	18.7	21.7
2008	18.8	17.4	20.0	17.4	15.4	18.8	20.4	18.7	21.6
2009	19.1	17.7	19.5	17.7	15.8	19.1	20.7	19.0	21.9
2010	19.1	17.7	20.3	17.7	15.8	19.1	20.6	18.8	22.0
At 75 years									
2006	11.7	10.6	12.5	11.1	9.6	12.0	13.0	11.7	13.7
2007	11.8	10.7	12.6	11.2	9.7	12.1	13.1	11.8	13.8
2008	11.8	10.7	12.6	11.3	9.8	12.2	13.0	11.7	13.8
2009	12.0	11.0	12.9	11.6	10.1	12.4	13.3	12.0	13.8
2010	12.0	11.0	12.8	11.6	10.1	12.5	13.2	11.7	14.1

[a]Data shown for 1900–1960 are for the nonwhite population.
[b]Death registration area only. The death registration area increased from 10 states and the District of Columbia (D.C.) in 1900 to the coterminous United States in 1933.
[c]Includes deaths of persons who were not residents of the 50 states and D.C.
[d]Hispanic origin was added to the U.S. standard death certificate in 1989 and was adopted by every state in 1997. To estimate life expectancy, age-specific death rates were corrected to address racial and ethnic misclassification, which underestimates deaths in the Hispanic population. To address the effects of age misstatement at the oldest ages, the probability of death for Hispanic persons older than 80 years is estimated as a function of non-Hispanic white mortality with the use of the Brass relational logit model.

Notes: Populations for computing life expectancy for 1991–1999 are 1990-based postcensal estimates of the U.S. resident population. Starting with *Health, United States, 2012*, populations for computing life expectancy for 2001–2009 were based on intercensal population estimates of the U.S. resident population. Populations for computing life expectancy for 2010 were based on 2010 census counts. In 1997, life table methodology was revised to construct complete life tables by single years of age that extend to age 100. Previously, abridged life tables were constructed for 5-year age groups ending with 85 years and over. In 2000, the life table methodology was revised. The revised methodology is similar to that developed for the 1999–2001 decennial life tables. In 2008, the life table methodology was further refined. Starting with 2003 data, some states allowed the reporting of more than one race on the death certificate. The multiple-race data for these states were bridged to the single-race categories of the 1977 Office of Management and Budget standards, for comparability with other states. The race groups, white and black include persons of Hispanic and non-Hispanic origin. Persons of Hispanic origin may be of any race.

SOURCE: "Table 18. Life Expectancy at Birth, at Age 65, and at Age 75, by Sex, Race, and Hispanic Origin: United States, Selected Years 1900–2010," in *Health, United States, 2012: With Special Feature on Emergency Care*, Centers for Disease Control and Prevention, National Center for Health Statistics, 2013, http://www.cdc.gov/nchs/data/hus/hus12.pdf (accessed October 8, 2013)

Obesity Association (AOA), observe that in the past, alcoholism was viewed as a personal choice or moral weakness, whereas in the 21st century it is considered a disease. They also note that eating disorders such as anorexia nervosa (intense fear of becoming fat even when dangerously underweight) and bulimia nervosa (recurrent episodes of binge eating followed by purging to prevent weight gain) are classified as diseases. In view of the size and scope of the obesity epidemic, proponents argue that the social and financial costs of allowing the problem of obesity to go unchecked will far exceed the costs associated with extending health care coverage for weight-reduction programs.

The AOA contends that obesity meets the criteria for disease because according to *Stedman's Medical Dictionary* (2005) a disease should have at least two of the following three features:

- Recognized etiologic (causative) agents

- Identifiable signs and symptoms

- Consistent anatomical alterations

The AOA describes etiologic agents for obesity as social, behavioral, cultural, physiological, metabolic, and genetic factors. The identifiable signs and symptoms of obesity include an excess accumulation of adipose tissue (fat); an increase in the size or number of fat cells; insulin resistance; decreased levels of high-density lipoprotein and norepinephrine; alterations in the activity of the sympathetic and parasympathetic nervous system; and elevated blood pressure, blood glucose, cholesterol, and triglyceride levels. The consistent anatomical alteration of obesity is the increase in body mass.

Opponents contend that although obesity increases the risk of developing many diseases, it is not an ailment in itself but an unhealthy consequence of poor lifestyle choices. They liken it to cigarette smoking, a risk factor that predisposes people to disease, and they dispute the notion that labeling obesity as a disease will have a beneficial effect on the ability of public health organizations to alter the course of the obesity epidemic. They maintain the public tends to view diseases as conditions that are contracted or contagious; and with disease comes

TABLE 2.2

Leading causes of death and numbers of deaths, according to sex and race, 1980 and 2010

[Data are based on death certificates]

Sex, race, Hispanic origin, and rank order	1980 Cause of death	Deaths	2010 Cause of death	Deaths
All persons				
Rank	All causes	1,989,841	All causes	2,468,435
1	Diseases of heart	761,085	Diseases of heart	597,689
2	Malignant neoplasms	416,509	Malignant neoplasms	574,743
3	Cerebrovascular diseases	170,225	Chronic lower respiratory diseases	138,080
4	Unintentional injuries	105,718	Cerebrovascular diseases	129,476
5	Chronic obstructive pulmonary diseases	56,050	Unintentional injuries	120,859
6	Pneumonia and influenza	54,619	Alzheimer's disease	83,494
7	Diabetes mellitus	34,851	Diabetes mellitus	69,071
8	Chronic liver disease and cirrhosis	30,583	Nephritis, nephrotic syndrome and nephrosis	50,476
9	Atherosclerosis	29,449	Influenza and pneumonia	50,097
10	Suicide	26,869	Suicide	38,364
Male				
Rank	All causes	1,075,078	All causes	1,232,432
1	Diseases of heart	405,661	Diseases of heart	307,384
2	Malignant neoplasms	225,948	Malignant neoplasms	301,037
3	Unintentional injuries	74,180	Unintentional injuries	75,921
4	Cerebrovascular diseases	69,973	Chronic lower respiratory diseases	65,423
5	Chronic obstructive pulmonary diseases	38,625	Cerebrovascular diseases	52,367
6	Pneumonia and influenza	27,574	Diabetes mellitus	35,490
7	Suicide	20,505	Suicide	30,277
8	Chronic liver disease and cirrhosis	19,768	Alzheimer's disease	25,364
9	Homicide	18,779	Nephritis, nephrotic syndrome and nephrosis	24,865
10	Diabetes mellitus	14,325	Influenza and pneumonia	23,615
Female				
Rank	All causes	914,763	All causes	1,236,003
1	Diseases of heart	355,424	Diseases of heart	290,305
2	Malignant neoplasms	190,561	Malignant neoplasms	273,706
3	Cerebrovascular diseases	100,252	Cerebrovascular diseases	77,109
4	Unintentional injuries	31,538	Chronic lower respiratory diseases	72,657
5	Pneumonia and influenza	27,045	Alzheimer's disease	58,130
6	Diabetes mellitus	20,526	Unintentional injuries	44,938
7	Atherosclerosis	17,848	Diabetes mellitus	33,581
8	Chronic obstructive pulmonary diseases	17,425	Influenza and pneumonia	26,482
9	Chronic liver disease and cirrhosis	10,815	Nephritis, nephrotic syndrome and nephrosis	25,611
10	Certain conditions originating in the perinatal period	9,815	Septicemia	18,743
White				
Rank	All causes	1,738,607	All causes	2,114,749
1	Diseases of heart	683,347	Diseases of heart	514,323
2	Malignant neoplasms	368,162	Malignant neoplasms	491,686
3	Cerebrovascular diseases	148,734	Chronic lower respiratory diseases	127,176
4	Unintentional injuries	90,122	Cerebrovascular diseases	109,119
5	Chronic obstructive pulmonary diseases	52,375	Unintentional injuries	104,945
6	Pneumonia and influenza	48,369	Alzheimer's disease	76,928
7	Diabetes mellitus	28,868	Diabetes mellitus	54,250
8	Atherosclerosis	27,069	Influenza and pneumonia	43,296
9	Chronic liver disease and cirrhosis	25,240	Nephritis, nephrotic syndrome and nephrosis	40,205
10	Suicide	24,829	Suicide	34,690
Black or African American				
Rank	All causes	233,135	All causes	286,959
1	Diseases of heart	72,956	Diseases of heart	69,083
2	Malignant neoplasms	45,037	Malignant neoplasms	65,930
3	Cerebrovascular diseases	20,135	Cerebrovascular diseases	15,965
4	Unintentional injuries	13,480	Diabetes mellitus	12,126
5	Homicide	10,172	Unintentional injuries	12,069
6	Certain conditions originating in the perinatal period	6,961	Nephritis, nephrotic syndrome and nephrosis	8,841
7	Pneumonia and influenza	5,648	Chronic lower respiratory diseases	8,715
8	Diabetes mellitus	5,544	Homicide	7,818
9	Chronic liver disease and cirrhosis	4,790	Septicemia	6,001
10	Nephritis, nephrotic syndrome and nephrosis	3,416	Alzheimer's disease	5,220

TABLE 2.2

Leading causes of death and numbers of deaths, according to sex and race, 1980 and 2010 [CONTINUED]

[Data are based on death certificates]

Notes: Starting with 2003 data, some states allowed the reporting of more than one race on the death certificate. The multiple-race data for these states were bridged to the single-race categories of the 1977 Office of Management and Budget standards for comparability with other states. The race groups, white, black, Asian or Pacific Islander, and American Indian or Alaska Native, include persons of Hispanic and non-Hispanic origin. Persons of Hispanic origin may be of any race.

SOURCE: Adapted from "Table 22. Leading Causes of Death and Numbers of Deaths, by Sex, Race, and Hispanic Origin: United States, 1980 and 2010," in *Health, United States, 2012: With Special Feature on Emergency Care*, Centers for Disease Control and Prevention, National Center for Health Statistics, 2013, http://www.cdc.gov/nchs/data/hus/hus12.pdf (accessed October 8, 2013)

TABLE 2.3

Health consequences of overweight and obesity

Premature death

- An estimated 300,000 deaths per year may be attributable to obesity.
- The risk of death rises with increasing weight.
- Even moderate weight excess (10 to 20 pounds for a person of average height) increases the risk of death, particularly among adults aged 30 to 64 years.
- Individuals who are obese (body mass index (BMI) > 30) have a 50 to 100% increased risk of premature death from all causes, compared to individuals with a healthy weight.

Heart disease

- The incidence of heart disease (heart attack, congestive heart failure, sudden cardiac death, angina or chest pain, and abnormal heart rhythm) is increased in persons who are overweight or obese (BMI > 25).
- High blood pressure is twice as common in adults who are obese than in those who are at a healthy weight.
- Obesity is associated with elevated triglycerides (blood fat) and decreased high density lipoprotein (HDL) cholesterol ("good cholesterol").

Diabetes

- A weight gain of 11 to 18 pounds increases a person's risk of developing type 2 diabetes to twice that of individuals who have not gained weight.
- Over 80% of people with diabetes are overweight or obese.

Cancer

- Overweight and obesity are associated with an increased risk for some types of cancer including endometrial (cancer of the lining of the uterus), colon, gall bladder, prostate, kidney, and postmenopausal breast cancer.
- Women gaining more than 20 pounds from age 18 to midlife double their risk of postmenopausal breast cancer, compared to women whose weight remains stable.

Breathing problems

- Sleep apnea (interrupted breathing while sleeping) is more common in obese persons.
- Obesity is associated with a higher prevalence of asthma.

Arthritis

- For every 2-pound increase in weight, the risk of developing arthritis is increased by 9 to 13%.
- Symptoms of arthritis can improve with weight loss.

Reproductive complications

Complications of pregnancy
- Obesity during pregnancy is associated with increased risk of death in both the baby and the mother and increases the risk of maternal high blood pressure by 10 times.
- In addition to many other complications, women who are obese during pregnancy are more likely to have gestational diabetes and problems with labor and delivery.
- Infants born to women who are obese during pregnancy are more likely to be high birthweight and, therefore, may face a higher rate of Cesarean section delivery and low blood sugar (which can be associated with brain damage and seizures).
- Obesity during pregnancy is associated with an increased risk of birth defects, particularly neural tube defects, such as spina bifida.
- Obesity in premenopausal women is associated with irregular menstrual cycles and infertility.

Additional health consequences

- Overweight and obesity are associated with increased risks of gall bladder disease, incontinence, increased surgical risk, and depression.
- Obesity can affect the quality of life through limited mobility and decreased physical endurance as well as through social, academic, and job discrimination.

Children and adolescents

- Risk factors for heart disease, such as high cholesterol and high blood pressure, occur with increased frequency in overweight children and adolescents compared to those with a healthy weight.
- Type 2 diabetes, previously considered an adult disease, has increased dramatically in children and adolescents. Overweight and obesity are closely linked to type 2 diabetes.
- Overweight adolescents have a 70% chance of becoming overweight or obese adults. This increases to 80% if one or more parent is overweight or obese.
- The most immediate consequence of overweight, as perceived by children themselves, is social discrimination.

SOURCE: "Overweight and Obesity: Health Consequences," in *The Surgeon General's Call to Action to Prevent and Decrease Overweight and Obesity*, U.S. Department of Health and Human Services, Office of the Surgeon General, 2001, http://www.surgeongeneral.gov/topics/obesity/calltoaction/fact_consequences.htm (accessed October 29, 2013)

---

a victim mentality, rather than an assumption of personal responsibility. Because many health professionals consider the assumption of personal responsibility as being crucial for the long-term success of obesity treatment, any action that releases people from assuming personal responsibility is counterproductive.

Furthermore, because people who are obese often function normally and can perform all the activities of daily living, opponents assert that their lives are not impaired or compromised as they might be by other chronic diseases. Some researchers, such as Silvia Migliaccio et al. of the Università Sapienza di Roma in "Is Obesity in Women Protective against Osteoporosis?" (*Diabetes, Metabolic Syndrome, and Obesity*, vol. 4, July 2011), also point to the fact that in a few instances obesity may even be protective by reducing the risk of osteoporosis.

Another concern is the lack of universally accepted, effective treatment for obesity. If obesity is classified as a disease, which treatment or therapies should be covered? For example, if exercise is deemed beneficial, then health insurers might be required to pay for gym memberships. Furthermore, some opponents believe it is not necessary to designate obesity as a disease to encourage Americans to seek treatment. They cite the more than $50 billion that is spent annually on weight-loss programs and services as evidence that Americans are not reluctant to seek treatment for obesity.

Although the debate has not been fully resolved, obesity is rapidly acquiring recognition as a disease. In 2002 the Internal Revenue Service ruled that for tax purposes obesity is a disease, allowing Americans for the first time to claim a deduction for some health care expenses that are related to obesity, just as they can for expenditures that are related to cancer, diabetes, heart disease, and other illnesses.

In 2004 the federal Medicare program discarded its long-standing position that obesity is not a disease, which effectively removed a major roadblock for people seeking coverage for treatment of obesity. After years of review, the Centers for Medicare and Medicaid Services, which administers the health program for older adults and people who are disabled, announced in *CMS Manual System: Pub. 100-03 Medicare National Coverage Determinations* (October 1, 2004, http://www.cms.hhs.gov/transmittals/downloads/R23NCD.pdf) that it eliminated the phrase "obesity itself cannot be considered an illness" from its policy that had been used to deny coverage for weight-loss treatment. Although the decision stopped short of declaring obesity a disease and did not automatically imply coverage for any specific treatment, it enabled individuals, physicians, and companies to apply to Medicare for reimbursement for a variety of weight-loss therapies. Medicare coverage for selected weight-loss procedures took effect in February 2006.

In June 2013 the American Medical Association (AMA) officially recognized obesity as a disease in an effort to increase attention to combating it and to encourage reimbursement for obesity treatment—drugs, surgery, and counseling. Andrew Pollack reports in "A.M.A. Recognizes Obesity as a Disease" (NYTimes.com, June 18, 2013) that the AMA statement characterizes obesity as a "multi-metabolic and hormonal disease state" that leads to unfavorable consequences, including type 2 diabetes and cardiovascular disease.

Because private insurance companies often use Medicare as a model for their coverage and benefits, the Medicare decision prompted them to expand coverage for weight-loss procedures. As of October 2013, private health insurance coverage for weight-loss therapies and surgical procedures varied widely. Nanci Hellmich reports in "Obamacare Requires Most Insurers to Tackle Obesity" (USAToday.com, July 4, 2013) that the Patient Protection and Affordable Care Act (ACA), the health care reform legislation that has been dubbed Obamacare, requires most insurance plans to help obese patients lose weight. Screening and counseling for obesity as well as U.S. Food and Drug Administration–approved drug treatment must be covered by the plans, however coverage for ongoing treatment varies. Some insurance plans provide counseling or coaching by telephone or in-person, others refer patients to weight-loss programs such as Weight Watchers.

In "Getting Paid for Treating Obesity, Now That It's a 'Disease'" (Medscape.com, July 17, 2013,), Leigh Page observes that the ACA offers slight improvements in coverage. Because obesity treatment is not defined in the ACA as an "essential health benefit" plans are not required to cover it. Nonetheless, at least 21 plans offered through state-based health insurance exchanges cover at least one kind of obesity treatment. Page reports that as of 2013, the California, Massachusetts, Michigan, and New Mexico exchanges covered weight-loss surgery and weight-loss programs while 17 exchanges covered surgery only.

THE GENETICS OF BODY WEIGHT AND OBESITY

Genetics, the study of single genes and their effects, explains how and why traits such as hair color and blood types run in families. In the early 21st century the scientific community agreed that body shape and body weight are also regulated traits, that genes govern much of this regulation, and that altering genetically predetermined set points for body weight is often difficult. Genomics, a discipline that emerged during the 1980s, is the study of more than single genes; it considers the functions and interactions of all the genes in the genome. In terms of understanding genetics as a risk factor for obesity, genomics has broader applicability than does genetics because it is likely that humans carry dozens of genes that are directly related to body size and that most obesity is multifactorial—resulting from the complex interactions of multiple genes and environmental factors.

TABLE 2.4

Obesity and genetics

What we know:	What we don't know:
Biological relatives tend to resemble each other in many ways, including body weight. Individuals with a family history of obesity may be predisposed to gain weight and interventions that prevent obesity are especially important.	Why are biological relatives more similar in body weight? What genes are associated with this observation? Are the same genetic associations seen in every family? How do these genes affect energy metabolism and regulation?
In an environment made constant for food intake and physical activity, individuals respond differently. Some people store more energy as fat in an environment of excess; others lose less fat in an environment of scarcity. The different responses are largely due to genetic variation between individuals.	Why are interventions based on diet and exercise more effective for some people than others? What are the biological differences between these high and low responders? How do we use these insights to tailor interventions to specific needs?
Fat stores are regulated over long periods of time by complex systems that involve input and feedback from fatty tissues, the brain, and endocrine glands like the pancreas and the thyroid. Overweight and obesity can result from only a very small positive energy input imbalance over a long period of time.	What elements of energy regulation feedback systems are different in individuals? How do these differences affect energy metabolism and regulation?
Rarely, people have mutations in single genes that result in severe obesity that starts in infancy. Studying these individuals is providing insight into the complex biological pathways that regulate the balance between energy input and energy expenditure.	Do additional obesity syndromes exist that are caused by mutations in single genes? If so, what are they? What are the natural history, management strategy, and outcome for affected individuals?
Obese individuals have genetic similarities that may shed light on the biological differences that predispose to gain weight. This knowledge may be useful in preventing or treating obesity in predisposed people.	How do genetic variations that are shared by obese people affect gene expression and function? How do genetic variation and environmental factors interact to produce obesity? What are the biological features associated with the tendency to gain weight? What environmental factors are helpful in countering these tendencies?
Pharmaceutical companies are using genetic approaches (pharmacogenomics) to develop new drug strategies to treat obesity.	Will pharmacologic approaches benefit most people affected with obesity? Will these drugs be accessible to most people?
The tendency to store energy in the form of fat is believed to result from thousands of years of evolution in an environment characterized by tenuous food supplies. In other words, those who could store energy in times of plenty were more likely to survive periods of famine and to pass this tendency to their offspring.	How can thousands of years of evolutionary pressure be countered? Can specific factors in the modern environment (other than the obvious) be identified and controlled to more effectively counter these tendencies?

SOURCE: "Obesity and Genetics: What We Know, What We Don't Know and What It Means," in *Genomics and Health*, Centers for Disease Control and Prevention, Office of Surveillance, Epidemiology, and Laboratory Services, Public Health Genomics, January 20, 2011, http://www.cdc.gov/genomics/resources/diseases/obesity/obesknow.htm (accessed October 8, 2013)

Because genomics is a relatively new discipline, many questions are still unanswered about how genes influence the ability to balance energy input and energy expenditure, and why individuals vary in their abilities to perform this critical body function. Table 2.4 summarizes what is known and what remains to be learned about variations in body weight, energy metabolism, and inherited obesity syndromes.

Single Mutant Genes Cause Obesity

Although most obesity in humans is not due to mutations (alterations or changes) in single genes, there are obesity syndromes caused by variations in single genes. According to Alexandra I. F. Blakemore and Philippe Froguel of the Imperial College of London, in "Investigation of Mendelian Forms of Obesity Holds out the Prospect of Personalized Medicine" (*Annals of the New York Academy of Sciences*, vol. 1214, no. 1, December 2010), these mutations occur in genes that encode proteins that are related to the regulation of food intake and account for approximately 5% of all obesity.

The Centers for Disease Control and Prevention (CDC) reports in "Genomics and Health: Genes and Obesity" (May 17, 2013, http://www.cdc.gov/genomics/resources/diseases/obesity/obesedit.htm) that since 2006 genome-wide association studies have found more than 50 genes associated with obesity, but most exert very small effects. Table 2.5 shows some of the gene variants associated with

obesity. One example is a mutation of the leptin gene (on chromosome 7) and its receptor. The circulating hormone leptin (leptos means thin) sends the brain a satiety signal to decrease appetite. Obese mice of the ob/ob strain (obese mice that are specially bred for research) produce no leptin and tend to overeat; when given leptin, the mice stop eating and lose weight. Experiments, however, have failed to replicate these findings in humans. Blood concentrations of leptin are usually elevated in obese people, suggesting that they may be insensitive or resistant to leptin, rather than leptin deficient. Most obese individuals appear to have normal genetic sequences for leptin and its receptor, although people with a demonstrable genetic leptin deficiency suffer from extreme obesity.

Melanocortin 4 receptor (MC4R) deficiency is the most commonly occurring monogenic (single gene) form of obesity. Inheriting one copy of certain variants of the gene causes obesity in some families. In "Melanocortin-4 Receptor Mutations in Obesity" (*Advances in Clinical Chemistry*, vol. 48, 2009), Ferruccio Santini et al. report that mutations in MC4R produce a distinct obesity syndrome that is inherited. The researchers observe that these mutant receptors play a pivotal role in the control of eating behavior—that the regulation of body weight in humans is sensitive to variations in the amount of functional MC4R and are present in about 6% of people who are obese.

TABLE 2.5

Selected genes variants associated with obesity

Gene symbol	Gene name	Gene product's role in energy balance
ADIPOQ	Adipocyte-, C1q-, and collagen domain-containing	Produced by fat cells, adiponectin promotes energy expenditure
FTO	Fat mass- and obesity-associated gene	Promotes food intake
LEP	Leptin	Produced by fat cells
LEPR	Leptin receptor	When bound by leptin, inhibits appetite
INSIG2	Insulin-induced gene 2	Regulation of cholesterol and fatty acid synthesis
MC4R	Melanocortin 4 receptor	When bound by alpha-melanocyte stimulating hormone, stimulates appetite
PCSK1	Proproteinconvertasesubtilisin/kexin type 1	Regulates insulin biosynthesis
PPARG	Peroxisome proliferator-activated receptor gamma	Stimulates lipid uptake and development of fat tissue

SOURCE: "Table. Selected Genes with Variants That Have Been Associated with Obesity," in *Genomics and Health*, Centers for Disease Control and Prevention, Office of Surveillance, Epidemiology, and Laboratory Services, Public Health Genomics, May 17, 2013, http://www.cdc.gov/genomics/resources/diseases/obesity/obesedit.htm#table (accessed October 8, 2013)

Blakemore and Froguel observe that recent research on genome-wide single nucleotide polymorphisms (SNPs) associated with obesity, particularly the role of the FTO (fat mass and obesity-associated) gene, has outpaced research concentrating on a single gene that determines the occurrence of obesity. The focus on the FTO gene may be warranted because common variants of the FTO gene, which are located on chromosome 16, may be implicated in as much as 22% of obesity, according to the CDC. The FTO gene is also associated with an increased risk for diabetes.

In "Pediatric Obesity: Etiology and Treatment" (*Endocrinology and Metabolism Clinics*, vol. 58, no. 5, October 2011), Melissa K. Crocker and Jack A. Yanovski of the U.S. Public Health Service summarize what is known about the genetic underpinnings of obesity. The researchers observe that "virtually all of the known genetic causes of obesity primarily increase energy intake. Genes regulating the leptin signaling pathway are particularly important for human energy homeostasis." They report that SNPs of many genes and chromosomal regions have been found to be associated with body weight or body composition; however, mechanisms explaining how such SNPs exert an influence on energy balance are often not fully understood. Crocker and Yanovski reiterate one of the challenges of clinical genetic research: "Even in studies including thousands of genotyped people, such SNPs can be linked to body weight only when they are relatively common in the population."

Multiple Gene Variants Involved in Body Weight and Obesity

Heritability studies seek to determine the proportion of variance of a particular trait that is attributable to genetic factors and the proportion that is attributable to environmental factors. Such studies indicate that genetic factors may account for as much as 75% of the variability in human body weight and approximately 33% of the variation in the overall BMI (body weight in kilograms divided by height in meters squared). Genetic factors affect variations in the resting metabolic rate, body fat distribution, and weight gain related to overfeeding, which explains in part why some individuals are more susceptible than others to weight gain or weight loss. To ensure survival in times of scarce food supplies, the human body has evolved to resist any loss of body fat. This biological drive to maintain weight is coordinated through central nervous system pathways, with the involvement of many neuropeptides. (Neuropeptides are released by neurons as intercellular messengers. Many neuropeptides are also hormones outside of the nervous system.) Evidence from twin, adoption, and family studies reveals that biological relatives exhibit similarities in the maintenance of body weight. First-degree relatives of moderately obese people are at three to four times the risk of obesity relative to the general population. First-degree relatives of severely obese people are at five times greater risk. Genetic predisposition to obesity does not mean that developing the condition is inevitable; however, research indicates that inherited genetic variation is an important risk factor for obesity.

Genetic factors have been implicated in the development of eating disorders such as anorexia and bulimia and appear to be involved in the extent to which diet and exercise are effective strategies for weight reduction. Furthermore, genetic variations among individuals may promote different food preferences and eating patterns that interact with environmental conditions to maintain healthy body weight or promote obesity.

These genetic risk factors tend to be familial but are not inherited in a simple manner; they may reflect many genetic variations, and each variation may contribute a small amount of risk and may interact with environmental elements to produce obesity. Tuomo Rankinen et al. present in "The Human Obesity Gene Map: The 2005 Update" (*Obesity*, vol. 14, no. 4, April 2006) the 12th update of the human obesity gene map, which was completed in October 2005. This map contains over

600 genes, markers, and chromosomal regions that are associated with or linked to human obesity. Besides offering direction for future efforts to prevent and treat obesity, mounting genetic evidence offers a compelling argument that obesity is not a personal failing and that in most cases obesity involves multiple genetic and environmental components that affect endocrine, metabolic, and regulatory mechanisms.

Extra Genes Point to a Genetic Cause of Thinness

Unlike obesity, few genetic variants associated with underweight have been identified. Sébastien Jacquemont et al. report in "Mirror Extreme BMI Phenotypes Associated with Gene Dosage at the Chromosome 16p11.2 Locus" (*Nature*, vol. 478, no. 7367, August 31, 2011) that duplication of a portion of chromosome 16 is associated with being very thin (BMI less than 18.5). The researchers analyzed the deoxyribonucleic acid of more than 95,000 people and find that more than half of children with this duplication had significantly lower than normal weight gain. Jacquemont et al. also note that people missing this gene have an increased risk for obesity.

Genetic Susceptibility and Environmental Influences

Although genetics may largely predetermine adult body weight absent specific environmental triggers or influences, genetic destiny in terms of body weight may not necessarily be realized. For example, an individual with a strong genetic predisposition for obesity will not become obese in the absence of sufficient food (caloric) intake. Similarly, when people who are genetically predisposed to normal body weight consume a largely high-fat diet, they may become overweight or obese because they may be more inclined to overeat. This is in part because the brain has difficulty conveying the satiety signal (the message to stop eating) when fatty foods are being consumed.

Besides caloric intake and physical activity, both of which are able to modify body weight, environmental influences before birth also significantly influence adult health and body weight. Research demonstrates that the pregnant mother's nutritional status affects the metabolism of her unborn child. Women who are severely malnourished during pregnancy stimulate the fetus to modify its metabolism to conserve and store energy, a survival practice that can promote overweight when the food supply is ample.

Societal and cultural norms can also cause environmental influences such as lifestyle and behavior to override genetic programming. For example, in the United States many young women with genetic predisposition to normal body weight or even overweight sharply limit their caloric intake and exercise vigorously to achieve "model thin"

bodies. Similarly, in cultures where overweight is perceived as an indication of prosperity and is admired and coveted, people may override genetic tendencies to be normal weight by increasing caloric intake in an effort to achieve the culturally established ideal.

HEALTH RISKS AND CONSEQUENCES OF OVERWEIGHT AND OBESITY

People who are overweight or obese are at higher risk of developing one or more serious medical conditions, and obesity is associated with increases in deaths from all causes. Overweight and obesity significantly increase the risk for hypercholesterolemia (high cholesterol), hypertension, heart disease, and stroke; type 2 diabetes; osteoarthritis and chronic joint pain; gallbladder disease; fatty liver disease; several types of cancers; and sleep apnea (interrupted breathing while sleeping) and sleep disorders.

According to Neil K. Mehta and Virginia W. Chang, in "Mortality Attributable to Obesity among Middle-Aged Adults in the United States" (*Demography*, vol. 46, no. 4, November 2009), there are divergent estimates of deaths attributable to obesity and the differences are largely explained by the studies' varying methodological approaches. For example, in 2004 one study analyzing data from 2000 reported that obesity was second only to smoking as a cause of preventable deaths and deemed obesity a contributing cause in 435,000 deaths per year. The following year other researchers estimated that fewer than 30,000 deaths in 2000 were attributable to overweight or obesity because they attributed 86,000 fewer deaths to overweight, which they considered to be protective against mortality. Mehta and Chang analyzed mortality data of middle-aged adults, a group that is experiencing improving mortality and increasing obesity. They find that being overweight or having class I obesity (BMI 30 to 35) is not associated with increased mortality risk compared with normal BMI but that class II/III (BMI 35 to 40 for class II and BMI greater than 40 for class III) obesity does confer significantly higher mortality—about 40% for females and 62% for males, compared with people with normal BMI.

The CDC observes in "Frequently Asked Questions about Calculating Obesity-Related Risk" (May 25, 2005, http://www.cdc.gov/PDF/Frequently_Asked_Questions _About_Calculating_Obesity-Related_Risk.pdf) that "because obesity has so many different effects on so many diseases, it is extremely difficult for doctors to identify obesity-related deaths reliably on death certificates. So, instead, scientists use complex modeling techniques to estimate deaths related to obesity," which in turn produce varying estimates of the annual number of obesity-related deaths. The CDC states that in the United States, an estimated 112,000 deaths per year are associated with obesity.

Hypercholesterolemia, Hypertension, Heart Disease, and Stroke

Overweight, obesity, and excess abdominal fat are directly related to cardiovascular risk factors, including high levels of total serum cholesterol, LDL cholesterol (low-density lipoprotein; a fatlike substance often called bad cholesterol because high levels increase the risk for heart disease), triglycerides, blood pressure, fibrinogen, and insulin, and low levels of HDL cholesterol (high-density lipoprotein; often called good cholesterol because high levels appear to protect against heart disease). The association between total serum cholesterol and coronary heart disease is largely due to LDL. A high-risk LDL cholesterol is greater than or equal to 160 milligrams per deciliter (mg/dL) with a 10 mg/dL rise in LDL cholesterol corresponding to approximately a 10% increase in risk. High-risk total serum cholesterol is greater than or equal to 240 mg/dL. The age-adjusted percentage of the population aged 20 years and older suffering from high serum cholesterol levels fell from 20.8% in 1988–94 to 13.7% in 2007–10. (See Table 2.6.) The overall decline in high total serum cholesterol occurred in response to the increasing use of effective cholesterol-lowering statin drugs.

The percentage of the population suffering from hypertension (people with elevated blood pressure and those taking antihypertensive medication) increased between 1988–94 and 2007–10, from 25.5% to 30.6% of the population. (See Table 2.7.) The highest rates for those aged 20 years and older during the 2007–10 period were reported among African American females (44.3%). Both men and women were increasingly likely to have hypertension as they aged. Hypertension is approximately three times more common in obese than in normal-weight people, and the relationship between weight and blood pressure is clearly one of cause and effect, because when weight increases, so does blood pressure, and when weight decreases, blood pressure falls.

The physiological processes that produce the hypertension associated with obesity include sodium retention and increases in vascular resistance, blood volume, and cardiac output (the volume of blood pumped, measured in liters per minute). Although it is not known precisely how weight-loss results in a decrease in blood pressure, it is known that weight loss is associated with a reduction in vascular resistance and total blood volume and cardiac output. Weight loss also results in an improvement in insulin resistance, a reduction in sympathetic nervous system activity, and the suppression of the renin-angiotensin-aldosterone system, a group of hormones that are responsible for the opening and narrowing of blood vessels and the retention of fluids.

Obesity increases the risk for coronary artery disease, which in turn increases the risk for future heart failure.

Congestive heart failure is not a disease but a condition that occurs when the heart is unable to pump enough blood to meet the needs of the body's tissues. When the heart fails, it is unable to pump out all the blood that enters its chambers. Congestive heart failure is a frequent complication of severe obesity and a major cause of death. The duration of obesity is a strong predictor of congestive heart failure because over time elevated total blood volume and high cardiac output cause the left ventricle of the heart to increase in size (known as left ventricular hypertrophy) beyond that expected from normal growth. Left ventricular hypertrophy is frequently identified in cardiac patients with obesity and in part results from hypertension, but abnormalities in left ventricular mass and function also occur in the absence of hypertension and may be related to the severity of obesity.

Inflammation in blood vessels and throughout the body is thought to increase the risk for heart disease and stroke (sudden injury to the brain due to a compromised blood and oxygen supply). People with more body fat have higher blood levels of substances such as plasminogen activator inhibitor-1, an enzyme produced in the kidneys that inhibits the conversion of plasminogen to plasmin and initiates fibrinolysis. Fibrinolysis leads to the breakdown of fibrin, which is responsible for the semisolid character of a blood clot that can occlude (block) blood vessels. This is the mechanism believed to account for the finding that obesity is associated with an increased risk of blood clot formation. Occluded arteries may produce myocardial infarction (heart attack) or stroke. Overweight increases the risk for ischemic stroke—resulting from a clot or blockage—but does not appear to increase the risk for hemorrhagic stroke (bleeding inside the brain), which, in general, is associated with more fatality. According to the National Heart, Lung, and Blood Institute (NHLBI), in *Clinical Guidelines on the Identification, Evaluation, and Treatment of Overweight and Obesity in Adults: The Evidence Report* (June 1998, http://www.nhlbi.nih.gov/guidelines/obesity/ob_gdlns.pdf), the risk of stroke increases as BMI rises. For example, the risk of ischemic stroke is 75% higher in women with a BMI greater than 27 and 137% higher in women with a BMI greater than 32, compared with women having a BMI less than 21.

In "Inflammation, a Link between Obesity and Cardiovascular Disease" (*Mediators of Inflammation*, August 2010), Zhaoxia Wang and Tomohiro Nakayama confirm that obesity is associated with increased morbidity and mortality from cardiovascular disease—heart disease, stroke and other vascular disease, and atherosclerosis (the deposit of fatty plaque in the walls of arteries that impede blood flow). The researchers posit that obesity induces inflammation, which accelerates atherosclerosis. Wang and Nakayama believe that advancing the understanding of inflammation and the relationship between obesity and cardiovascular disease will help enhance the biological, physical, and functional changes that are associated with obesity.

TABLE 2.6

Cholesterol levels among persons 20 years of age and older, by selected characteristics, selected years 1988–2010

[Data are based on interviews and laboratory data of a sample of the civilian noninstitutionalized population]

Sex, age, race and Hispanic origin[a], and percent of poverty level	1988–1994	1999–2002	2003–2006	2007–2010
20 years and over, age-adjusted[b]	Percent of population with high serum total cholesterol (greater than or equal to 240 mg/dL)[e]			
Both sexes[c]	20.8	17.3	16.3	13.7
Male	19.0	16.4	15.1	12.6
Female	22.0	17.8	17.1	14.4
Not Hispanic or Latino:				
White only, male	18.8	16.5	15.5	12.2
White only, female	22.2	18.1	18.0	15.3
Black or African American only, male	16.9	12.4	10.9	10.8
Black or African American only, female	21.4	17.7	13.3	11.5
Mexican male	18.5	17.4	17.6	15.1
Mexican female	18.7	13.8	14.4	13.6
Percent of poverty level:[d]				
Below 100%	20.6	18.3	18.1	14.4
100%–199%	20.6	19.1	16.7	15.0
200%–399%	20.8	18.9	15.8	14.4
400% or more	19.5	14.4	15.9	12.3
20 years and over, crude				
Both sexes[c]	19.6	17.3	16.4	14.1
Male	17.7	16.5	15.2	12.9
Female	21.3	18.0	17.5	15.2
Not Hispanic or Latino:				
White only, male	18.0	16.9	15.7	12.6
White only, female	22.5	19.1	18.9	16.7
Black or African American only, male	14.7	12.2	10.8	10.9
Black or African American only, female	18.2	16.1	12.5	11.3
Mexican male	15.4	15.0	15.7	14.7
Mexican female	14.3	10.7	12.6	12.3
Percent of poverty level:[d]				
Below 100%	17.6	16.4	16.8	12.8
100%–199%	19.8	18.2	16.0	14.6
200%–399%	19.3	18.7	15.8	14.6
400% or more	19.9	15.5	17.1	13.7
Male				
20–44 years	12.5	14.2	14.1	11.1
20–34 years	8.2	9.8	9.5	7.6
35–44 years	19.4	19.7	20.5	16.2
45–64 years	27.2	22.2	19.1	17.7
45–54 years	26.6	23.6	20.8	18.7
55–64 years	28.0	19.9	16.0	16.3
65–74 years	21.9	13.7	10.9	7.5
75 years and over	20.4	10.2	9.6	6.8
Female				
20–44 years	9.4	10.4	11.3	8.4
20–34 years	7.3	8.9	10.3	5.8
35–44 years	12.3	12.4	12.7	11.9
45–64 years	33.4	23.0	23.9	21.3
45–54 years	26.7	21.4	19.7	17.7
55–64 years	40.9	25.6	30.5	25.6
65–74 years	41.3	32.3	24.2	20.6
75 years and over	38.2	26.5	18.6	20.2

[a]Persons of Mexican origin may be of any race. Starting with 1999 data, race-specific estimates are tabulated according to the 1997 Revisions to the Standards for the Classification of Federal Data on Race and Ethnicity and are not strictly comparable with estimates for earlier years. The two non-Hispanic race categories shown in the table conform to the 1997 Standards. Starting with 1999 data, race-specific estimates are for persons who reported only one racial group. Prior to data year 1999, estimates were tabulated according to the 1977 Standards. Estimates for single-race categories prior to 1999 included persons who reported one race or, if they reported more than one race, identified one race as best representing their race.

[b]Age-adjusted to the 2000 standard population using five age groups: 20–34 years, 35–44 years, 45–54 years, 55–64 years, and 65 years and over. Age-adjusted estimates may differ from other age-adjusted estimates based on the same data and presented elsewhere if different age groups are used in the adjustment procedure.

[c]Includes persons of all races and Hispanic origins, not just those shown separately.

[d]Percent of poverty level is based on family income and family size. Persons with unknown percent of poverty level are excluded (8% in 2007–2010).

[e]High serum total cholesterol is defined as greater than or equal to 240 mg/dL (6.20 mmol/L), regardless of whether the respondent reported taking cholesterol-lowering medications.

SOURCE: Adapted from "Table 68. Cholesterol among Adults Aged 20 and Over, by Selected Characteristics: United States, Selected Years 1988–1994 through 2007–2010," in *Health, United States, 2012: With Special Feature on Emergency Care*, Centers for Disease Control and Prevention, National Center for Health Statistics, 2013, http://www.cdc.gov/nchs/data/hus/hus12.pdf (accessed October 8, 2013)

TABLE 2.7

Hypertension and elevated blood pressure among persons 20 years of age and older, by selected characteristics, selected years 1988–2010

[Data are based on interviews and physical examinations of a sample of the civilian noninstitutionalized population]

Sex, age, race and Hispanic origin[a], and percent of poverty level	Hypertension[b, c] (high blood pressure and/or taking antihypertensive medication)				Uncontrolled high blood pressure among persons with hypertension[d]			
	1988–1994	1999–2002	2003–2006	2007–2010	1988–1994	1999–2002	2003–2006	2007–2010
20 years and over, age-adjusted[e]				Percent of population				
Both sexes[f]	25.5	30.0	31.3	30.6	77.2	70.6	63.3	55.8
Male	26.4	28.8	31.8	31.3	83.2	73.3	65.0	61.4
Female	24.4	30.6	30.3	29.6	68.5	61.8	53.6	46.3
Not Hispanic or Latino:								
White only, male	25.6	27.6	31.2	31.1	82.6	70.3	63.3	57.3
White only, female	23.0	28.5	28.3	28.1	67.0	63.6	47.5	44.2
Black or African American only, male	37.5	40.6	42.2	40.5	84.0	74.3	70.2	71.5
Black or African American only, female	38.3	43.5	44.1	44.3	71.1	67.2	59.0	51.0
Mexican male	26.9	26.8	24.8	28.6	87.9	89.5	70.7	71.6
Mexican female	25.0	27.9	28.6	27.8	77.6	71.5	66.1	56.4
Percent of poverty level:[g]								
Below 100%	31.7	33.9	35.0	33.8	75.0	71.2	69.8	54.5
100%–199%	26.6	33.5	34.1	33.4	76.0	73.4	68.2	60.4
200%–399%	24.7	30.2	31.9	31.7	76.2	67.8	63.9	51.9
400% or more	22.6	26.4	28.9	28.5	81.5	70.3	56.8	56.2
20 years and over, crude								
Both sexes[f]	24.1	30.2	32.1	32.2	73.9	67.3	58.0	49.3
Male	23.8	27.6	31.3	31.7	79.3	67.1	58.4	52.3
Female	24.4	32.7	32.9	32.8	68.8	67.4	58.8	46.4
Not Hispanic or Latino:								
White only, male	24.3	28.3	32.4	33.7	78.0	64.0	56.2	48.7
White only, female	24.6	32.8	33.4	33.4	67.8	66.9	58.2	44.6
Black or African American only, male	31.1	35.9	38.8	37.6	83.3	71.3	65.9	62.3
Black or African American only, female	32.5	41.9	42.8	44.4	70.0	67.5	55.5	49.2
Mexican male	16.4	16.5	16.6	19.9	86.5	86.9	66.9	66.2
Mexican female	15.9	18.8	20.0	21.4	80.6	74.5	68.6	58.6
Percent of poverty level:[g]								
Below 100%	25.7	30.3	28.8	27.5	74.0	71.3	67.3	54.4
100%–199%	26.7	34.8	36.8	36.2	75.1	70.7	63.2	54.5
200%–399%	22.4	29.9	33.1	34.2	73.4	64.4	58.0	46.3
400% or more	22.0	26.8	29.2	30.6	74.3	63.8	53.4	45.1
Male								
20–44 years	10.9	12.1	14.2	12.5	90.5	79.7	71.1	67.9
20–34 years	7.1	8.1*	9.2	6.8	92.6	89.9	83.1	82.5
35–44 years	17.1	17.1	21.1	20.7	89.0	73.3	63.6	60.8
45–64 years	34.2	36.4	41.2	41.2	73.1	61.4	57.0	50.6
45–54 years	29.2	31.0	36.2	35.5	76.2	66.4	59.3	54.4
55–64 years	40.6	45.0	50.2	49.5	70.3	55.9	53.9	46.7
65–74 years	54.4	59.6	64.1	64.1	74.3	59.1	45.9	42.2
75 years and over	60.4	69.0	65.0	71.7	82.5	74.3	59.7	50.7
Female								
20–44 years	6.5	8.3	6.9	8.3	63.4	58.3	49.1	44.4
20–34 years	2.9	2.7*	2.2*	3.8	82.2	56.9	47.9*	52.6
35–44 years	11.2	15.1	12.6	14.2	56.8	58.6	49.4	41.6
45–64 years	32.8	40.0	43.4	39.7	62.1	60.5	55.5	42.9
45–54 years	23.9	31.8	36.2	31.2	58.5	61.1	57.4	38.9
55–64 years	42.6	53.9	54.4	50.4	64.3	60.0	53.6	46.1
65–74 years	56.2	72.7	70.8	69.3	68.7	73.5	58.5	44.9
75 years and over	73.6	83.1	80.2	81.3	81.9	78.1	70.3	56.0

Figure 2.1 shows the process, known as a treatment algorithm, that is used to assess and treat overweight individuals, based on their body weight, abdominal fat, and the risk factors for cardiovascular morbidity and mortality.

Type 2 Diabetes

Diabetes is a disease that affects the body's use of food, causing blood glucose (sugar levels in the blood) to become too high. Normally, the body converts sugars, starches, and proteins into a form of sugar called glucose. The blood then carries glucose to all the cells throughout the body. In the cells, with the help of the hormone insulin, the glucose is either converted into energy for use immediately or stored for the future. Beta cells of the pancreas, a small organ located behind the stomach, manufacture the insulin. The process of turning food into energy via glucose (blood sugar) is important because the body depends on glucose for every function.

TABLE 2.7

Hypertension and elevated blood pressure among persons 20 years of age and older, by selected characteristics, selected years 1988–2010 [CONTINUED]

[Data are based on interviews and physical examinations of a sample of the civilian noninstitutionalized population]

*Estimates are considered unreliable.
[a]Persons of Mexican origin may be of any race. Starting with 1999 data, race-specific estimates are tabulated according to the 1997 Revisions to the Standards for the Classification of Federal Data on Race and Ethnicity and are not strictly comparable with estimates for earlier years. The two non-Hispanic race categories shown in the table conform to the 1997 Standards. Starting with 1999 data, race-specific estimates are for persons who reported only one racial group. Prior to data year 1999, estimates were tabulated according to the 1977 Standards. Estimates for single-race categories prior to 1999 included persons who reported one race or, if they reported more than one race, identified one race as best representing their race.
[b]Hypertension is defined as having measured high blood pressure and/or taking antihypertensive medication. High blood pressure is defined as having measured systolic pressure of at least 140 mmHg or diastolic pressure of at least 90 mmHg. Those with high blood pressure also may be taking prescribed medicine for high blood pressure. Those taking antihypertensive medication may not have measured high blood pressure but are still classified as having hypertension.
[c]Respondents were asked, "Are you now taking prescribed medicine for your high blood pressure?"
[d]Uncontrolled high blood pressure among persons with hypertension is defined as measured systolic pressure of at least 140 mmHg or diastolic pressure of at least 90 mmHg, among those with measured high blood pressure or reporting taking antihypertensive medication.
[e]Age-adjusted to the 2000 standard population using five age groups: 20–34 years, 35–44 years, 45–54 years, 55–64 years, and 65 years and over. Age-adjusted estimates in this table may differ from other age-adjusted estimates based on the same data and presented elsewhere if different age groups are used in the adjustment procedure.
[f]Includes persons of all races and Hispanic origins, not just those shown separately.
[g]Percent of poverty level is based on family income and family size. Persons with unknown percent of poverty level are excluded (8% in 2007–2010).
Notes: Percentages are based on the average of blood pressure measurements taken. In 2007–2010, 81% of participants had three blood pressure readings. Excludes pregnant women.

SOURCE: "Table 64. Hypertension among Adults Aged 20 and over, by Selected Characteristics: United States, Selected Years 1988–1994 through 2007–2010," in *Health, United States, 2012: With Special Feature on Emergency Care*, Centers for Disease Control and Prevention, National Center for Health Statistics, 2013, http://www.cdc.gov/nchs/data/hus/hus12.pdf (accessed October 8, 2013)

With diabetes, the body can convert food to glucose, but there is a problem with insulin. In one type of diabetes (insulin-dependent diabetes or type 1), the pancreas does not manufacture enough insulin, and in another type (noninsulin dependent or type 2), the body has insulin but cannot use the insulin effectively (this latter condition is called insulin resistance). When insulin is either absent or ineffective, glucose cannot get into the cells to be used for energy. Instead, the unused glucose builds up in the bloodstream and circulates through the kidneys. If a person's blood-glucose level rises high enough, the excess glucose "spills" over into the urine, causing frequent urination. This, in turn, leads to an increased feeling of thirst as the body tries to compensate for the fluid that is lost through urination.

Type 2 diabetes is most often seen in adults and is the most common type of diabetes in the United States. In this type, the pancreas produces insulin, but it is not used effectively because the body resists responding to it. Heredity may be a predisposing factor in the genesis of type 2 diabetes, but because the pancreas continues to produce insulin, the disease is considered more of a problem of insulin resistance, in which the body is not using the hormone efficiently.

Because diabetes deprives body cells of the glucose needed to function properly, several complications can develop to threaten the lives of diabetics. The healing process of the body is slowed or impaired and the risk of infection increases. Complications of diabetes include higher risk and rates of heart disease; circulatory problems, especially in the legs, are often severe enough to require surgery or even amputation; diabetic retinopathy, a condition that can cause blindness; kidney disease that may require dialysis; dental problems; and problems with pregnancy.

The National Institutes of Health's Weight-Control Information Network observes in *Do You Know Some of the Health Risks of Being Overweight?* (December 2012, http://win.niddk.nih.gov/Publications/health_risks.htm) that about 80% of people with type 2 diabetes are overweight, and in people who are prone to type 2 diabetes, becoming overweight can trigger the onset of the disease. It is not known precisely how overweight contributes to the causation of this disease. One hypothesis is that being overweight causes cells to change, making them less effective at using glucose. This then stresses the cells that produce insulin, causing them to fail gradually. Maintaining a healthy weight and keeping physically fit can usually prevent or delay the onset of type 2 diabetes.

From 1997 to March 2013 the percentage of Americans diagnosed with diabetes rose from 5.1% to 9.2%. (See Figure 2.2.) These numbers may significantly underestimate the true prevalence of diabetes in the United States in view of National Health and Nutrition Examination Survey findings that show sizable numbers of adults have undiagnosed diabetes.

"DIABESITY" AND "DOUBLE DIABETES." The recognition of obesity-dependent diabetes prompted scientists and physicians to coin a new term to describe this condition: diabesity. The term was first used during the 1990s and has gained widespread acceptance. Although diabesity is attributed to the same causes as type 2 diabetes (insulin resistance and pancreatic cell dysfunction), researchers are beginning to link the inflammation that is associated

FIGURE 2.1

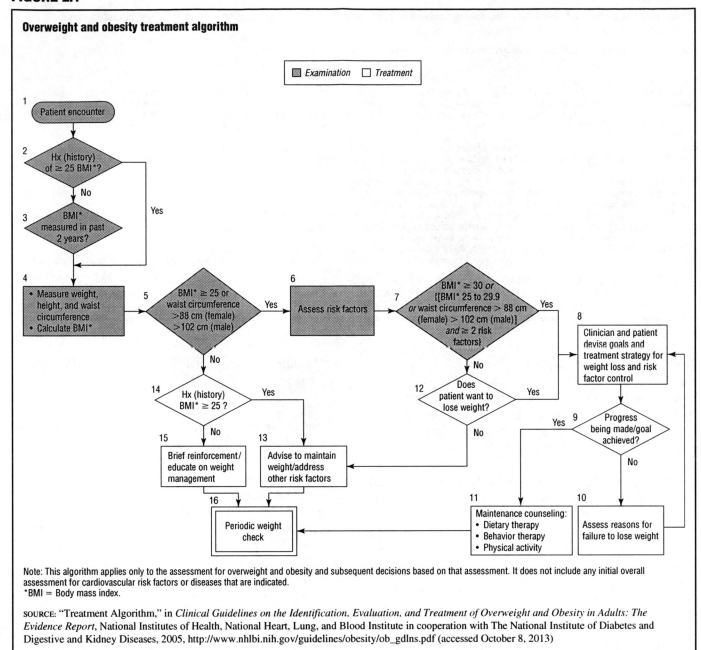

Overweight and obesity treatment algorithm

Note: This algorithm applies only to the assessment for overweight and obesity and subsequent decisions based on that assessment. It does not include any initial overall assessment for cardiovascular risk factors or diseases that are indicated.
*BMI = Body mass index.

SOURCE: "Treatment Algorithm," in *Clinical Guidelines on the Identification, Evaluation, and Treatment of Overweight and Obesity in Adults: The Evidence Report*, National Institutes of Health, National Heart, Lung, and Blood Institute in cooperation with The National Institute of Diabetes and Digestive and Kidney Diseases, 2005, http://www.nhlbi.nih.gov/guidelines/obesity/ob_gdlns.pdf (accessed October 8, 2013)

with obesity to the development of diabetes and cardiovascular disease.

Qudsia Anjum of the International Medical Center in Rabigh, Saudi Arabia, contends in "Diabesity—A Future Pandemic" (*Journal of Pakistan Medical Association*, vol. 61, no. 4, April 2011) that the diabesity epidemic is the "tip of the iceberg; the impending threat is yet to be dealt. The combination and interdependence of diabetes and obesity imposes a therapeutic challenge to the clinicians." Anjum observes that global estimates of diabetes project an increase from 171 million in 2000 to 366 million in 2030. The increasing prevalence of diabesity has prompted the development of new treatment strategies to address both

problems. In "Emerging Therapies in the Treatment of 'Diabesity': Beyond GLP-1" (*Trends in Pharmacological Sciences*, vol. 32, no. 1, January 2011), George Tharakan, Tricia Tan, and Stephen Bloom of the Imperial College of London explain that although weight-loss surgery has proven to be an effective treatment for diabesity, "finding a pharmaceutical alternative that mimics the benefits of surgery without surgical complications has become the 'holy grail' of the twenty-first century."

Another recent phenomenon is the growing number of patients diagnosed with both type 1 and type 2 diabetes simultaneously. Dubbed "double diabetes," it has been reported in both children and adults. Paolo Pozzilli et al.

FIGURE 2.2

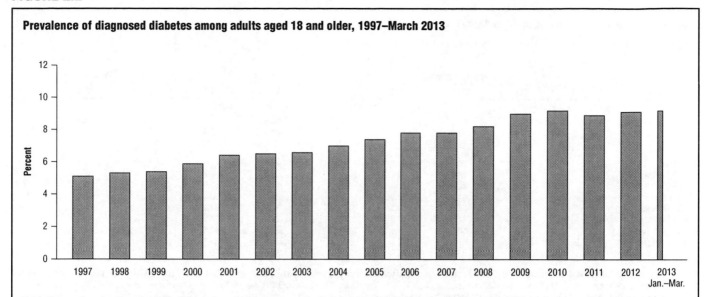

Prevalence of diagnosed diabetes among adults aged 18 and older, 1997–March 2013

Notes: Data are based on household interviews of a sample of the civilian noninstitutionalized population. Prevalence of diagnosed diabetes is based on self-report of ever having been diagnosed with diabetes by a doctor or other health professional. Persons reporting "borderline" diabetes status and women reporting diabetes only during pregnancy were not coded as having diabetes in the analyses. The analyses excluded persons with unknown diabetes status (about 0.1% of respondents each year).

SOURCE: Brian W. Ward, Jeannine S. Schiller, and Gulnur Freeman, "Figure 14.1. Prevalence of Diagnosed Diabetes among Adults Aged 18 Years and over: United States, 1997–March 2013," in *Early Release of Selected Estimates Based on Data from the January–March 2013 National Health Interview Survey*, Centers for Disease Control and Prevention, National Center for Health Statistics, September 2013, http://www.cdc.gov/nchs/data/nhis/earlyrelease/earlyrelease201309_14.pdf (accessed October 8, 2013)

explain in "Obesity, Autoimmunity, and Double Diabetes in Youth" (*Diabetes Care*, vol. 34, suppl. 2, May 2011) that the increase in double diabetes, also known as type 1.5, has gained the attention of the medical community. People with double diabetes have characteristics of both type 1 and type 2 diabetes. When children and adolescents with type 1 diabetes become overweight or obese, they are at increased risk for double diabetes. Pozzilli et al. do not believe that double diabetes is a new or emerging form of diabetes; they opine that it reflects the increasing prevalence of obesity.

Osteoarthritis and Joint Injury

Being only 10 pounds overweight increases the force on the knee by 30–60 pounds with each step.... Even small amounts of weight loss reduce the risk of developing knee OA [osteoarthritis]. Preliminary studies suggest weight loss decreases pain substantially in those with knee OA.

—Susan Bartlett, "Osteoarthritis Weight Management" (2010)

The word *arthritis* literally means joint inflammation. The name applies to more than 100 related diseases that are known as rheumatic diseases. A joint is any point where two bones meet. When a joint becomes inflamed, swelling, redness, pain, and loss of motion occur. In the most serious forms of the disease, the loss of motion can be physically disabling. Arthritis is the leading cause of disability and the leading cause of limitation of activity among working-age

adults (aged 18 to 64 years) in the United States. In 2010, 20.6% of adults aged 18 to 44 years, 42.9% of those aged 45 to 64 years, and 49.6 of people aged 65 years and older said they suffered from joint pain in the 30 days preceding the survey. (See Table 2.8.)

People who are overweight or obese are at increased risk for osteoarthritis, which is not an inflammatory arthritis. Osteoarthritis, sometimes called degenerative arthritis, causes the breakdown of bones and cartilage (connective tissue attached to bones) and usually causes pain and stiffness in the fingers, knees, feet, hips, and back. Extra weight places extra pressure on joints and cartilage, causing them to erode. Furthermore, people with more body fat may have higher blood levels of substances that cause inflammation. Inflammation at the joints may increase the risk for osteoarthritis.

According to the CDC, in "Announcements: Arthritis Awareness Month—May 2013" (*Morbidity and Mortality Weekly Report*, vol. 62, no. 17, May 3, 2013), an estimated 50 million adults in the United States suffer from arthritis. The CDC observes in "Obesity Trends in Adults with Arthritis" (August 1, 2011, http://www.cdc.gov/arthritis/resources/spotlights/obesity-trends.htm) that the prevalence of obesity among adults with arthritis is on average 54% higher than among adults without arthritis. For example, among obese adults in 2009, more (35.2%) reported suffering from arthritis than not suffering from the disease (23.6%). (See Figure 2.3.)

TABLE 2.8

Joint pain reported by persons aged 18 and older, by age, 2002, 2009, and 2010

[Data are based on household interviews of a sample of the civilian noninstitutionalized population]

Characteristic	Any joint pain[a]			Knee pain[a]			Shoulder pain[a]		
	2002	2009	2010	2002	2009	2010	2002	2009	2010
	Percent of adults reporting joint pain in past 30 days								
18 years and over, age-adjusted[b, c]	29.5	32.0	32.1	16.5	19.5	19.6	8.6	9.0	9.0
18 years and over, crude[c]	29.5	33.0	33.3	16.5	20.2	20.3	8.7	9.3	9.4
Age									
18–44 years	19.3	20.7	20.6	10.5	12.4	12.6	4.9	5.3	5.2
18–24 years	14.2	14.8	15.2	8.3	8.8	9.8	3.4	3.0	3.5
25–44 years	21.0	22.8	22.6	11.2	13.7	13.6	5.4	6.1	5.8
45–64 years	37.5	41.8	42.9	20.4	26.2	26.1	12.3	12.4	13.2
45–54 years	34.3	37.5	39.3	18.4	23.8	23.5	10.5	11.0	12.0
55–64 years	42.3	47.3	47.3	23.4	29.4	29.3	15.1	14.2	14.8
65 years and over	47.2	50.6	49.6	28.6	30.3	30.5	14.1	14.9	13.6
65–74 years	46.0	47.9	49.5	27.6	28.9	30.2	14.0	14.2	13.5
75 years and over	48.7	53.8	49.8	29.7	31.9	30.9	14.1	15.7	13.7

[a]Starting with 2002 data, respondents were asked, "During the past 30 days, have you had any symptoms of pain, aching, or stiffness in or around a joint?" Respondents were instructed not to include the back or neck. To facilitate their response, respondents were shown a card illustrating the body joints. Respondents reporting more than one type of joint pain were included in each response category. This table shows the most commonly reported joints.
[b]Estimates are age-adjusted to the year 2000 standard population using five age groups: 18–44 years, 45–54 years, 55–64 years, 65–74 years, and 75 years and over.
[c]Includes all other races not shown separately, unknown education level, and unknown disability status.

SOURCE: "Table 53. Joint Pain among Adults 18 Years of Age and over, by Selected Characteristics: United States, Selected Years 2002–2010," in *Health, United States, 2011: With Special Feature on Socioeconomic Status and Health,* Centers for Disease Control and Prevention, National Center for Health Statistics, 2012, http://www.cdc.gov/nchs/data/hus/2011/053.pdf (accessed October 8, 2013)

FIGURE 2.3

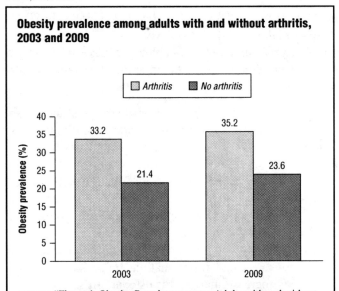

Obesity prevalence among adults with and without arthritis, 2003 and 2009

SOURCE: "Figure 1. Obesity Prevalence among Adults with and without Arthritis," in *Obesity Trends in Adults with Arthritis*, Centers for Disease Control and Prevention, National Center for Chronic Disease Prevention and Health Promotion, Division of Population Health, http://www.cdc.gov/arthritis/resources/spotlights/obesity-trends.htm (accessed October 8, 2013)

In "Role of Body Weight in Osteoarthritis" (March 27, 2012, http://www.hopkinsarthritis.org/patient-corner/disease-management/role-of-body-weight-in-osteoarthritis/), Susan Bartlett of Johns Hopkins University indicates that obese women have about four times the risk of knee osteoarthritis, compared with women of healthy weight, and for obese men the risk is five times greater. The CDC observes that even modest weight loss of just 11 pounds (5 kg) can reduce the risk for knee osteoarthritis among women by 50% and may also reduce the mortality risk in people with osteoarthritis by half.

By 2013 the relationship between weight loss and improvements in the symptoms of knee pain due to arthritis was clear and definitive enough to warrant classifying it as an effective treatment for this condition. According to Erika Ringdahl and Sandesh Pandit of the University of Missouri School of Medicine, in "Treatment of Knee Osteoarthritis" (*American Family Physician*, vol. 83, no. 11, June 1, 2011), obesity is the strongest modifiable risk factor for knee osteoarthritis. Weight loss is one of the standard nonsurgical treatments for overweight and obese patients suffering from osteoarthritis of the knee because it acts to reduce pain and improve physical function.

Gallbladder Disease

Gallstones are small, hard pellets that can form when bile in the gallbladder (a muscular saclike organ that lies under the liver in the right side of the abdomen) precipitates (becomes solid out of the bile solution). Bile contains water, cholesterol, fats, bile salts, proteins, and bilirubin. The gallbladder stores and concentrates the bile produced in the liver that is not needed immediately for digestion. Bile is released from the gallbladder into the small intestine in response to food. The pancreatic duct

FIGURE 2.4

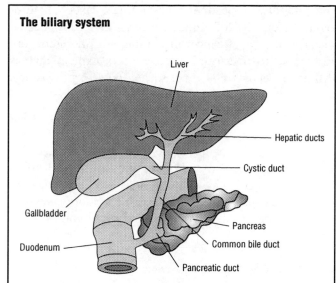

The biliary system

Liver

Hepatic ducts

Cystic duct

Gallbladder

Pancreas

Duodenum

Common bile duct

Pancreatic duct

The gallbladder and the ducts that carry bile and other digestive enzymes from the liver, gallbladder, and pancreas to the small intestine are called the biliary system.

SOURCE: "The Gallbladder and the Ducts That Carry Bile and Other Digestive Enzymes from the Liver, Gallbladder, and Pancreas to the Small Intestine Are Called the Biliary System," in *Gallstones*, National Institutes of Health, National Institute of Diabetes and Digestive and Kidney Diseases, National Digestive Diseases Information Clearinghouse, July 2007, http://digestive.niddk.nih.gov/ddiseases/pubs/gallstones/index.htm (accessed October 9, 2013)

joins the common bile duct at the small intestine, adding enzymes to aid in digestion. (See Figure 2.4.) If bile contains too much cholesterol, bile salts, or bilirubin, under certain conditions it can harden into stones. Most gallstones are formed primarily from cholesterol.

The National Digestive Diseases Information Clearinghouse of the National Institute of Diabetes and Digestive and Kidney Diseases explains in "Gallstones" (September 11, 2013, http://digestive.niddk.nih.gov/ddiseases/pubs/gallstones/) that when gallstones block the flow of bile they can produce inflammation in the gallbladder, liver, and pancreas. When blockage persists, the consequences may be severe infection, which if left untreated may not only be painful but also deadly. When gallstones produce such symptoms, the treatment is generally a surgical procedure, called cholecystectomy, in which the gallbladder is removed. People who are not candidates for surgery may be given prescription drugs to dissolve gallstones; however, it is likely that gallstones will recur in people treated with drugs.

People who are overweight have an increased risk for developing gallstones because the liver overproduces cholesterol and deposits it in the bile, which then becomes supersaturated. The National Digestive Diseases Information Clearinghouse indicates that the risk of gallstones is higher among people who are overweight or obese and among people who fast or lose a large amount of weight

very quickly. Rapid weight loss or weight cycling (the repeated loss and regain of body weight) further increases cholesterol production in the liver, with resulting supersaturation and risk for gallstone formation.

In "Gastrointestinal System and Obesity" (*Critical Care Clinics*, vol. 26, no. 4, October 2010), Doyle D. Ashburn and Mary Jane Reed confirm that obesity increases the risk for development of cholesterol gallstones. The researchers theorize that this occurs in response to the activity of adipose tissue in and around the internal organs. Insulin resistance leads to an excess of insulin called hyperinsulinemia that in turn increases cholesterol excretion from the liver and results in the abnormal function of the gallbladder. These conditions create an environment conducive to stone formation. Although some gallstones produce no symptoms, others cause serious and even life-threatening medical conditions.

Fatty Liver Disease

Fatty liver is defined as an excess accumulation of fat in the liver, usually exceeding 5% of the total liver weight. More than 50% of the excess fat deposit in the liver is triglyceride. The enlargement of the liver is caused by the reduction of fatty acid oxidation (fat metabolism) in the liver, resulting in an excess accumulation of fat. It causes injury and inflammation in the liver and may lead to severe liver damage, cirrhosis (buildup of scar tissue that blocks proper blood flow in the liver), or liver failure. Arthur J. McCullough of the Cleveland Clinic in Cleveland, Ohio, observes in "Epidemiology of the Metabolic Syndrome in the USA" (*Journal of Digestive Diseases*, vol. 12, no. 5, October 2011) that nonalcoholic fatty liver disease (NAFLD) is now recognized as a component of metabolic syndrome, which includes hypertension, diabetes, and elevated triglycerides. Metabolic syndrome is a major risk factor for the development of nonalcoholic steatohepatitis, the most severe form of NAFLD. McCullough estimates that 25% of people in the United States have metabolic syndrome and as such also suffer from NAFLD.

People with diabetes or with higher than normal blood sugar levels (but not yet in the diabetic range) are more likely to have fatty liver disease than those with normal blood sugar levels. It is not known why some people who are overweight or diabetic get fatty liver and others do not. Losing weight reduces the buildup of fat in the liver and prevents further injury; however, weight loss should not exceed 2.2 pounds (1 kg) per week because more rapid weight loss may exacerbate the disease.

In "Nonalcoholic Fatty Liver Disease and the Metabolic Syndrome: Clinical Implications and Treatment" (*Nutrition in Clinical Practice*, vol. 28, no. 1, February 2013), Robert S. Rahimi and Carmen Landaverde predict that the prevalence of NAFLD is anticipated to increase as the prevalence of obesity increases. They observe that along with obesity, specific nutritional trends such as increased consumption of high-fructose corn syrup and animal fats also may be implicated in the rise of NAFLD.

Cancer

Cancer encompasses a group of diseases that are characterized by the uncontrolled growth and spread of abnormal cells. These cells may grow into masses of tissue called malignant tumors. The dangerous aspect of cancer is that cancer cells invade and destroy normal tissue.

The spread of cancer cells occurs either by local growth of the tumor or by some of the cells becoming detached and traveling through the blood and lymph systems to start additional tumors in other parts of the body. Metastasis (the spread of cancer cells) may be confined to a region of the body, but if left untreated (and often despite treatment), the cancer cells can spread throughout the entire body, eventually causing death. It is perhaps the rapid, invasive, and destructive nature of cancer that makes it, arguably, the most feared of all diseases, although it is second to heart disease as the leading cause of death in the United States. (See Table 2.2.)

Kyla King reports in "Obesity: A Preventable Cancer Risk? Promoting Change with Sensitivity" (WestMichigan Reader.com, March 28, 2011) that in the United States overweight and obesity are responsible for as many as 14% of cancer deaths in men and 20% of cancer deaths in women. King also observes that people with cancer who are overweight or obese face additional challenges, in that surgery may be more complicated and doses of anticancer drugs must be adjusted.

Overweight increases the risk of developing several types of cancer, including cancers of the colon, esophagus, gallbladder, kidney, pancreas, liver, and prostate, as well as uterine (specifically cancer of the lining of the uterus) and postmenopausal breast cancer. Excessive weight gain during adult life increases the risk for several of these cancers. For example, according to the American Cancer Society, in *Cancer Prevention and Early Detection: Facts and Figures, 2013* (2013, http://www.cancer .org/acs/groups/content/@epidemiologysurveillance/ documents/document/acspc-037535.pdf), overweight and obesity contribute to between 14% and 20% of all cancer-related deaths, and between one-quarter and one-third of all cancer cases in the United States may be attributed to poor diet, physical inactivity, overweight, and obesity. The American Cancer Society states that losing weight may reduce the risk of developing some cancers such as breast cancer and that diets high in processed and red meat and low in fruits, vegetables, and whole grains are associated with increased cancer risk.

In "Obesity and Cancer Risk: Recent Review and Evidence" (*Current Oncology Reports*, vol. 13, no 1,

February 2011), Karen Basen-Engquist and Maria Chang report that 9% of postmenopausal breast cancer, 11% of colon cancer, 25% of kidney cancer, 37% of esophageal cancer, and 39% of cancer of the lining of the uterus are attributable to obesity. The researchers explain that as BMI increases by 1 pound per square foot (5 kg per sq m), cancer mortality increases by 10%.

It is not yet known exactly how being overweight increases cancer risk, recurrence, or mortality. It may be that fat cells make or influence hormones such as estrogen, progesterone, and androgens and insulin that affect cell growth and lead to cancer. It is also possible that eating habits—such as a high-fat, high-calorie diet—or physical inactivity that promote overweight contribute to cancer risk.

Sleep Apnea and Sleep Disorders

Sleep apnea is a condition in which breathing becomes shallow or stops completely for short periods during sleep. A pause in breathing can last about 10 to 20 seconds or longer, and pauses can occur 20 times or more an hour. Sleep apnea increases the risk of developing high blood pressure, heart attack, or stroke. Untreated sleep apnea can increase the risk of diabetes and daytime sleepiness, which can increase the risk for work-related accidents and automobile accidents.

The most common type of sleep apnea, and the type that is linked to overweight and obesity, is obstructive sleep apnea. During sleep there is insufficient airflow into the lungs through the mouth and nose, and the amount of oxygen in the blood may drop because the airway is transiently occluded. The NHLBI notes in "Who Is at Risk for Sleep Apnea?" (July 10, 2012, http://www.nhlbi.nih.gov/health/ health-topics/topics/sleepapnea/atrisk.html) that millions of Americans have obstructive sleep apnea and that "about half of the people who have this condition are overweight."

Obesity, particularly upper-body obesity, is a risk factor for sleep apnea and is related to its severity. Most people with sleep apnea have a BMI greater than 30. In general, men whose neck circumference is 17 inches (43.2 cm) or greater and women with a neck circumference of 16 inches (40.6 cm) or greater are at higher risk for sleep apnea. Large neck girth in both men and women who snore is highly predictive of sleep apnea because people with large neck girth store more fat around their neck, which may compromise their airway. A smaller airway can make breathing difficult or stop it altogether. In addition, fat stored in the neck and throughout the body can produce substances that cause inflammation, and inflammation in the neck may be a risk factor for sleep apnea. Weight loss usually resolves or significantly improves sleep apnea by decreasing neck size and reducing inflammation.

Too little sleep is also linked to obesity. Anne G. Wheaton et al. of the CDC note in "Relationship between

Body Mass Index and Perceived Insufficient Sleep among U.S. Adults: An Analysis of 2008 BRFSS Data" (*BMC Public Health*, vol. 10, no. 11, May 2011) that people who are overweight or obese report that they sleep less per week than their normal-weight counterparts. The researchers analyzed data from 384,541 participants in the 2008 Behavioral Risk Factor Surveillance System, which asked survey respondents, "During the past 30 days, for about how many days have you felt you did not get enough rest or sleep?" The researchers find a strong association between reported insufficient sleep and BMI-based weight categories from normal weight through obese class III among both men and women. For example, 35% of people with class III obesity said they had 14 or more days of insufficient sleep, compared with 25% of normal-weight people. Wheaton et al. suggest that "the possible effect of excess weight on sleep should be considered by developers of programs to address sleep disorders and that the possible effect of insufficient sleep on weight should be considered by developers of weight-reduction programs."

Other research suggests that sleep deprivation may be related to craving high calorie foods most likely to promote weight gain. In "The Impact of Sleep Deprivation on Food Desire in the Human Brain" (*Nature Communications*, August 6, 2013), Stephanie M. Greer, Andrea N. Goldstein, and Matthew P. Walker compare food choices made by people who received adequate sleep and those who were sleep deprived. They find that high-calorie foods such as chocolate and potato chips were significantly more desirable when people were sleep-deprived and on average, sleep-deprived study subjects consumed about 600 more calories than well-rested subjects. Greer, Goldstein, and Walker opine that a "combination of altered brain activity and decision-making may help explain why people who sleep less also tend to be overweight or obese."

Women's Reproductive Health

Besides increased risk of breast cancer and cancer of the lining of the uterus, women who are overweight or obese may suffer from infertility (difficulty or inability to conceive a child) and other gynecological or pregnancy-related medical problems. Obesity is associated with menstrual irregularities such as abnormally heavy menstrual periods and amenorrhea (cessation of menstruation), and has been found to affect ovulation, response to fertility treatment, pregnancy rates, and pregnancy outcomes.

Lea S. Vilmann et al. note in "Development of Obesity and Polycystic Ovary Syndrome in Adolescents" (*Hormone Research in Pediatrics*, vol. 78, nos. 5–6, November 2012) that obesity is linked to polycystic ovarian syndrome (PCOS), an endocrine condition that afflicts approximately 15% of women of reproductive age. PCOS is characterized by the accumulation of cysts (fluid-filled sacs) on the ovaries, chronic anovulation (absent ovulation), and other metabolic disturbances. Symptoms include excess facial and body hair, acne, obesity, irregular menstrual cycles, insulin resistance, and infertility. A key characteristic of PCOS is hyperandrogenism—excessive production of male hormones (androgens), particularly testosterone, by the ovaries— which is responsible for the acne, male-pattern hair growth, and baldness seen in women with PCOS. Hyperandrogenism has been linked to insulin resistance and hyperinsulinemia, both of which are common in PCOS. Women with PCOS have an increased risk of early-onset heart disease, hypertension, diabetes, and reproductive cancers and a higher incidence of miscarriage and infertility. In overweight women, modest weight loss (as little as 5%) through diet and exercise may correct hyperandrogenism and restore ovulation and fertility.

Vilmann et al. report that between 18% and 26% of adolescent females have PCOS, and the risk of developing this condition is highest among obese adolescents. Signs of PCOS have even been observed in preadolescent girls who are obese. They conclude that "it is of great importance to detect girls who are obese in adolescence (and even younger), because counseling and treatment in an early stage of the metabolic disturbances may prevent the future deleterious effects on their health."

Obesity during pregnancy is associated with increased morbidity for both the expectant mother and the unborn child. Obese pregnant women are significantly more likely to suffer from hypertension and gestational diabetes (glucose intolerance of variable severity that begins during pregnancy and generally resolves after birth) than normal-weight expectant mothers. Obesity is also associated with difficulties in managing labor and delivery, leading to premature births and higher rates of cesarean section (delivery of a fetus by surgical incision through the abdominal wall and uterus). Risks associated with anesthesia are higher in obese women, as there is a greater tendency toward hypoxemia (abnormal lack of oxygen in the blood) and greater difficulty administering local or general anesthesia.

The children of women who are obese during pregnancy are at increased risk of birth defects—congenital malformations, particularly of neural tube defects. Neural tube defects are abnormalities of the brain and spinal cord that result from the failure of the neural tube to develop properly during early pregnancy. The neural tube is the embryonic nerve tissue that eventually develops into the brain and the spinal cord.

Women who are obese before pregnancy also appear to have a higher risk of stillbirth and of having an infant die soon after birth. Peter W. Tennant, Judith Rankin, and Ruth Bell of Newcastle University note in "Maternal

Body Mass Index and the Risk of Fetal and Infant Death: A Cohort Study from the North of England" (*Human Reproduction*, vol. 26, no. 6, April 2011) that early pregnancy obesity (BMI greater than or equal to 30) carries significant health implications. Tennant, Rankin, and Bell find that obese mothers were at increased risk for gestational diabetes and that their infants were at increased risk for stillbirth, early infant death, and birth defects. It is not yet known how obesity increases the risk of stillbirth and early infant death, but one possible explanation may be that obesity influences the hormonal system and the metabolism of blood fats that in turn may compromise blood flow to the placenta (an organ that forms during pregnancy and functions as a filter between the mother and fetus).

Babies born to overweight and obese women are at greater risk of having heart defects. Suzanne M. Gilboa et al. report in "Association between Prepregnancy Body Mass Index and Congenital Heart Defects" (*American Journal of Obstetrics and Gynecology*, vol. 202, no. 1, January 2010) the results of a study of 6,440 infants born with congenital heart defects and 5,673 infants without birth defects. The researchers find that when compared with babies born to normal-weight women, there was a significant increase in many types of heart defects in babies born to overweight and obese women. Gilboa et al. looked at 25 types of heart defects and found associations with obesity for 10 of them. Five of these 10 types were also associated with overweight prior to pregnancy. Women who were overweight but not obese prior to and during pregnancy had approximately a 15% increased risk of delivering a baby with certain heart defects.

WEIGHT GAIN DURING PREGNANCY. Weight gain during pregnancy is expected and beneficial. The fetus, expanded blood volume, the enlarged uterus, breast tissue growth, and other products of conception generate approximately 13 to 17 pounds (5.9 to 7.7 kg) of extra weight. Weight gain beyond this anticipated amount is largely maternal adipose tissue that is often retained after pregnancy. The challenge health professionals face when developing recommendations about weight gain during pregnancy is achieving a balance between gains intended to produce high-birth-weight infants, who may then require delivery by cesarean section, and low-birth-weight infants with a higher infant mortality rate. Analysis of data from the CDC's Pregnancy Nutrition Surveillance System shows that extremely overweight women benefit from reduced weight gain during pregnancy to help decrease the risk for high-birth-weight infants. Table 2.9 shows the recommended amount of weight gain during pregnancy based on prepregnancy BMI.

Raul Artal and Amy Flick opine in "Obesity and Weight Gain in Pregnancy" (*Contemporary OB/GYN*, July 1, 2013) that no pregnancy weight gain in women with BMI of 30 or even modest weight loss may reduce

TABLE 2.9

Recommended weight gain during pregnancy

BMI	Kilograms	Pounds
<19.8	12.5 to 18	28 to 40
>19.8 to 26	11.5 to 16	25 to 35
>26 to 29	7 to 11.5	15 to 25
>29	≤6	≤13

SOURCE: "Weight Gain during Pregnancy," in *Guidelines on Overweight and Obesity: Electronic Textbook*, National Institutes of Health, National Heart, Lung, and Blood Institute in cooperation with The National Institute of Diabetes and Digestive and Kidney Diseases, 1998, http://www.nhlbi.nih.gov/guidelines/obesity/e_txtbk/ratnl/22111.htm (accessed October 11, 2013)

some risks such as infants who are large for their gestational age, cesarean delivery, and preeclampsia (high blood pressure and excess protein in the urine). Artal and Flick assert, "Physical activity, weight maintenance, and even weight reduction have not proven harmful in obese pregnant patients according to studies in the recent literature." They also point out that infants of obese women are at significantly increased risk for being born with neural tube defects, congenital heart disease, and other anomalies.

Metabolic Syndrome

McCullough estimates in "Epidemiology of the Metabolic Syndrome in the USA" that approximately 25% of Americans exhibit a cluster of medical conditions that are characterized by insulin resistance and the presence of obesity, abdominal fat, high blood sugar and triglycerides, high blood cholesterol, and high blood pressure. This constellation of symptoms, called metabolic syndrome, was first defined in *Third Report of the National Cholesterol Education Program (NCEP) Expert Panel on Detection, Evaluation, and Treatment of High Blood Cholesterol in Adults (Adult Treatment Panel III)* (September 2002, http://www.nhlbi.nih.gov/guidelines/cholesterol/atp3full.pdf). The report concludes that for most affected people, metabolic syndrome results from poor diet and insufficient physical activity.

The diagnosis of metabolic syndrome, which is also known as syndrome X, requires that people meet at least three of the following criteria:

- Waistline measurement (waist circumference) of 40 inches (102 cm) or more for men and 35 inches (89 cm) or more for women

- Blood pressure of 130/85 millimeters of mercury (mmHg) or higher

- Fasting blood glucose level greater than 100 mg/dL

- Serum triglyceride level above 150 mg/dL

- HDL level less than 40 mg/dL for men or under 50 mg/dL for women

According to the American Heart Association, three groups of people are the most likely to be diagnosed with metabolic syndrome: diabetics, people with hypertension and hyperinsulinemia, and people who have suffered heart attacks and have hyperinsulinemia without glucose intolerance.

Although research shows that the signs of metabolic syndrome are common among family members, until 2003 a definitive genetic link had not been identified. Ruth J. F. Loos et al. demonstrate in "Genome-Wide Linkage Scan for the Metabolic Syndrome in the HERITAGE Family Study" (*Journal of Clinical Endocrinology and Metabolism*, vol. 88, no. 12, December 2003) the existence of genetic regions that may signal a predisposition to metabolic syndrome. The researchers find evidence of genetic linkages to metabolic syndrome in both African American and white patients.

By 2013 additional genetic links had been identified. For example, Yi Zhang et al. report in "A Comprehensive Analysis of Adiponectin QTLs Using SNP Association, SNP Cis-Effects on Peripheral Blood Gene Expression and Gene Expression Correlation Identified Novel Metabolic Syndrome (MetS) Genes with Potential Role in Carcinogenesis and Systemic Inflammation" (*BMC Medical Genomics*, vol. 6, no. 14, April 2013) that an evaluation of linkages for traits that are associated with metabolic syndrome finds multiple regions genes that correlate with these traits.

The exact origins of metabolic syndrome are not fully known; regardless, affected individuals experience a series of biochemical changes that, in time, lead to the development of potentially harmful medical conditions. The biochemical changes begin when insulin loses its ability to cause cells to absorb glucose from the blood (insulin resistance). As a result, glucose levels remain high after food is consumed and the pancreas, sensing a high glucose level in the blood, continues to secrete insulin. The loss of insulin sensitivity may be genetic or may be in response to high fat levels with fatty deposits in the pancreas.

Moderate weight loss, in the range of 5% to 10% of body weight, can help restore the body's sensitivity to insulin and greatly reduce the chance that the syndrome will progress into a more serious illness. Increased physical activity alone has also been shown to improve insulin sensitivity.

By 2013 it was widely accepted that metabolic syndrome included vascular risk factors that were associated with cognitive decline and even the development of dementia. In "Low Cerebral Blood Flow Is Associated with Lower Memory Function in Metabolic Syndrome" (*Obesity*, vol. 21, no. 7, May 2013), Alex C. Birdsill et al. assert that, although it is not understood how or why metabolic syndrome causes cognitive impairment, early identification and treatment of people who are at risk may offer new ways to delay the onset of cognitive decline and dementia syndromes or to prevent the progression of these syndromes. The researchers believe that reducing cardiovascular risk factors that can compromise blood flow to the brain, can reduce the risk of cognitive decline.

REDEFINING METABOLIC SYNDROME. In an effort to standardize diagnosis, prevention, screening, and treatment, the International Diabetes Federation presents in *The IDF Consensus Worldwide Definition of the Metabolic Syndrome* (2006, http://www.idf.org/webdata/docs/ IDF_Meta_def_final.pdf) a new worldwide definition of metabolic syndrome. The diagnostic criteria are central obesity, which is defined as a waist circumference that is equal to or more than 37 inches (94 cm) for males and 31.5 inches (80 cm) for females of European descent, and ethnic-specific measurements for Chinese, Japanese, and South Asians, along with two of the following: triglycerides of at least 150 mg/dL; low HDL cholesterol, which is defined as less than 40 mg/dL in males and less than 50 mg/dL in females; blood pressure of at least 130/85 mmHg; fasting hyperglycemia, which is defined as glucose that is equal to or greater than 100 mg/dL; previous diagnosis of diabetes; or impaired glucose tolerance. This definition of metabolic syndrome, which includes diabetes or prediabetes, abdominal obesity, unfavorable lipid profile, and hypertension, triples the risk of myocardial infarction and stroke and doubles mortality from these conditions. It also increases the risk of developing type 2 diabetes, if not already present, fivefold.

SOME QUESTION THE DIAGNOSIS OF METABOLIC SYNDROME. In 2010 the World Health Organization joined the American Diabetes Association and the European Association for the Study of Diabetes in questioning the utility of the diagnosis of metabolic syndrome. Representatives of these organizations say they feel the syndrome is neither a distinct disease nor well established by scientific research. Rakesh M. Parikh and Viswanathan Mohan state in "Changing Definitions of Metabolic Syndrome" (*Indian Journal of Endocrinology and Metabolism*, vol. 16, no. 1, January–February 2012) that there are different definitions of metabolic syndrome, which creates confusion when comparing prevalence rates. Parikh and Mohan propose a simple clinical definition and explain that metabolic syndrome should be considered a screening tool that is used "to identify people at high risk of metabolic complications and cardiovascular disease so that further detailed investigations can be performed. This definition translates into a very simple message to the community 'If your waist size is more than half of your height, you should consult your doctor.'"

CHAPTER 3

THE INFLUENCES OF MENTAL HEALTH AND CULTURE ON WEIGHT AND EATING DISORDERS

That diet and appetite are closely linked to psychological health and emotional well-being is widely recognized. Psychological factors often influence eating habits. Many people overeat when they are bored, stressed, angry, depressed, or anxious. Psychological distress can aggravate weight problems by triggering impulses to overeat. Emotional discomfort drives many people to overeat as a way to relieve anxiety and improve mood. Some people revert to the so-called comfort foods of their youth—the meals or treats that were offered to them when they were sick or the foods that evoke memories of the carefree days of childhood. Others rely on chocolate and other sweets, which actually contain chemicals that are known to have a soothing effect on mood. Over time, the associations between emotions, food, and eating can become firmly fixed.

Emotional arousal may also sabotage healthy self-care efforts such as resolutions to diet and exercise. Anxiety and depression can produce feelings of helplessness and hopelessness about efforts to lose weight that undermine the best intentions, prompt detrimental food choices and inactivity, and over time cause many people to give up trying entirely. Because overweight and obesity often contribute to emotional stress and psychological disorders, a cycle develops that couples increasing weight gain with progressively more severe emotional difficulties.

Emotional disturbance alone is rarely the causative factor of overweight or obesity. However, for people with a genetic susceptibility or predisposition to obesity and exposure to environmental factors that promote obesity, emotional and psychological stress can trigger or exacerbate the problem. Even efforts to lose weight can backfire, serving to increase rather than to alleviate emotional stress. For example, people who fail to lose weight or those who succeed in losing weight only to regain it may suffer from frustration and diminished feelings of competence and self-worth. Similarly, being overweight or obese and feeling self-conscious about it or suffering from weight-based discrimination or prejudice can be ongoing sources of stress and frustration. Feelings of helplessness, frustration, and continuous emotional stress can cause or worsen mental health problems such as anxiety and depression.

Many mental health and medical professionals view overweight as both a cause and a consequence of disturbances in physical and mental health. Although it may be important to determine whether a metabolic disturbance caused an individual to become overweight or resulted from excessive weight gain, or whether depression triggered behaviors leading to obesity or resulted from problems associated with obesity, it is often impossible to distinguish whether overweight is a symptom of another disorder or the causative factor.

THE ORIGINS OF EATING DISORDERS

Despite the challenges of compromised self-esteem and societal prejudice, the National Institute of Diabetes and Digestive and Kidney Diseases indicates that most overweight people have about the same number of psychological problems as people of average weight. Nevertheless, the Weight-Control Information Network explains in "Binge Eating Disorder" (December 2012, http://win.niddk.nih.gov/publications/binge.htm) that although eating disorders affect normal-weight individuals, people who are mildly obese and try to lose weight repetitively may suffer from eating disorders such as binge eating, and most people with binge-eating disorders are overweight or obese. People with the most severe eating disorders are more likely to have symptoms of depression and low self-esteem. Binge eaters have lost control of their eating behaviors and consume abnormal quantities of food in short periods. Binge-eating disorders are thought to be even more common in people who are severely obese.

Although depression and stress may contribute to a substantial percentage of cases of obesity, they are considered the leading causes of eating disorders. Most mental health professionals concur that the origins of eating disorders can be traced to behavioral or psychological difficulties. Anger and impulsive behavior have been associated with binge-eating disorders, but even mild mental health or social problems such as shyness or lack of self-confidence can lead to social withdrawal, isolation, and a sedentary lifestyle that promotes weight gain and ultimately obesity.

Jerica M. Berge et al. of the University of Minnesota report in "Family Life Cycle Transitions and the Onset of Eating Disorders: A Retrospective Grounded Theory Approach" (*Journal of Clinical Nursing*, vol. 21, nos. 9–10, July 12, 2011) that eating disorders may be precipitated by transitional events in family life, such as school transitions, the death of a family member, relationship changes, illness or hospitalization, home or job changes, and abuse or sexual assault. The risk for eating disorders is greatest when there is a lack of needed support during these stressful life transitions.

At first glance, eating disorders appear to center on preoccupations with food and weight; however, mental health professionals believe these disorders are often about more than simply food. Besides psychological factors that may predispose people to eating disorders, including diminished self-esteem, depression, anxiety, loneliness, or feelings of lack of control, a variety of interpersonal and social factors have been implicated as causal factors for these disorders. Interpersonal issues that may increase the risk for developing eating disorders include troubled family and personal relationships; difficulty expressing emotions; a history of physical or sexual abuse; or the experience of being teased, taunted, or ridiculed about body size, shape, or weight.

Twin and family studies suggest that the predisposition to develop an eating disorder also has a genetic origin. In "The Genetics of Eating Disorders" (*Annual Review of Clinical Psychology*, vol. 9, March 2013), Sara E. Trace et al. report that genetic factors account for about 40% to 60% of eating disorders.

Social factors that may contribute to eating disorders include sharply restricted, rigid definitions of beauty that exclude people who do not conform to a particular body weight and shape; cultures that glorify thinness and overemphasize the importance of obtaining a "perfect body"; and cultures that judge and value people based on external physical appearance rather than on internal qualities such as character, intellect, generosity, and kindness. Appearance-driven concerns, rather than health needs, continue to motivate many obese individuals to lose weight. Societal pressures reinforce these appearance-driven concerns by portraying obese individuals in a negative manner.

A related consideration that further complicates pinpointing the origins of eating disorders is the extent to which temperament interacts with genetic predisposition and interpersonal and social factors to promote eating disorders. Researchers and mental health professionals observe that temperamental tendencies such as perfectionism, compulsivity, impulsivity, and other behavioral, cognitive, and emotional leanings seem to predispose to eating disorders.

Binge-Eating Disorders

Binge eating is a common problem among people who are overweight and obese. Besides consuming unusually large amounts of food in a single sitting, binge eaters generally suffer from low mood and low alertness, and experience uncontrollable compulsions to eat. They experience food cravings before binge episodes and feelings of discontent, dissatisfaction, and restlessness following binges.

An estimated 2.8% of adults will have a binge-eating disorder at some point during their lifetime. (See Figure 3.1.) In "Director's Blog: Spotlight on Eating Disorders" (February 24, 2012, http://www.nimh.nih.gov/about/director/2012/spotlight-on-eating-disorders.shtml), Thomas Insel, the director of the National Institute of Mental Health (NIMH), reports that the lifetime rate among women is higher (3.5%, compared with 2% among men). In "Eating Disorders among Adults—Binge Eating Disorder" (2014, http://www.nimh.nih.gov/statistics/1EAT_ADULT_RB.shtml), the NIMH indicates that binge-eating disorder is the most common eating disorder.

FIGURE 3.1

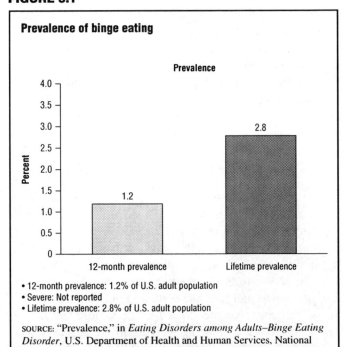

Prevalence of binge eating

Prevalence

- 12-month prevalence: 1.2% of U.S. adult population
- Severe: Not reported
- Lifetime prevalence: 2.8% of U.S. adult population

SOURCE: "Prevalence," in *Eating Disorders among Adults–Binge Eating Disorder*, U.S. Department of Health and Human Services, National Institute of Mental Health, undated, http://www.nimh.nih.gov/statistics/EAT_ADULT_RB.shtml (accessed October 11, 2013)

The prevalence of binge eating declines with advancing age; people aged 18 to 59 years are more likely to suffer from it than people aged 60 years and older.

Although the disorder is more common in people who are overweight or obese, normal-weight people also develop the disorder. People who suffer from binge eating often:

- Feel that eating is out of their ability to control

- Eat amounts of food most people would think are unusually large

- Eat much more quickly than usual during binge episodes

- Eat until the point of physical discomfort

- Consume large amounts of food, even when they are not hungry

- Eat alone because they feel embarrassed about the amount of food they eat

- Feel disgusted, depressed, or guilty after overeating

Until recently some eating disorders were not officially recognized as mental disorders. For example, whereas anorexia nervosa was included in the first edition of the Diagnostic and Statistical Manual of Mental Disorders (DSM), the definitive manual that classifies and establishes criteria for mental disorders in 1952, binge eating disorder was not included until the fifth edition of the DSM in 2012. Inclusion in the DSM is important because it promotes awareness, recognition, and treatment of the disorder.

Some Dieters Are Consumed by Eating Disorders

In the 21st century Americans are preoccupied with body image. They are constantly bombarded with images of thin, beautiful young women and lean, muscular men in magazines, on billboards, on the Internet, on television, and in movies. Advertising implies that to be thin and beautiful is to be happy. Many prominent weight-loss programs reinforce this suggestion. Well-balanced, low-fat food plans or other diets that restrict carbohydrates or calories combined with exercise can help many overweight people achieve a healthier weight and lifestyle. Dieting to achieve a healthy weight is quite different from dieting obsessively to become "model thin," which can have consequences that range from mildly harmful to life-threatening. Table 3.1 enumerates the health consequences of eating disorders.

According to the NIMH, dieting plays a role in the onset of two serious eating disorders: anorexia nervosa and bulimia. Preteens, teens, and college-age women are at special risk. In fact, the National Women's Health Resource Center states in "Eating Disorders" (August 26, 2013, http://www.healthywomen.org/condition/eating-disorders) that between 85% and 95% of people who

TABLE 3.1

Health consequences of eating disorders

- Eating disorders are serious, potentially life-threatening conditions that affect a person's emotional and physical health.
- Eating disorders are not just a "fad" or a "phase." People do not just "catch" an eating disorder for a period of time. They are real, complex, and devastating conditions that can have serious consequences for health, productivity, and relationships.
- People struggling with an eating disorder need to seek professional help. The earlier a person with an eating disorder seeks treatment, the greater the likelihood of physical and emotional recovery.

Health consequences of anorexia nervosa: In anorexia nervosa's cycle of self-starvation, the body is denied the essential nutrients it needs to function normally. Thus, the body is forced to slow down all of its processes to conserve energy, resulting in serious medical consequences:
- Abnormally slow heart rate and low blood pressure, which mean that the heart muscle is changing. The risk for heart failure rises as the heart rate and blood pressure level sink lower and lower.
- Reduction of bone density (osteoporosis), which results in dry, brittle bones.
- Muscle loss and weakness.
- Severe dehydration, which can result in kidney failure.
- Fainting, fatigue, and overall weakness.
- Dry hair and skin; hair loss is common.
- Growth of a downy layer of hair called lanugo all over the body, including the face, in an effort to keep the body warm.

Health consequences of bulimia nervosa: The recurrent binge-and-purge cycles of bulimia can affect the entire digestive system and can lead to electrolyte and chemical imbalances in the body that affect the heart and other major organ functions. Some of the health consequences of bulimia nervosa include:
- Electrolyte imbalances that can lead to irregular heartbeats and possibly heart failure and death. Electrolyte imbalance is caused by dehydration and loss of potassium and sodium from the body as a result of purging behaviors.
- Potential for gastric rupture during periods of bingeing.
- Inflammation and possible rupture of the esophagus from frequent vomiting.
- Tooth decay and staining from stomach acids released during frequent vomiting.
- Chronic irregular bowel movements and constipation as a result of laxative abuse.
- Peptic ulcers and pancreatitis.

Health consequences of binge eating disorder: Binge eating disorder often results in many of the same health risks associated with clinical obesity. Some of the potential health consequences of binge eating disorder include:
- High blood pressure.
- High cholesterol levels.
- Heart disease as a result of elevated triglyceride levels.
- Secondary diabetes.
- Gallbladder disease.

SOURCE: "Health Consequences of Eating Disorders," National Eating Disorders Association, 2002, http://www.nationaleatingdisorders.org/health-consequences-eating-disorders (accessed October 11, 2013)

develop anorexia or bulimia are women. Researchers, however, are beginning to report rising rates of anorexia and bulimia among men. Studies suggest that for every 10 women with an eating disorder, one male is afflicted.

A 2011 survey of high school students found that 17.4% of teenaged girls and 7.2% of teenaged boys said they had not eaten for 24 or more hours, and 6.3% of teenaged girls and 3.8% of teenaged boys reported other behaviors that may be symptoms of eating disorders, such as taking laxatives to lose weight or keep from gaining weight. (See Table 3.2.) In 2011, 5.9% of teenaged girls and 4.2% of teenaged boys said they took diet pills, powders or liquids without a doctor's advice to lose weight and 6% of teenaged girls and 2.5% of teenaged boys admitted that they vomited or took laxatives to lose or maintain their weight. (See Table 3.2 and Table 3.3.)

TABLE 3.2

Percentage of high school students engaging in dangerous dieting behaviors, 2011

| | Did not eat for 24 or more hours to lose weight or to keep from gaining weight | | | Took diet pills, powders, or liquids to lose weight or to keep from gaining weight | | |
| | Female | Male | Total | Female | Male | Total |
Category	%	%	%	%	%	%
Race/ethnicity						
White*	17.5	6.7	11.9	5.8	3.7	4.7
Black*	15.1	8.0	11.6	4.1	4.3	4.2
Hispanic	18.8	7.8	13.2	7.8	5.0	6.4
Grade						
9	18.8	6.3	12.4	5.5	3.6	4.6
10	17.4	6.8	11.9	4.5	4.2	4.3
11	17.3	8.6	12.9	6.8	5.1	5.9
12	15.6	7.1	11.3	6.8	4.0	5.4
Total	**17.4**	**7.2**	**12.2**	**5.9**	**4.2**	**5.1**

*Non-Hispanic.
Notes: To lose weight or to keep from gaining weight during the 30 days before the survey without a doctor's advice.

SOURCE: Danice K. Eaton et al., "Table 105. Percentage of Students Who Did Not Eat for 24 or More Hours and Who Took Diet Pills, Powders, or Liquids, by Sex, Race/Ethnicity, and Grade—United States, Youth Risk Behavior Survey, 2011," in "Youth Risk Behavior Surveillance—United States, 2011," *MMWR*, vol. 61, no. 4, June 8, 2012, http://www.cdc.gov/mmwr/pdf/ss/ss6104.pdf (accessed October 11, 2013)

TABLE 3.3

Percentage of high school students who vomited or took laxatives to lose or maintain weight, 2011

[During the 30 days before the survey]

| | Female | Male | Total |
Category	%	%	%
Race/ethnicity			
White*	6.5	1.8	4.1
Black*	2.9	3.0	3.0
Hispanic	7.2	3.3	5.2
Grade			
9	5.9	2.4	4.1
10	5.9	2.3	4.1
11	5.8	2.9	4.3
12	6.4	2.5	4.4
Total	**6.0**	**2.5**	**4.3**

*Non-Hispanic.

SOURCE: Danice K. Eaton et al., "Table 107. Percentage of High School Students Who Vomited or Took Laxatives to Lose Weight or to Keep from Gaining Weight, by Sex, Race/Ethnicity, and Grade—United States, Youth Risk Behavior Survey, 2011," in "Youth Risk Behavior Surveillance—United States, 2011," *MMWR*, vol. 61, no. 4, June 8, 2012, http://www.cdc.gov/mmwr/pdf/ss/ss6104.pdf (accessed October 11, 2013)

Anorexia Nervosa

Anorexia nervosa involves severe weight loss (a minimum of 15% below normal body weight). Anorexic people literally starve themselves, although they may be very hungry. For reasons that researchers do not yet fully understand, anorexics become terrified of gaining weight. Both food and weight become obsessions. They often develop strange eating habits, refuse to eat with other people, and exercise strenuously to burn calories and prevent weight gain. Anorexic individuals continue to believe they are overweight even when they are dangerously thin.

This condition often begins when a young woman who is slightly overweight or normal weight starts to diet to lose weight. After achieving the desired weight loss, she redoubles her efforts to lose more weight, and dieting becomes an obsession that may eclipse other interests. Affected individuals take pleasure in how well they can avoid food consumption and measure their self-worth by their ability to lose weight. Eating and weight gain are perceived as weaknesses and personal failures.

The medical complications of anorexia are similar to starvation. When the body attempts to protect its most vital organs, the heart and the brain, it goes into "slow gear." Menstrual periods stop, and breathing, pulse, blood pressure, and thyroid function slow down. The nails and hair become brittle, the skin dries, and the lack of body fat produces an inability to withstand cold temperatures. Depression, weakness, and a constant obsession with food are also symptoms of the disease. In addition, personality changes may occur. The person suffering from anorexia may have outbursts of anger and hostility or may withdraw socially. In the most serious cases, death can result.

Scientists often describe eating disorders as addictions, and Mario Speranza et al. support this notion in "An Investigation of Goodman's Addictive Disorder Criteria in Eating Disorders" (*European Eating Disorders Review*, vol. 20, no. 3, May 2012). The researchers find that common addictive personality traits are present in many people suffering from eating disorders and substance use–related disorders. Speranza et al. conclude that "a subgroup of individuals with an eating disorder experiences their disorder as an addiction and may deserve specific therapeutic attention."

Bulimia

People who suffer from bulimia eat compulsively and then purge (get rid of the food) through self-induced vomiting, use of laxatives, diuretics, strict diets, fasts, exercise, or a combination of several of these compensatory behaviors. Bulimia often begins when a person is disgusted with the excessive amount of "bad" food consumed and vomits to rid the body of the calories.

Many bulimics are at a normal body weight or above because of their frequent binge-purge behavior, which can occur from once or twice per week to several times per day. Those bulimics who maintain normal weight may manage to keep their eating disorder a secret for years. As with anorexia, bulimia usually begins during adolescence or early adulthood. According to the NIMH, the average age of onset is 20, but many bulimics do not seek help until they are in their 30s or 40s. Figure 3.2 shows the prevalence and demographics of bulimia nervosa as well as the utilization of treatment and services.

Binge eating and purging are dangerous. In rare cases bingeing can cause esophageal ruptures, and purging can result in life-threatening cardiac (heart) conditions because the body loses vital minerals. The acid in vomit wears down tooth enamel and the lining of the esophagus, throat, and mouth and can cause scarring on the hands when fingers are pushed down the throat to induce vomiting. The esophagus may become inflamed, and glands in the neck may become swollen.

Bulimics often talk of being "hooked" on certain foods and needing to feed their "habits." This addictive behavior carries over into other areas of their life, including the likelihood of alcohol and drug abuse. Many bulimics suffer from coexisting medical or mental health problems, such as severe depression, which increases their risk for suicide.

CAUSES OF EATING DISORDERS

As described earlier, research indicates that there is a genetic component to susceptibility to eating disorders. For example, in the general population the chance of developing anorexia is about one out of 200, but when a family member has the disorder, the risk increases to one out of 30. Twin studies demonstrate that when one twin is affected, there is a 50% chance the other will develop an eating disorder. Cynthia M. Bulik et al. calculated heritability estimates for anorexia nervosa and bulimia nervosa and published the estimates of their genetic correlation in "Understanding the Relation between Anorexia Nervosa and Bulimia Nervosa in a Swedish National Twin Sample" (*Biological Psychiatry*,

FIGURE 3.2

Bulimia prevalence, demographics, and treatment

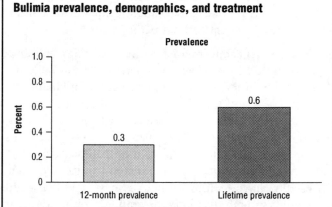

Prevalence

• 12-month prevalence: 0.3% of U.S. adult population
• Severe: Not reported
• Lifetime prevalence: 0.6% of U.S. adult population

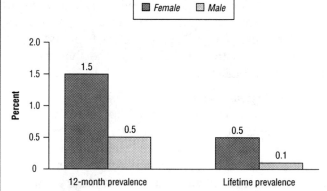

Demographics (for lifetime prevalence)

• Sex:
• Race: Not reported
• Age: People ages 18–29, 30–44, and 45–59 were all significantly more likely than 60+ year olds to suffer from bulimia nervosa

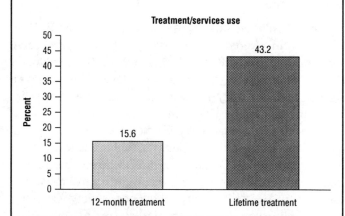

Treatment/services use

• 12-month treatment for bulimia nervosa: 15.6% of those with disorder are receiving treatment
• Lifetime treatment for bulimia nervosa: 43.2% of those with disorder are receiving treatment

Average age-of-onset: 20 years old

SOURCE: "Bulimia Nervosa," in *Eating Disorders among Adults—Bulimia Nervosa*, U.S. Department of Health and Human Services, National Institute of Mental Health, undated, http://www.nimh.nih.gov/statistics/pdf/NCS-R_Bulimia_Nervosa.pdf (accessed October 11, 2013)

vol. 67, no. 1, January 1, 2010). Consistent with the findings of other researchers, Bulik et al. find an overlap of genetic and unique environmental factors that influence the development of both eating disorders.

Besides a genetic predisposition, bulimics and anorexics seem to have different temperaments. Bulimics are likely to be impulsive (acting without thought of the consequences) and are more likely to abuse alcohol and drugs. Anorexics tend to be perfectionists, good students, and competitive athletes. They usually keep their feelings to themselves and rarely disobey their parents. However, bulimics and anorexics do share certain traits: they lack self-esteem, have feelings of helplessness, and fear gaining weight. In both disorders, the eating problems appear to develop as a way of handling stress and anxiety.

Bulimics consume huge amounts of food (often junk food) in search of comfort and stress relief. The bingeing, however, results in feelings of guilt and depression. By contrast, anorexics restrict food to gain a sense of control and mastery over some aspect of their lives. Controlling their weight seems to offer two advantages: they can take control of their body, and they can gain approval from others.

Psychological theories that explain the origins of bulimia include conflicted relationships between mothers and daughters, attempts to control one's own body in the face of seemingly uncontrollable family or other interpersonal relationships, or ambivalence about sexual development and attention. The latter theory has also been used to explain overweight and obesity in teenage girls and young women—as protection from or defense against attention from males who make them fearful or uncomfortable.

In "Childhood Anxiety Associated with Low BMI in Women with Anorexia Nervosa" (*Behaviour Research and Therapy*, vol. 48, no. 1, January 2010), Jocilyn E. Dellava et al. look at risk factors for developing anorexia nervosa and low body mass index (BMI; body weight in kilograms divided by height in meters squared) after they interviewed 326 women and their mothers who participated in the Genetics of Anorexia Nervosa Study. The researchers find that women with anorexia nervosa who had been especially fearful or anxious as children were at greater risk for dangerously low BMI and that childhood anxiety was associated with caloric restriction. Dellava et al. posit that "measures of anxiety and factors associated with anxiety-proneness in childhood may index children at risk for restrictive behaviors and extremely low BMIs in [anorexia nervosa]." In another study, Pamela K. Keel and K. Jean Forney of Florida State University consider risk factors for developing eating disorders and report their findings in "Psychosocial Risk Factors for Eating Disorders" (*International Journal of Eating Disorders*, vol. 46, no. 5, July 2013). The researchers find that idealizing thinness coupled with negativity and perfectionism contribute to the development of eating disorders as do peer influences.

OCCURRENCE OF EATING DISORDERS

Sonia A. Swanson et al. of the NIMH analyzed eating disorders using data from the National Comorbidity Survey Replication Adolescent Supplement, a nationally representative sample of adolescents aged 13 to 18 years in the United States. In "Prevalence and Correlates of Eating Disorders in Adolescents: Results from the National Comorbidity Survey Replication Adolescent Supplement" (*Archives of General Psychiatry*, vol. 68, no. 7, July 2011), the researchers note that the lifetime prevalence rates of anorexia nervosa, bulimia nervosa, and binge eating disorder were 0.3%, 0.9%, and 1.6%, respectively, and their 12-month prevalence rates were 0.2%, 0.6%, and 0.9%, respectively. The majority of adolescents with an eating disorder also met criteria for at least one other mental disorder, and nearly all adolescents with anorexia nervosa reported social problems. Adolescents with eating disorders were also at increased risk for other self-destructive and suicidal behavior. Swanson et al. conclude that "the prevalence of these disorders is higher than previously expected in this age range, and the patterns of comorbidity, role impairment, and suicidality indicate that eating disorders represent a major public health concern."

The Eating Disorders Coalition for Research, Policy, and Action notes in the fact sheet "Facts about Eating Disorders: What the Research Shows" (2013, http://www.eatingdisorderscoalition.org/documents/EatingDisorder-Facts.pdf) that at least 14 million Americans are affected by eating disorders and that anorexia is the third most common illness among adolescents. The coalition observes that the incidence of eating disorders is increasing in younger age groups and is becoming more common in diverse ethnic and sociocultural groups. Eating disorders account for 4% of children's hospitalizations.

According to Swanson et al., the prevalence of eating disorders among adults ranges from 0.5% to 1% for anorexia nervosa and from 0.5% to 3% for bulimia nervosa. In *Textbook of Psychiatric Epidemiology* (2011), the editors Ming Tsuang, Mauricio Tohen, and Peter B. Jones observe that the lifetime prevalence of anorexia nervosa across studies from North America, Europe, Australia, and New Zealand ranges from 0.9% to 2.2%; for bulimia nervosa the range is from 1.5% to 4.6%; and for binge eating disorder the range is from 0.6% to 3.5%. Research reveals that males are much less likely to suffer from eating disorders, with their lifetime prevalence of anorexia nervosa ranging from 0.1% to 0.4% and bulimia nervosa of about 0.5%. When all other eating disorders are added, between 8.7% and 15.9% of women will suffer from an eating disorder during their lifetime.

Eating disorders are often associated with various impulsive behaviors. In "Obsessive-Compulsive Disorder, Impulse Control Disorders, and Drug Addiction: Common Features and Potential Treatments" (*Drugs*, vol. 71, no. 7, May 7, 2011), Leonardo F. Fontenelle et al. examine the relationship between compulsive, impulsive, and addictive behaviors. They find a relationship between these behaviors and posit that impulsive or addictive features of eating disorders might be effectively treated with drugs that address the quality of the underlying drives and the involvement of neural systems such as those that act to reduce or prevent relapse of addiction.

According to Walter Kaye et al. of the University of California, San Diego, in "Does a Shared Neurobiology for Foods and Drugs of Abuse Contribute to Extremes of Food Ingestion in Anorexia and Bulimia Nervosa?" (*Biological Psychiatry*, vol. 73, no. 9, May 2013), there is a significant association between eating disorders and substance use disorders, in that high rates of substance abuse (alcohol and illicit drugs) are reported by people with bulimia while those with anorexia appear to be protected from substance abuse. The researchers explain that people with bulimia may share vulnerabilities to specific chemicals in the brain. Kaye et al. report that imaging studies of the brain provide insights into the inhibition and self-control characteristic of anorexia and the diminished self-control in bulimia that also may increase the risk of substance abuse.

TREATMENT OF EATING DISORDERS

Generally, physicians treat the medical complications of the disorder, whereas nutritionists advise the affected individuals about specific diet and eating plans. Psychotherapy is usually necessary to help people with eating disorders face their underlying problems and emotional issues. The initial challenge is to convince them to seek and obtain treatment; after they start treatment, the challenge then becomes helping them to stay in the program. Many anorexics deny their illness, and getting and keeping anorexic patients in treatment can be difficult. Treating bulimia is also difficult. Many bulimics are easily frustrated and want to leave treatment if their symptoms are not quickly relieved.

Several approaches are used to treat eating disorders. Cognitive-behavioral therapy (CBT) teaches people how to monitor their eating and change unhealthy eating habits. It also teaches them how to change the way they respond to stressful situations. CBT is based on the premise that thinking influences emotions and behavior—that feelings and actions originate with thoughts. CBT posits that it is possible to change the way people feel and act even if their circumstances do not change. It teaches the advantages of feeling calm when faced with undesirable situations. CBT clients learn that they will confront undesirable events and circumstances whether they become troubled about them or not. When they are troubled about events or circumstances, they have two problems: the troubling event or circumstance, and the troubling feelings about the event or circumstance. Clients learn that when they do not become troubled about trying events and circumstances, they can reduce the number of problems they face by half.

Interpersonal psychotherapy (IPT) helps people look at their relationships with friends and family and make changes to resolve problems. IPT is short-term therapy that has demonstrated effectiveness for the treatment of depression. According to the International Society for Interpersonal Psychotherapy, IPT emphasizes that mental health and emotional problems occur within an interpersonal context. For this reason the therapy aims to intervene specifically in social functioning to relieve symptoms.

Group therapy has been found helpful for bulimics, who are relieved to find that they are not alone or unique in their eating behavior. A combination of behavioral therapy and family systems therapy is often the most effective with anorexics. Family systems therapy considers the family as the unit of treatment and focuses on relationships and communication patterns within the family rather than on the personality traits or symptoms displayed by individual family members. Problems are addressed by modifying the system rather than by trying to change an individual family member. People with eating disorders who also suffer from depression may benefit from antidepressant and antianxiety medications to help relieve coexisting mental health problems.

Recovery from eating disorders is uneven and the lack of consensus about the criteria for recovery further confounds efforts to assess how people fare as a result of treatment. Greta Noordenbos of Leiden University explains in "When Have Eating Disordered Patients Recovered and What Do the DSM-IV Criteria Tell about Recovery?" (*Eating Disorders*, vol. 19, no. 3, May 2011) that varying criteria result in a wide range of estimates of recovered patients. Noordenbos laments that "outcome studies not only use different criteria for recovery, but also quite different instruments, rendering their results incomparable. The same problem occurs among studies of predictors for recovery from eating disorders. Without consensus on criteria for recovery, it is not clear which goals of treatment are important to realize full recovery."

In "Facts about Eating Disorders," the Eating Disorders Coalition for Research, Policy, and Action characterizes recovery as a process that frequently entails multiple rehospitalizations, limited ability to work or attend school, and limited capacity for interpersonal relationships. With treatment, which can take months to years, about one-third of people with an eating disorder recover after an initial episode, one-third fluctuates between recovery and relapse, and the remaining third suffer chronic deterioration.

Eating disorders are difficult to treat effectively because many sufferers resist entering treatment and/or fail to complete treatment programs. Because attrition (dropping out of treatment) is a known problem, Karen Farchaus Stein et al. report in "An Eating Disorder Randomized Clinical Trial and Attrition: Profiles and Determinants of Dropout" (*International Journal of Eating Disorders*, vol. 44, no. 4, May 2011) their efforts to determine whether attrition is related to changes in symptoms during treatment, including participants' perceptions of dissatisfaction with their body. To do this, the researchers compared the perceptions of dropouts to those of participants who remained in treatment for six months.

Stein et al. find that both dropouts and those who remained in treatment experienced decreases in the drive for thinness, body dissatisfaction, and bulimia during the treatment phase, but that women who dropped out of treatment had a greater decrease in body dissatisfaction after one month of treatment than those who remained. The researchers theorize that a decrease in symptoms along with changes in self-perception, such as diminished body dissatisfaction, discourage participants from continuing in treatment. Stein et al. opine that "attention to treatment response from the earliest phases of intervention through follow-up may help to identify those at greatest risk of dropping and lead to strategies for promoting participant retention."

New Directions in Research and Treatment

According to the NIMH, in "Eating Disorders," the results of its research are aiding both the understanding of eating disorders and their treatment. Research on intervening in the binge-eating cycle demonstrates that initiating structured patterns of eating enables people with eating disorders to experience less hunger, less deprivation, and fewer negative feelings about food and eating. When the two key predictors of bingeing (hunger and negative feelings) are reduced, the frequency of binges declines.

Continued study of the human genome promises the identification of additional susceptibility genes (genes that indicate an individual's increased risk for developing eating disorders) that will help develop more effective treatments for these disorders. Other research is investigating the relationship between brain functions and emotional and social behavior related to eating disorders and the role of the brain in feeding behavior. Scientists have learned that both appetite and energy expenditure are regulated by a highly complex network of nerve cells and intercellular messengers called neuropeptides. The role of sex hormones, known as gonadal steroids, in the development of eating disorders is suggested by gender and the onset of puberty as a risk for these disorders. These discoveries

provide insight into the biochemical mechanisms of eating disorders and offer potential direction for the development of new drugs and treatments for these disorders.

In "Update on Course and Outcome in Eating Disorders" (*International Journal of Eating Disorders*, vol. 43, no. 3, April 2010), Pamela K. Keel and Tiffany A. Brown of Florida State University review 26 studies that describe inpatient and outpatient treatment of eating disorders and the outcomes (how patients fared) as a result of treatment. The researchers find that inpatient treatment and the co-occurrence of serious psychiatric disorders were significant predictors of poor outcomes. Keel and Brown note that although treatment may serve to stabilize or reduce the progression of symptoms and minimize the medical consequences and complications of eating disorders for many people, it is not yet known if treatment (or if a specific type of treatment) increases the number of people who fare well long term. Furthermore, little is known about the other factors that predict good or poor results of treatment.

In "Virtual Reality for Enhancing the Cognitive Behavioral Treatment of Obesity with Binge Eating Disorder: Randomized Controlled Study with One-Year Follow-Up" (*Journal of Medical Internet Research*, vol. 15, no. 6, June 2013), Gian Luca Cesa et al. looked at how people suffering from obesity and binge eating disorder fared following treatment with CBT that included a virtual reality program. The virtual reality presented environments and situations related to the triggering disordered eating or relapse such as home, supermarket, pub, and restaurant, enabling patients to practice eating and emotional management as well as decision-making and problem-solving skills. By practicing these skills in the virtual reality environment, patients learned to develop specific strategies for avoiding and/or coping with triggering situations. When Cesa et al. compared this novel approach to CBT alone, they found it was more effective in terms of preventing weight regain and improving weight loss after one-year follow-up.

The considerable proportion of people with eating disorders who do not fare well in treatment, along with the high mortality rates that are associated with these disorders, prompts questions about factors that may influence recovery. In view of the genetic component in the genesis and progression of eating disorders, it seems likely that there may be genetic variants that contribute to the prospects for recovery. Identifying these variants may lead to more personalized treatment that includes more effective psychotherapies and/or pharmacological interventions for the most treatment-resistant patients.

In "Genetic Association of Recovery from Eating Disorders: The Role of GABA Receptor SNPs" (*Neuropsychopharmacology*, vol. 36, no. 11, October 2011), Cinnamon S. Bloss et al. tested more than 5,000 single nucleotide polymorphisms (SNPs) in approximately

350 genes to determine whether any of these SNPs were associated with recovery from eating disorders. SNPs associated with g-aminobutyric acid (a neurotransmitter that acts to inhibit the central nervous system, exerting a calming effect) were overrepresented among people with eating disorders. Bloss et al. conclude that their findings "could provide new insights into the development of more effective interventions for the most treatment-resistant patients." In "Association between Serotonin Transporter Gene Polymorphism and Eating Disorders Outcome: A Six-Year Follow-Up Study" (*American Journal of Medical Genetics*, vol. 159B, no. 5, July 2012), Giovanni Castellini et al. of the University of Florence find that a specific variant of the serotonin transporter (5-HTT) gene not only increases the risk of suffering from both eating disorders and depression but also influences the long-term outcomes of patients with anorexia.

PREVENTING EATING DISORDERS

Conventional public health definitions describe primary prevention as the prevention of new cases and secondary prevention as the prevention of recurrence of a disease or prevention of its progression. Primary prevention measures fall into two categories: actions to protect against disease and disability and actions to promote health such as good nutrition and hygiene, adequate exercise and rest, and avoidance of environmental and health risks. Health promotion also includes education about other interdependent dimensions of health known as wellness. Examples of health promotion programs aimed at preventing eating disorders include programs to enhance self-esteem, nutrition education classes, and programs that support children and teens to resist unhealthy pressures to conform to unrealistic body weight.

Secondary prevention programs are intended to identify and detect disease in its earliest stages, when it is most likely to be successfully treated. With early detection and diagnosis, it may be possible to cure the disease, slow its progression, prevent or minimize complications, and limit disability. Secondary prevention of eating disorders includes efforts to identify affected individuals to intervene early and prevent the development of serious and potentially life-threatening consequences.

Tertiary prevention programs aim to improve the quality of life for people with various diseases by limiting complications and disabilities, reducing the severity and progression of the disease, and providing rehabilitation (therapy to restore function and self-sufficiency). Unlike primary and secondary prevention, tertiary prevention involves actual treatment for the disease, and in the case of eating disorders it is conducted primarily by medical and mental health practitioners rather than by public health or social service agencies. An example of tertiary prevention is a program that monitors people with eating disorders to ensure that they maintain appropriate body weight and adhere to healthy diets and other prescribed medication or treatment. Because the treatment of eating disorders is not always effective or lasting, many health professionals contend that initiatives directed at controlling or eliminating the disorders by treating each affected individual or by training enough professionals as interventionists are ill advised. Instead, they advocate redirecting time, energy, and resources to primary and secondary prevention efforts.

Table 3.4 lists the basic principles for the prevention of eating disorders prepared by the National Eating Disorders Association (NEDA). These principles underscore the complexity of addressing eating disorders and the need for comprehensive, community-wide prevention programs that address the social and cultural issues promoting the rise of these disorders. The NEDA also urges parents to spearhead efforts to prevent eating disorders by

TABLE 3.4

Eating disorders prevention

What is eating disorders prevention?

Prevention is any systematic attempt to change the circumstances that promote, initiate, sustain, or intensify problems like eating disorders.

- **Primary prevention** refers to programs or efforts that are designed to prevent the occurrence of eating disorders before they begin. Primary prevention is intended to help promote healthy development.
- **Secondary prevention** (sometimes called "targeted prevention") refers to programs or efforts that are designed to promote the early identification of an eating disorder—to recognize and treat an eating disorder before it spirals out of control. The earlier an eating disorder is discovered and addressed, the better the chance for recovery.

Basic principles for the prevention of eating disorders

1. Eating disorders are serious and complex problems. We need to be careful to avoid thinking of them in simplistic terms, like "anorexia is just a plea for attention," or "bulimia is just an addiction to food." Eating disorders arise from a variety of physical, emotional, social, and familial issues, all of which need to be addressed for effective prevention and treatment.
2. Eating disorders are not just a "woman's problem" or "something for the girls." Males who are preoccupied with shape and weight can also develop eating disorders as well as dangerous shape control practices like steroid use. In addition, males play an important role in prevention. The objectification and other forms of mistreatment of women by others contribute directly to two underlying features of an eating disorder: obsession with appearance and shame about one's body.
3. Prevention efforts will fail, or worse, inadvertently encourage disordered eating, if they concentrate solely on warning the public about the signs, symptoms, and dangers of eating disorders. Effective prevention programs must also address:
   - Our cultural obsession with slenderness as a physical, psychological, and moral issue.
   - The roles of men and women in our society.
   - The development of people's self-esteem and self-respect in a variety of areas (school, work, community service, hobbies) that transcend physical appearance.
4. Whenever possible, prevention programs for schools, community organizations, etc., should be coordinated with opportunities for participants to speak confidentially with a trained professional with expertise in the field of eating disorders, and, when appropriate, receive referrals to sources of competent, specialized care.

SOURCE: Michael Levine and Margo Maine, "Eating Disorders Can Be Prevented!" National Eating Disorders Association, 2005, http://www.dukehealth.org/repository/dukehealth/2009/10/12/09/51/04/6591/Eating%20Disorder%20Can%20Be%20Prevented.pdf (accessed October 14, 2013)

practicing positive, healthy attitudes and behaviors and encouraging children to resist media stereotypes about body shape and weight. Furthermore, it outlines the philosophies and actions parents can adopt and the behaviors they can model to help their children cultivate healthy attitudes about food, eating, exercise, and body weight. Table 3.5 outlines 10 steps parents can take to help prevent eating disorders, and Table 3.6 presents 10 steps family, friends, and the public-at-large can take to help prevent eating disorders.

Changing Social and Cultural Norms

The cultural idealization of thinness as a standard of female beauty and worth and the societal acceptance of dieting as a female ritual have been widely cited as sociocultural causes of eating disorders. The widespread misperception that the body is readily reshaped and that one can, and should, strive to change its size and form to correspond with aesthetic preferences also contributes to distorted perceptions and unrealistic expectations.

Media images that create, reflect, communicate, and reinforce cultural definitions of attractiveness, especially female beauty, are often acknowledged as factors that contribute to the rise of eating disorders. They exert powerful influences on values, attitudes, and practices for body image, diet, and activity. The role of the media, in conjunction with the fashion and entertainment industries, in promoting unrealistic standards of female beauty and unhealthy eating habits has been named as a causative factor for body dissatisfaction, unhealthy dieting behavior, and the rise of eating disorders.

Although media messages portraying thinness as a desirable attribute do not directly cause eating disorders, they help create the context in which people learn to place a value on the size and shape of their body. To the extent that media advertising defines cultural values

TABLE 3.5

Ten things parents can do to prevent eating disorders

1. Consider your thoughts, attitudes, and behaviors toward your own body and the way that these beliefs have been shaped by the forces of weightism and sexism. Then educate your children about
   (a) the genetic basis for the natural diversity of human body shapes and sizes, and
   (b) the nature and ugliness of prejudice.
   - Make an effort to maintain positive, healthy attitudes & behaviors. Children learn from the things you say and do!
2. Examine closely your dreams and goals for your children and other loved ones. Are you overemphasizing beauty and body shape, particularly for girls?
   - Avoid conveying an attitude which says in effect, "I will like you more if you lose weight, don't eat so much, look more like the slender models in ads, fit into smaller clothes, etc."
   - Decide what you can do and what you can stop doing to reduce the teasing, criticism, blaming, staring, etc. that reinforce the idea that larger or fatter is "bad" and smaller or thinner is "good."
3. Learn about and discuss with your sons and daughters (a) the dangers of trying to alter one's body shape through dieting, (b) the value of moderate exercise for health, and (c) the importance of eating a variety of foods in well-balanced meals consumed at least three times a day.
   - Avoid categorizing foods into "good/safe /no-fat or low-fat" vs. "bad/dangerous/ fattening."
   - Be a good role model in regard to sensible eating, exercise, and self-acceptance.
4. Make a commitment not to avoid activities (such as swimming, sunbathing, dancing, etc.) simply because they call attention to your weight and shape. Refuse to wear clothes that are uncomfortable or that you don't like but wear simply because they divert attention from your weight or shape.
5. Make a commitment to exercise for the joy of feeling your body move and grow stronger, not to purge fat from your body or to compensate for calories eaten.
6. Practice taking people seriously for what they say, feel, and do, not for how slender or "well put together" they appear.
7. Help children appreciate and resist the ways in which television, magazines, and other media distort the true diversity of human body types and imply that a slender body means power, excitement, popularity, or perfection.
8. Educate boys and girls about various forms of prejudice, including weightism, and help them understand their responsibilities for preventing them.
9. Encourage your children to be active and to enjoy what their bodies can do and feel like. Do not limit their caloric intake unless a physician requests that you do this because of a medical problem.
10. Do whatever you can to promote the self-esteem and self-respect of all of your children in intellectual, athletic, and social endeavors. Give boys and girls the same opportunities and encouragement. Be careful not to suggest that females are less important than males, e.g., by exempting males from housework or child care. A well-rounded sense of self and solid self-esteem are perhaps the best antidotes to dieting and disordered eating.

SOURCE: Michael Levine, "10 Things Parents Can Do to Help Prevent Eating Disorders," National Eating Disorders Association, 2005, http://www.niu .edu/csdc/counseling/docs/10PARENT.PDF (accessed October 10, 2013)

TABLE 3.6

Ten ways family and friends can help to prevent eating disorders

- Learn all you can about anorexia nervosa, bulimia nervosa, and binge eating disorder. Genuine awareness will help you avoid judgmental or mistaken attitudes about food, weight, body shape, and eating disorders.
- Discourage the idea that a particular diet, weight, or body size will automatically lead to happiness and fulfillment.
- Choose to challenge the false belief that thinness, weight loss and/or muscularity are desirable, while body fat and weight gain are shameful, or indicate laziness, worthlessness, or immorality.
- Avoid categorizing foods as "good/safe" vs. "bad/dangerous." Remember, we all need to eat a balanced variety of foods.
- Decide to avoid judging others and yourself on the basis of body weight or shape. Turn off the voices in your head that tell you that a person's body weight or muscularity says anything about their character, personality, or value as a person.
- Avoid conveying an attitude that says, "I will like you better if you lose weight, don't eat so much, or change your body shape."
- Become a critical viewer of the media and its messages about self-esteem and body image. Talk back to the television when you hear a comment or see an image that promotes a certain body ideal at all costs. Rip out (or better yet, write to the editor about) advertisements or articles in magazines that make you feel bad about your body shape or size.
- If you think someone has an eating disorder, express your concerns in a forthright, caring manner. Gently but firmly encourage the person to seek trained professional help.
- Be a model of healthy self-esteem and body image. Recognize that others pay attention and learn from the way you talk about yourself and your body. Choose to talk about yourself with respect and appreciation. Choose to value yourself based on your goals, accomplishments, talents, and character. Refrain from letting the way you feel about your body weight and shape determine the course of your day. Embrace the natural diversity of human bodies and celebrate your body's unique shape and size.
- Support local and national nonprofit eating disorders organizations—like the National Eating Disorders Association—by volunteering your time or giving a tax-deductible donation.

SOURCE: "What Can You Do to Help Prevent Eating Disorders?" National Eating Disorders Association, 2013, http://www.nationaleatingdisorders.org/what-can-you-do-help-prevent-eating-disorders (accessed October 14, 2013)

about that which is beautiful and desirable, the media have potent power over the development of self-esteem and body image. Even if the media were to present more diverse and realistic images of people, this change would be unlikely to immediately reduce or eliminate eating disorders. Many observers, however, believe it would reduce the pressures to conform to one ideal, lessen feelings of body dissatisfaction, and ultimately decrease the potential for eating disorders.

EMPHASIS ON REALISTIC BODIES IN SKIN CARE ADVERTISING CAMPAIGN. In June 2005 Dove, a skin and hair care division of the Unilever company, launched the "Campaign for Real Beauty," which featured a purportedly unretouched photo of six smiling women of various sizes and ethnicities posing in plain white underwear to promote a skin-firming cream. The women, who were not professional models, ranged from a slim size 6 to a curvy size 14 and graced print advertisements and billboards. The campaign generated considerable discussion and debate in the media.

According to the article "Dove Ads with 'Real' Women Get Attention" (Associated Press, July 29, 2005), Philippe Harousseau, the Dove marketing director, described the campaign as responsive to "our belief that beauty comes in different shapes, sizes, and ages. Our mission is to make more women feel beautiful every day by broadening the definition of beauty." Industry observers wondered whether the company was in fact broadening the definition of beauty and improving women's body image and self-esteem or simply launching a provocative advertising campaign. Although the company did not disclose just how much the advertisements helped promote its products, it conceded that the campaign was beneficial for all Dove products, not just the firming creams.

The article notes that the ads were not, however, universally well received. For example, the *Chicago Sun-Times* columnist Richard Roeper characterized the women as "chunky," which earned him angry letters from about a thousand readers. Some skeptics asserted that although they endorsed the notion of the ads featuring real women who felt good about their body, they believed the ads sent contradictory messages (e.g., promoting a product to reduce the curves the models were flaunting). The most impassioned detractors accused the company of appearing hypocritical because the ads aimed to profit from "improving" the same curves the campaign exhorted women to celebrate.

The Dove advertising campaign ended in early 2011, but by that time it had prompted some attitudinal change. The campaign coined the term *Dove beauties*, which referred to attractive women with healthy bodies as opposed to model-thin frames. It also inspired some other advertisers and editors to use more average-sized models instead of relying solely on extremely thin models.

For example, in September 2009 *Glamour* magazine ran an unretouched, nearly nude photo of the plus-sized model Lizzi Miller (1989–), in which her rounded belly was clearly visible. The photo touched a nerve with readers who were generally overjoyed to see the photograph of a clearly happy, self-confident young woman who was not extremely thin. Readers and others in the media pleaded for more images of beautiful women of all sizes, and the magazine complied with its November 2009 issue, which featured photos of seven models who were all several sizes larger than the typical thin model.

Among the models was Crystal Renn (1986–), the coauthor (with Marjorie Ingall) of *Hungry: A Young Model's Story, of Appetite Ambition, and the Ultimate Embrace of Curves* (2009), a memoir that describes her as having an eating disorder. When she acknowledged her disorder and began to eat healthily, her career as a fashion model took off. Renn became a healthy, successful plus-sized model and advocate for media recognition and celebration of women of all sizes. In September 2011, however, the poster girl for curvier plus-sized models debuted a new, much thinner look. According to Sarah Bull and Laura Schreffler in "Plus-Size Past: Former 'Big' Model Crystal Renn Shows Full Extent of Weight Loss in Slinky Gold Dress at Metropolitan Opera" (DailyMail.co.uk, September 29, 2011), Renn denied that her weight loss was attributable to pressure from the fashion industry. Renn claimed she was happy with her body, opining, "I think the most important thing that we all need to know, whether you're a model, you're a normal person walking around, you're an editor, you're a photographer, you're anybody out in the world—it's about individual health."

In "Waif Goodbye! Average-Size Female Models Promote Positive Body Image and Appeal to Consumers" (*Psychology and Health*, vol. 26, no. 10, October 2011), Phillippa C. Diedrichs and Christina Lee of the University of Queensland examine the effectiveness of advertising using average-sized models compared with thin models. Among men and women, the average-sized models were associated with a more positive body image than the thin models. Based on their findings, Diedrichs and Lee conclude that "average-size female models can promote positive body image and appeal to consumers."

ATTEMPTS TO ADOPT HEALTHY STANDARDS IN THE MODELING INDUSTRY. After the deaths of dangerously thin models Luisel Ramos (1984–2006) and Ana Carolina Reston (1985–2006) in late 2006, Spain banned the use of models with a BMI of less than 18, and according to Eric Wilson in "Health Guidelines Suggested for Models" (NYTimes.com, January 6, 2007) the Chamber of Fashion in Milan proposed that models be at least 16 years old with a minimum BMI of 18.5. (BMI below 18.5 is considered underweight. See Table 1.5 in chapter 1.)

In January 2007 the Council of Fashion Designers of America proposed a series of actions intended to safeguard models' health. The recommendations included developing workshops for models and their families about eating disorders and supplying healthy meals, snacks, and water backstage and at shoots and provide nutrition and fitness education.

Despite efforts to encourage designers to use models of a healthy weight in 2013, models that appeared abnormally thin continued to dominate the runway. The editorial "Plus Size Bodies, What Is Wrong with Them Anyway?" (Plus-Model-Mag.com, January 2012) reports that most models have BMIs consistent with anorexia. The editorial laments, "Twenty years ago the average fashion model weighed 8% less than the average woman. Today, she weighs 23% less."

In "H&M CEO Karl-Johan Persson on Anorexic Models, Bangladeshi Factory Workers" (Metro.us, May 28, 2013), Elisabeth Braw quotes Karl-Johan Persson (1975–), the chief executive officer of the international clothing retailer H&M, who admitted, "Some of our models have been too skinny." Persson vowed to "show diversity in our advertising and not give people the impression that girls have to look a particular way."

CHAPTER 4
DIET, NUTRITION, AND WEIGHT ISSUES AMONG CHILDREN AND ADOLESCENTS

One of the most disturbing observations about overweight and obesity in the United States is the epidemic of supersized (overweight and obese) kids. The National Center for Health Statistics reports in *Health, United States, 2012* (2013, http://www.cdc.gov/nchs/data/hus/hus12.pdf) that in 2007–10 nearly three times as many American children aged six to 11 years and more than three times as many children aged 12 to 19 years were seriously overweight than were overweight in 1976–80. (See Table 4.1.) Between 1988–94 and 2007–10, the prevalence of overweight among children and adolescents increased from 7.2% to 11.1% for children aged two to five years and from 11.3% to 18.8% for children aged six to 11 years. Among teenagers aged 12 to 19 years, the percentage nearly doubled, from 10.5% to 18.2%.

With children and teens as well as with adults, the body mass index (BMI; body weight in kilograms divided by height in meters squared) is used to determine underweight, healthy weight, overweight, and at risk for overweight. Children's body fatness changes over the years as they grow, and girls and boys differ in their body fatness as they mature. In light of these differences, the BMI for children (also referred to as BMI-for-age) is gender and age specific. For example, Figure 4.1 shows BMI percentiles for boys aged two to 20 years and demonstrates how different BMI numbers are interpreted for a 10-year-old boy. Figure 4.2 shows that children of different ages (and genders) may have the same BMI number, but that number will fall into a different percentile for each child, classifying a 10-year-old boy as overweight and a 15-year-old boy as at a healthy weight.

Overweight is defined as at or above the age- and gender-specific 95th percentile on the BMI. (See Table 4.2.) Still, even children at the 85th percentile are considered at risk for overweight- and obesity-induced illnesses and overweight throughout their adult life.

Overweight children are much more likely to become overweight adults, and those children who are likely to become overweight and obese can be identified when they are toddlers and preschoolers. Laura E. Pryor et al. indicate in "Developmental Trajectories of Body Mass Index in Early Childhood and Their Risk Factors: An Eight-Year Longitudinal Study" (*Archives of Pediatric and Adolescent Medicine*, vol. 165, no. 10, October 2011) that by plotting age against BMI an "atypically elevated BMI trajectory" is identifiable at age three and a half. They also find that two maternal risk factors (high maternal BMI and smoking during pregnancy) were associated with the sharply rising trajectory predictive of overweight and obesity.

Joan Lo et al. find in "PS3-20: Prevalence of Obesity and Extreme Obesity in Children Aged Three to Five Years" (*Clinical Medicine & Research*, vol. 11, no. 3, September 2013) that obesity, and even severe obesity, are evident in children as young as three to five years of age. A review of the medical records of nearly 43,000 children found that 12.4% of boys and 10% of girls had BMI equal to or greater than the 95th percentile. The 3.9% of young children with BMI equal to or greater than the 99th percentile were considered extremely obese.

Although the Centers for Disease Control and Prevention (CDC) reports in "Progress on Childhood Obesity" (*CDC Vital Signs*, August 2013, http://www.cdc.gov/VitalSigns/ChildhoodObesity/index.html#info graphic) that one in eight preschoolers is obese, some progress in reversing this trend is evident. From 2008 to 2010, 19 states and territories had significant decreases in obesity among children aged two to four years. During this period, obesity among young children increased in just three states: Colorado, Pennsylvania, and Tennessee. (See Figure 4.3.)

TABLE 4.1

Obesity among children and teens, selected years 1963–2010

[Data are based on physical examinations of a sample of the civilian noninstitutionalized population]

Sex, age, race and Hispanic origin[a], and percent of poverty level	1963–1965 1966–1970[b]	1971–1974	1976–1980[c]	1988–1994	1999–2002	2003–2006	2007–2010
2–5 years				Percent of population			
Both sexes[d]	—	—	—	7.2	10.3	12.5	11.1
Not Hispanic or Latino:							
White only	—	—	—	5.2	8.7	10.8	9.0
Black or African American only	—	—	—	7.7	8.8	14.9	15.0
Mexican	—	—	—	12.3	13.1	16.7	14.6
Boys	—	—	—	6.1	10.0	12.8	11.9
Not Hispanic or Latino:							
White only	—	—	—	4.5*	8.2*	11.1	8.8
Black or African American only	—	—	—	7.7	8.0*	13.3	15.7
Mexican	—	—	—	12.4	14.1	18.8	19.1
Girls	—	—	—	8.2	10.6	12.2	10.2
Not Hispanic or Latina:							
White only	—	—	—	5.9	9.0*	10.4	9.2*
Black or African American only	—	—	—	7.6	9.6	16.6	14.2*
Mexican	—	—	—	12.3	12.2*	14.5	9.9*
Percent of poverty level:[e]							
Below 100%	—	—	—	9.7	10.9	14.3	13.2
100%–199%	—	—	—	7.2	13.8*	12.7	11.8
200%–399%	—	—	—	5.6	7.6*	11.9	13.9
400% or more	—	—	—	*	*	10.0*	5.8*
6–11 years							
Both sexes[d]	4.2	4.0	6.5	11.3	15.9	17.0	18.8
Boys	4.0	4.3*	6.6	11.6	16.9	18.0	20.7
Not Hispanic or Latino:							
White only	—	—	6.1	10.7	14.0	15.5	18.6
Black or African American only	—	—	6.8	12.3	17.0	18.6	23.3
Mexican	—	—	13.3	17.5	26.5	27.5	24.3
Girls	4.5	3.6*	6.4	11.0	14.7	15.8	16.9
Not Hispanic or Latina:							
White only	—	—	5.2	9.8*	13.1	14.4	14.0
Black or African American only	—	—	11.2	17.0	22.8	24.0	24.5
Mexican	—	—	9.8	15.3	17.1	19.7	22.4
Percent of poverty level:[e]							
Below 100%	—	—	—	11.4	19.1	22.0	22.2
100%–199%	—	—	—	11.1	16.4	19.2	20.7
200%–399%	—	—	—	11.7	15.3	16.7	18.9
400% or more	—	—	—	*	12.9	9.2	12.5*
12–19 years							
Both sexes[d]	4.6	6.1	5.0	10.5	16.0	17.6	18.2
Boys	4.5	6.1	4.8	11.3	16.7	18.2	19.4
Not Hispanic or Latino:							
White only	—	—	3.8	11.6	14.6	17.3	17.1
Black or African American only	—	—	6.1	10.7	18.8	18.4	21.2
Mexican	—	—	7.7	14.1	24.7	22.1	27.9
Girls	4.7	6.2	5.3	9.7	15.3	16.8	16.9
Not Hispanic or Latina:							
White only	—	—	4.6	8.9	12.6	14.5	14.6
Black or African American only	—	—	10.7	16.3	23.5	27.7	27.1
Mexican	—	—	8.8	13.4*	19.6	19.9	18.0
Percent of poverty level:[e]							
Below 100%	—	—		15.8	19.8	19.3	24.3
100%–199%	—	—	—	11.2	15.1	18.4	20.1
200%–399%	—	—	—	9.4	15.7	19.3	16.3
400% or more	—	—	—	*	13.9	12.6	14.0

The prevalence of overweight and obesity among adolescents is of particular concern because overweight and obese adolescents are at even greater risk than overweight children of becoming overweight or obese adults. Natalie S. The et al. of the University of North Carolina, Chapel Hill, observe in "Association of Adolescent Obesity with Risk of Severe Obesity in Adulthood" (*JAMA*, vol. 304, no. 18, November 2010) that previous studies have shown that obesity in childhood continues into adolescence and adulthood. The researchers find that there is strong persistence of severe obesity from adolescence to young adulthood and that obese adolescents are significantly more likely to become severely obese in adulthood. The et al. recommend that "primary prevention efforts should focus on the prevention of obesity prior to adolescence, while secondary prevention efforts should focus on the identification and treatment of high-risk groups in adolescence, including overweight and obese adolescents."

TABLE 4.1

Obesity among children and teens, selected years 1963–2010 [CONTINUED]

[Data are based on physical examinations of a sample of the civilian noninstitutionalized population]

—Data not available.
*Estimates are considered unreliable.
[a]Persons of Mexican origin may be of any race. Starting with 1999 data, race-specific estimates are tabulated according to the 1997 *Revisions to the Standards for the Classification of Federal Data on Race and Ethnicity* and are not strictly comparable with estimates for earlier years. The two non-Hispanic race categories shown in the table conform to the 1997 Standards. Starting with 1999 data, race-specific estimates are for persons who reported only one racial group. Prior to data year 1999, estimates were tabulated according to the 1977 Standards. Estimates for single-race categories prior to 1999 included persons who reported one race or, if they reported more than one race, identified one race as best representing their race.
[b]Data for 1963–1965 are for children aged 6–11; data for 1966–1970 are for adolescents aged 12–17, not 12–19.
[c]Data for Mexican-origin persons are for 1982–1984.
[d]Includes persons of all races and Hispanic origins, not just those shown separately.
[e]Percent of poverty level is based on family income and family size. Persons with unknown percent of poverty level are excluded (7% in 2007–2010).
Notes: Obesity is defined as body mass index (BMI) at or above the sex- and age-specific 95th percentile BMI cutoff points from the 2000 CDC Growth Charts: United States. Kuczmarski RJ, Ogden CL, Guo SS, Grummer-Strawn LM, Flegal KM, Mei Z, Wei R, Curtin LR, Roche AF, Johnson CL. 2000 CDC Growth Charts for the United States: methods and development. Starting with *Health United States, 2010,* the terminology describing weight for height among children changed from prior editions. The term "obesity" now refers to children who were formerly labeled as overweight. This is a change in terminology only and not measurement; the previous definition of overweight is now the definition of obesity. Ogden CL, Flegal KM. Changes in terminology for childhood overweight and obesity. Age is at time of examination at the mobile examination center. Crude rates, not age-adjusted rates, are shown. Excludes pregnant females starting with 1971–1974. Pregnancy status not available for 1963–1965 and 1966–1970.

SOURCE: "Table 69. Obesity among Children and Adolescents Aged 2–19 Years, by Selected Characteristics: United States, Selected Years 1963–1965 through 2007–2010," in *Health, United States, 2012: With Special Feature on Emergency Care,* Centers for Disease Control and Prevention, National Center for Health Statistics, 2013, http://www.cdc.gov/nchs/data/hus/hus12.pdf (accessed October 8, 2013)

In "The Utility of Childhood and Adolescent Obesity Assessment in Relation to Adult Health" (*Medical Decision Making*, vol. 33, no. 2, February 2013), Jeremy D. Goldhaber-Fiebert et al. sought to identify the portion of adult obesity and related chronic conditions associated with childhood obesity, and the usefulness of assessing childhood obesity at different ages. The researchers find that consistent with other studies, most obese adults were normal-weight children, and many obese children become nonobese adults. The predictive value of BMI assessment in younger children is relatively poor; however, BMI stabilizes in preteen and teen years, so using childhood BMI as an indicator of future obesity risk may be more useful in older children. The CDC reports in "Basics about Childhood Obesity" (April 27, 2012, http://www.cdc.gov/obesity/childhood/basics.html) that among five- to 17-year-olds, "70% of obese children had at least one [cardiovascular disease] risk factor, and 39% had two or more."

PREVALENCE OF OVERWEIGHT AND OBESE TEENS BY SEX, GRADE, RACE, AND ETHNICITY

The Youth Risk Behavior Surveillance System (YRBSS) is a national school-based survey conducted by the CDC. It examines health-risk behaviors among youth and young adults, including unhealthy dietary behaviors, physical inactivity, and overweight.

The 2011 YRBSS found that throughout the United States, 15.2% of students were overweight. (See Table 4.3.) The prevalence of overweight was higher among Hispanic males (16.9%) and among non-Hispanic white males (14.7%) than among non-Hispanic African American males (12.8%). For females, the prevalence of overweight was higher among non-Hispanic African Americans (19.6%) and Hispanics (18%) than among non-Hispanic whites (13.8%). Overall, the prevalence of overweight was higher among Hispanics (17.4%) and non-Hispanic African Americans (16.2%) and then among non-Hispanic white students (14.2%).

The prevalence of overweight was higher among ninth-grade students (17.3%) than among 12th-grade students (14.7%) and higher among ninth-grade females (16.3%) than among 10th-grade (14.5%), 11th-grade (15.2%), and 12th-grade (15.4%) females. (See Table 4.3.) The prevalence of overweight ranged from 10.7% to 19.5% across state surveys and from 11.6% to 22.7% across urban school district surveys. (See Table 4.4.)

The 2011 YRBSS found that 13% of high school students were obese. (See Table 4.3.) The prevalence of obesity was higher among male students (16.1%) than among female students (9.8%). It was also higher among non-Hispanic African American females (18.2%) and Hispanic females (14.1%) than among non-Hispanic white females (7.7%) and higher among Hispanic males (19.2%) and non-Hispanic African American males (17.7%) than among non-Hispanic white males (15%). Overall, there were higher rates of obesity among non-Hispanic African American (18.2%) and Hispanic (14.1%) students than among non-Hispanic white (11.5%) students.

The prevalence of obesity was higher among 11th-grade males (17.7%) than ninth-grade males (15.8%), 10th-grade males (15.5%), and 12th-grade males (15.1%) than among ninth-grade females (11.4%), 10th-grade females (9.8%), 11th-grade females (8%), and 12th-grade females (9.8%). (See Table 4.3.)

FIGURE 4.1

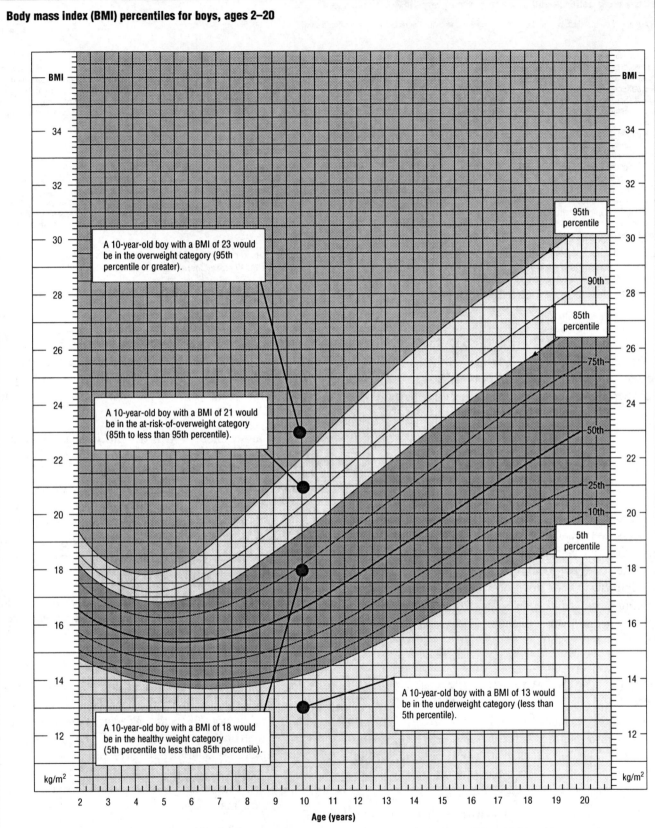

Body mass index (BMI) percentiles for boys, ages 2–20

A 10-year-old boy with a BMI of 23 would be in the overweight category (95th percentile or greater).

A 10-year-old boy with a BMI of 21 would be in the at-risk-of-overweight category (85th to less than 95th percentile).

A 10-year-old boy with a BMI of 18 would be in the healthy weight category (5th percentile to less than 85th percentile).

A 10-year-old boy with a BMI of 13 would be in the underweight category (less than 5th percentile).

Age (years)

SOURCE: "Body Mass Index-for-Age Percentiles: Boys, 2 to 20 Years," in *About BMI for Children and Teens*, Centers for Disease Control and Prevention, National Center for Chronic Disease Prevention and Health Promotion, Division of Nutrition, Physical Activity, and Obesity, January 27, 2009, http://cdc.gov/nccdphp/dnpa/bmi/childrens_BMI/about_childrens_BMI.htm (accessed October 15, 2013)

FIGURE 4.2

The interpretation of body mass index (BMI) varies by age

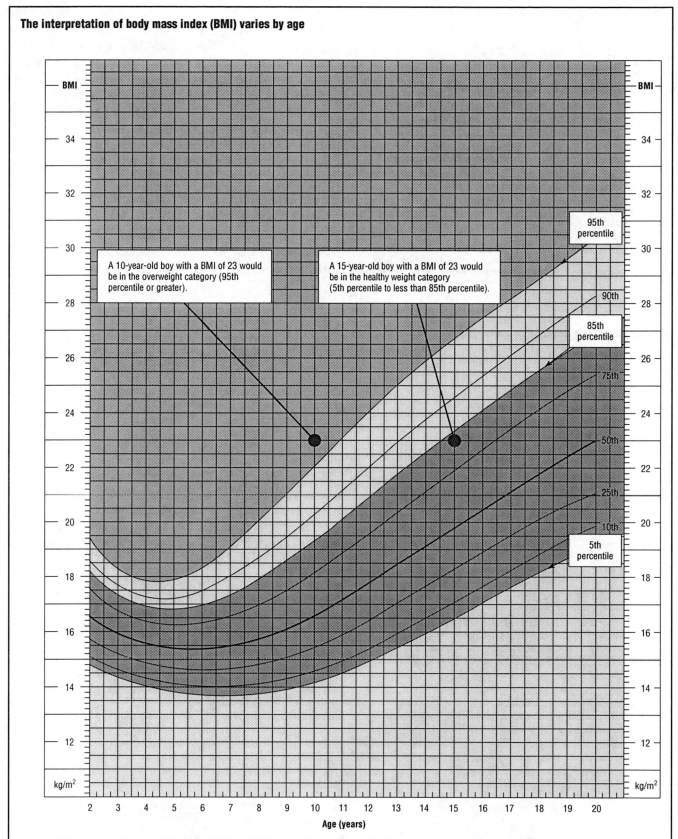

SOURCE: "Weight Status Category," in *About BMI for Children and Teens*, Centers for Disease Control and Prevention, National Center for Chronic Disease Prevention and Health Promotion, Division of Nutrition, Physical Activity, and Obesity, January 27, 2009, http://www.cdc.gov/nccdphp/dnpa/bmi/childrens_BMI/about_childrens_BMI.htm (accessed October 15, 2013)

The 2011 YRBSS finding of significant percentages of overweight and obese teens in lower grades suggests the likelihood of yet another generation of overweight adults who may be at risk for subsequent overweight- and obesity-related health problems. According to Y. Claire Wang et al. in "Health and Economic Burden of the Projected Obesity Trends in the USA and the UK" (*Lancet*, vol. 378, no. 9793, August 2011), forecasts based on the National Health and Nutrition Examination Surveys predict that if the current trends continue, three out of four Americans will be overweight or obese by 2020 and by 2030 there will be 65 million more obese American adults. In children, at the current rate, the prevalence of overweight is likely to nearly double by 2030.

WHY ARE SO MANY CHILDREN AND TEENS OVERWEIGHT?

Most children are overweight for the same reason as their adult counterparts: they consume more calories than they expend. Infants and toddlers appear to be effective

TABLE 4.2

Weight status categories by BMI-for-age percentiles

Weight status category	Percentile range
Underweight	Less than the 5th percentile
Healthy weight	5th percentile to less than the 85th percentile
At risk of overweight	85th to less than the 95th percentile
Overweight	Equal to or greater than the 95th percentile

BMI = Body mass index.

SOURCE: "Weight Status Category," in *About BMI for Children and Teens*, Centers for Disease Control and Prevention, National Center for Chronic Disease Prevention and Health Promotion, Division of Nutrition, Physical Activity, and Obesity, January 27, 2009, http://www.cdc.gov/nccdphp/dnpa/bmi/childrens_BMI/about_childrens_BMI.htm (accessed October 15, 2013)

FIGURE 4.3

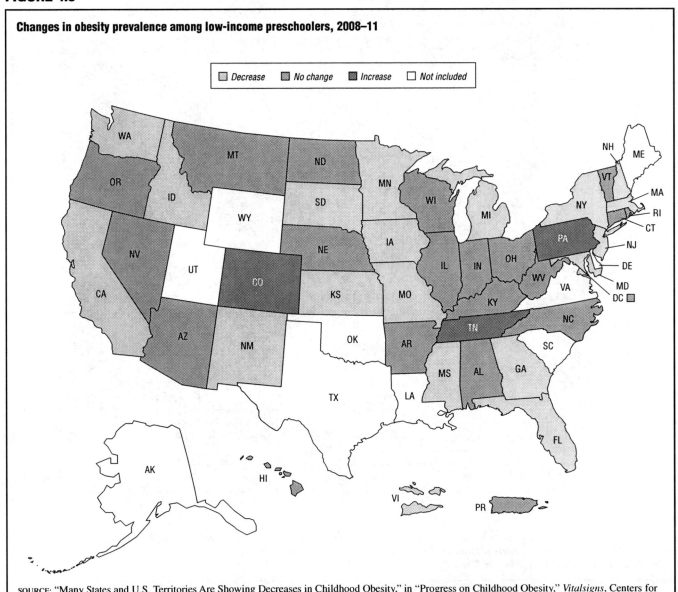

Changes in obesity prevalence among low-income preschoolers, 2008–11

SOURCE: "Many States and U.S. Territories Are Showing Decreases in Childhood Obesity," in "Progress on Childhood Obesity," *Vitalsigns*, Centers for Disease Control and Prevention, August 2013, http://www.cdc.gov/VitalSigns/ChildhoodObesity/index.html#infographic (accessed October 16, 2013)

TABLE 4.3

Percentages of overweight and obese high school students, by sex, race/ethnicity, and grade, 2011

	Obese			Overweight		
	Female	Male	Total	Female	Male	Total
Category	%	%	%	%	%	%
Race/ethnicity						
White*	7.7	15.0	11.5	13.8	14.7	14.2
Black*	18.6	17.7	18.2	19.6	12.8	16.2
Hispanic	8.6	19.2	14.1	18.0	16.9	17.4
Grade						
9	11.4	15.8	13.6	16.3	18.2	17.3
10	9.8	15.5	12.8	14.5	14.3	14.4
11	8.0	17.7	12.9	15.2	13.4	14.3
12	9.8	15.1	12.5	15.4	14.0	14.7
Total	**9.8**	**16.1**	**13.0**	**15.4**	**15.1**	**15.2**

*Non-Hispanic.

Notes: Obese measured as students who were ≥95th percentile for body mass index, based on sex- and age-specific reference data from the 2000 Centers for Disease Control (CDC) growth charts. Overweight measured as students who were ≥85th percentile but <95th percentile for body mass index, based on sex- and age-specific reference data from the 2000 CDC growth charts.

SOURCE: Adapted from Danice K. Eaton et al., "Table 101. Percentage of High School Students Who Were Obese and Who Were Overweight, by Sex, Race/Ethnicity, and Grade—United States, Youth Risk Behavior Survey, 2011," in "Youth Risk Behavior Surveillance—United States, 2011," *MMWR*, vol. 61, no. 4, June 8, 2012, http://www.cdc.gov/mmwr/pdf/ss/ss6104.pdf (accessed October 11, 2013)

regulators of caloric consumption, taking in only the calories needed for growth and development. By the time children are school age, this self-regulatory mechanism has weakened and when offered larger portions, they will eat them.

Heredity and environment play key roles in determining a child's risk of becoming overweight or obese. The American Academy of Child and Adolescent Psychiatry notes in "Obesity in Children and Teens" (March 2011, http://www.aacap.org/cs/root/facts_for_families/obesity_in_children_and_teens) that if one parent is obese, then there is a 50% chance that a child will be obese, and when both parents are obese, a child has an 80% chance of being obese. Although there is mounting evidence of genetic predisposition and susceptibility to overweight and obesity, childhood obesity is still considered largely an environmental problem—the result of behaviors, attitudes, and preferences learned early in life. Children's relationships with food develop in response to family and cultural values and practices as well as to the influences of school, peers, and the media.

The question remains: Which environmental factors have given rise to the increasing prevalence of overweight children and teens during the past three decades? Many observers point to a reliance on fat-laden convenience and fast foods, along with time spent watching television, playing video games, and surfing the Internet, instead of being outdoors and getting physical activity.

The Federal Interagency Forum on Child and Family Statistics reports in *America's Children: Key National Indicators of Well-Being, 2013* (2013, https://www.nichd.nih.gov/publications/pubs/Documents/Americas_Children_2013_DRAFT.pdf) that the diet quality score, a measure of how well children's diets meet federal diet quality standards, for children aged two to 17 years was 50 out of a possible 100. The forum asserts that children's diet scores would improve by increasing consumption of vegetables, especially dark greens and beans, replacing refined grains with whole grains, substituting seafood for some meat and poultry, and decreasing the intake of salt, solid fats, and added sugars.

In "Patterns of Physical Activity, Sedentary Behavior, and Diet in U.S. Adolescents" (*Journal of Adolescent Health*, vol. 53, no. 2, August 2013), Ronald J. Iannotti and Jing Wang of the National Institute of Child Health and Human Development (NICHD) report the results of a survey of more than 9,000 adolescents aged 11 to 16 years. Participants were asked about their physical activity, the amount of time they spent in front of a computer screen or other electronic screen, and the amount of healthful and unhealthful foods they consumed. They also were asked about symptoms of depression and their satisfaction with their bodies.

Based on their responses, Iannotti and Wang classified participants as unhealthful (26%), healthful (27%), and typical (47%). They find that the typical adolescents were least likely to exercise five or more days each week or to eat fruits and vegetables at least once a day. They were more likely to spend time in front of screens than the healthful group, and less likely to do so than the unhealthful group. They occasionally ate fruits and vegetables but also infrequently consumed sweets, chips, fries, or soda. These typical adolescents were more likely than those in the other two groups to be overweight or obese and to be dissatisfied with their bodies.

TABLE 4.4

Percentages of overweight and obese high school students by sex and selected cities and states, 2011

	Obese			Overweight		
	Female	Male	Total	Female	Male	Total
Site	%	%	%	%	%	%
State surveys						
Alabama	14.3	19.7	17.0	16.3	15.3	15.8
Alaska	8.8	14.0	11.5	14.7	14.1	14.4
Arizona	6.9	14.6	10.9	12.6	15.1	13.9
Arkansas	10.3	19.8	15.2	16.3	14.4	15.4
Colorado	2.6	11.7	7.3	8.2	13.0	10.7
Connecticut	8.4	16.5	12.5	11.7	16.5	14.1
Delaware	9.5	14.9	12.2	19.7	14.1	16.9
Florida	7.7	15.2	11.5	13.4	13.8	13.6
Georgia	11.7	18.2	15.0	14.9	16.6	15.8
Hawaii	8.7	17.7	13.2	13.2	13.6	13.4
Idaho	6.9	11.4	9.2	12.4	14.3	13.4
Illinois	7.1	15.9	11.6	15.7	13.2	14.5
Indiana	11.5	17.8	14.7	18.5	12.5	15.5
Iowa	10.1	16.2	13.2	14.5	14.5	14.5
Kansas	8.0	12.3	10.2	12.8	14.9	13.9
Kentucky	12.1	20.6	16.5	16.6	14.3	15.4
Louisiana	13.8	18.6	16.1	22.1	16.8	19.5
Maine	7.7	15.0	11.5	13.0	15.0	14.0
Maryland	10.5	13.4	12.0	15.3	15.5	15.4
Massachusetts	6.2	13.5	9.9	14.0	15.1	14.6
Michigan	8.1	15.8	12.1	15.4	15.2	15.3
Mississippi	13.5	18.2	15.8	18.1	14.9	16.5
Montana	5.4	11.4	8.5	11.6	14.0	12.9
Nebraska	8.0	15.0	11.6	13.6	13.5	13.6
New Hampshire	9.4	14.6	12.1	14.4	13.8	14.1
New Jersey	7.4	14.7	11.0	15.1	15.3	15.2
New Mexico	7.8	17.5	12.8	14.1	14.7	14.4
New York	8.0	13.9	11.0	14.9	14.6	14.7
North Carolina	10.9	14.8	12.9	16.4	15.5	15.9
North Dakota	7.4	14.4	11.0	15.1	13.9	14.5
Ohio	11.8	17.4	14.7	13.3	17.2	15.3
Oklahoma	15.5	17.9	16.7	15.2	17.5	16.3
Rhode Island	8.4	13.2	10.8	14.9	14.9	14.9
South Carolina	8.4	18.1	13.3	18.4	14.3	16.3
South Dakota	7.5	12.0	9.8	14.3	13.9	14.1
Tennessee	12.4	17.9	15.2	17.5	17.1	17.3
Texas	11.9	19.0	15.6	18.3	13.8	16.0
Utah	4.8	12.2	8.6	10.7	13.6	12.2
Vermont	6.4	13.2	9.9	11.4	14.5	13.0
Virginia	10.7	11.4	11.1	16.5	18.0	17.2
West Virginia	9.5	19.5	14.6	15.3	16.1	15.7
Wisconsin	6.8	13.9	10.4	15.0	14.9	15.0
Wyoming	7.0	14.9	11.1	12.6	11.5	12.0
Median	8.4	15.0	12.0	14.9	14.6	14.7
Range	2.6–15.5	11.4–20.6	7.3–17.0	8.2–22.1	11.5–18.0	10.7–19.5
Large urban school district surveys						
Boston, MA	14.2	14.4	14.3	17.0	18.9	18.0
Broward County, FL	6.7	12.1	9.5	12.9	14.5	13.7
Charlotte-Mecklenburg, NC	11.9	13.6	12.8	15.2	14.6	14.9
Chicago, IL	11.8	19.5	15.5	21.9	14.2	18.2
Dallas, TX	13.0	17.6	15.3	19.9	21.0	20.4
Detroit, MI	19.0	18.7	18.9	24.8	20.4	22.7
District of Columbia	15.5	13.4	14.5	19.5	16.4	18.0
Duval County, FL	9.1	14.7	11.9	17.1	13.5	15.3
Houston, TX	11.4	15.7	13.6	19.1	16.6	17.8
Los Angeles, CA	6.3	19.8	13.3	18.0	15.9	16.9
Memphis, TN	18.4	18.5	18.4	19.7	13.7	16.8
Miami-Dade County, FL	9.6	16.0	12.7	15.2	14.8	15.0
Milwaukee, WI	15.0	18.9	17.0	23.5	13.4	18.4
New York City, NY	9.1	14.1	11.6	16.4	14.6	15.5
Orange County, FL	7.4	12.6	10.0	11.7	12.3	12.0
Palm Beach County, FL	6.8	11.8	9.3	13.0	14.5	13.8
Philadelphia, PA	15.0	19.7	17.3	21.6	13.8	17.7

Not surprisingly, the unhealthful group ate the most sweets, chips, fries, and soft drinks. They were more likely than the other groups to spend more than two hours per day in front of screens. Adolescents in the unhealthful group were more likely to be underweight and to report needing to put on weight. They also were more likely to report symptoms of depression and of poor physical health.

TABLE 4.4

Percentages of overweight and obese high school students by sex and selected cities and states, 2011 [CONTINUED]

	Obese			Overweight		
	Female	**Male**	**Total**	**Female**	**Male**	**Total**
Site	**%**	**%**	**%**	**%**	**%**	**%**
San Bernardino, CA	12.4	18.0	15.2	19.2	17.3	18.2
San Diego, CA	6.9	15.5	11.4	13.4	18.5	16.0
San Francisco, CA	6.1	8.8	7.4	10.4	12.7	11.6
Seattle, WA	6.2	9.5	7.9	13.2	13.6	13.4
Median	11.4	15.5	13.3	17.1	14.6	16.8
Range	6.1–19.0	8.8–19.8	7.4–18.9	10.4–24.8	12.3–21.0	11.6–22.7

Note: Obese measured as students who were ≥95th percentile for body mass index, based on sex- and age-specific reference data from the 2000 Centers for Disease Control (CDC) growth charts. Overweight measured as students who were ≥85th percentile but <95th percentile for body mass index, based on sex- and age-specific reference data from the 2000 CDC growth charts.

SOURCE: Adapted from Danice K. Eaton et al., "Table 102. Percentage of High School Students Who Were Obese and Who Were Overweight, by Sex—Selected U.S. Sites, Youth Risk Behavior Survey, 2011," in "Youth Risk Behavior Surveillance—United States, 2011," *MMWR*, vol. 61, no. 4, June 8, 2012, http://www.cdc.gov/mmwr/pdf/ss/ss6104.pdf (accessed October 11, 2013)

Nearly two-thirds of youth in the healthful group said they exercised at least five days per week. These students were least likely to spend time in front of a screen and were most likely to report eating fruits and vegetables at least once a day. They also were least likely to consume sweets, soda, chips, and fries. They reported the fewest depressive symptoms and had the highest scores in life satisfaction.

The 2011 YRBSS found that nearly one-third (31.1%) of high school students used computers or played video games for three or more hours per day and that 32.4% watched television for three or more hours per day. (See Table 4.5.)

Eating alone, in front of a television or computer, children are more likely to overeat because they are lonely, bored, or susceptible to advertising cues. Overcome with guilt because they are not home to prepare meals, some working parents may intensify the problem by indulging their children with too many food treats. However, stay-at-home parents do not necessarily convey healthier attitudes about food, eating, and nutrition than parents who work outside the home. Both groups may use food, especially sweets, to reward good behavior or may pressure children to clean their plates. Although these suppositions remain unproven, it is known that parents with eating disorders, obsessive dieters, and those with unhealthful eating habits are powerful, negative role models for children.

HOW HIGH SCHOOL STUDENTS EAT

The 2011 YRBSS found that only 22.4% of students had eaten fruit or drank 100% fruit juice at least three times per day during the seven days preceding the survey. (See Table 4.6.) About one-third (34%) of students reported eating fruits or drinking fruit juice two or more times per day. Nearly two-thirds (62.3%) of students ate vegetables one or more times per day but 5.7% did not

eat any vegetables. (See Table 4.7.) Just 15.3% of students ate vegetables three or more times per day. (See Table 4.8.)

Even fewer students (14.9%) had drunk at least three glasses of milk per day than had eaten the recommended servings of fruits and vegetables during the seven days preceding the survey. (See Table 4.9.) The prevalence of having consumed at least three glasses of milk per day was more than two times higher among male (20%) than among female (9.3%) students.

Less than one-third (29.2%) of high school students surveyed in the 2011 YRBSS described themselves as "slightly" or "very" overweight. More teenaged girls (34.8%) than teenaged boys (23.9%) considered themselves overweight. Almost half (46%) of the students said they were trying to lose weight, but nearly twice as many female teens (61.2%) as male teens (31.6%) reported making an effort to lose weight.

Is Fast Food to Blame?

In "Trends in Energy Intake among U.S. Children by Eating Location and Food Source, 1977–2006" (*Journal of the American Dietetic Association*, vol. 111, no. 8, August 2011), Jennifer M. Poti and Barry M. Popkin of the University of North Carolina, Chapel Hill, indicate that children's increased food consumption between 1977 and 2006 was associated with a major increase in food that was eaten away from home. The researchers analyzed data from 29,217 children aged two to 18 years from the 1977–78 Nationwide Food Consumption Survey, the 1989–91 and 1994–98 Continuing Survey of Food Intakes by Individuals, and the 2003–06 National Health and Nutrition Examination Surveys. They find that the percentage of daily energy (as measured in calories) children ate away from home increased from 23.4% to 33.9% between 1977 and 2006. During the same period there were significant increases in children's

TABLE 4.5

Percentages of high school students who used computers, played video games, or watched television for 3 or more hours/day, by sex, race/ethnicity, and grade, 2011

| | Used computers 3 or more hours/day | | | Watched television 3 or more hours/day | | |
| | Female | Male | Total | Female | Male | Total |
Category	%	%	%	%	%	%
Race/ethnicity						
White*	22.6	33.3	28.1	23.9	27.3	25.6
Black*	35.2	41.1	38.1	54.9	54.4	54.6
Hispanic	28.3	36.3	32.4	37.2	38.4	37.8
Grade						
9	29.5	35.5	32.5	33.8	33.9	33.9
10	26.7	36.1	31.6	31.7	35.3	33.6
11	24.6	36.7	30.7	30.4	32.3	31.4
12	25.0	32.4	28.8	29.9	30.9	30.4
Total	**26.6**	**35.3**	**31.1**	**31.6**	**33.3**	**32.4**

*Non-Hispanic.
Note: For something that was not school work on an average school day.

SOURCE: Adapted from Danice K. Eaton et al., "Table 95. Percentage of High School Students Who Played Video or Computer Games or Used a Computer for 3 or More Hours/Day and Who Watched 3 or More Hours/Day of Television, by Sex, Race/Ethnicity, and Grade—United States, Youth Risk Behavior Survey, 2011," in "Youth Risk Behavior Surveillance—United States, 2011," *MMWR*, vol. 61, no. 4, June 8, 2012, http://www.cdc.gov/mmwr/pdf/ss/ss6104.pdf (accessed October 11, 2013)

TABLE 4.6

Percentages of high school students who ate fruit or drank fruit juice 2 or more times/day, by sex, race/ethnicity, and grade, 2011

| | Ate fruit or drank 100% fruit juices two or more times/day[a] | | | Ate fruit or drank 100% fruit juices three or more times/day[a] | | |
| | Female | Male | Total | Female | Male | Total |
Category	%	%	%	%	%	%
Race/ethnicity						
White[b]	30.6	34.8	32.8	17.4	22.3	20.0
Black[b]	34.5	40.0	37.2	25.6	30.3	27.9
Hispanic	30.9	40.0	35.6	21.8	27.6	24.8
Grade						
9	30.7	39.3	35.1	19.4	27.2	23.4
10	33.3	37.4	35.4	22.0	26.3	24.2
11	31.2	34.0	32.6	19.5	21.7	20.7
12	29.3	34.9	32.2	18.1	23.2	20.7
Total	**31.2**	**36.5**	**34.0**	**19.8**	**24.8**	**22.4**

[a]During the 7 days before the survey.
[b]Non-Hispanic.

SOURCE: Adapted from Danice K. Eaton et al., "Table 78. Percentage of High School Students Who Ate Fruit or Drank 100% Fruit Juices, by Sex, Race/Ethnicity, and Grade—United States, Youth Risk Behavior Survey, 2011," in "Youth Risk Behavior Surveillance—United States, 2011," *MMWR*, vol. 61, no. 4, June 8, 2012, http://www.cdc.gov/mmwr/pdf/ss/ss6104.pdf (accessed October 11, 2013)

consumption of fast food eaten at home and store-bought food eaten away from home. Poti and Popkin conclude that "foods prepared away from home, including fast food eaten at home and store-prepared food eaten away from home, are fueling the increase in total energy intake."

Echoing the sentiments of many health professionals, the Committee on Nutrition of the European Society for Paediatric Gastroenterology, Hepatology, and Nutrition named fast-food consumption as a contributing factor to childhood obesity. In "Role of Dietary Factors and Food Habits in the Development of Childhood Obesity:

A Commentary by the ESPGHAN Committee on Nutrition" (*Journal of Pediatric Gastroenterology and Nutrition*, vol. 52, no. 6, June 2011), Carlo Agostino et al. observe that fast foods offer large portions of high-energy-dense foods that are low in fiber and high in saturated and trans fats, glycemic load (a ranking system for carbohydrate content in food based on its glycemic index [a measure of a food's ability to raise blood glucose] and the portion size), and tastiness, which may promote not only a lifelong preference for foods high in fat, salt, and sugar but also excessive weight gain. Agostino et al. reviewed the relevant literature and conclude that

TABLE 4.7

Percentages of high school students who ate no vegetables and who ate vegetables 1 or more times/day, by sex, race/ethnicity, and grade, 2011

[During the 7 days before the survey]

	Did not eat vegetables			Ate vegetables one or more times/day		
	Female	Male	Total	Female	Male	Total
Category	%	%	%	%	%	%
Race/ethnicity						
White*	2.4	5.5	4.0	66.1	65.3	65.7
Black*	8.6	11.1	9.9	52.7	55.9	54.3
Hispanic	8.1	8.2	8.2	53.8	58.9	56.4
Grade						
9	5.0	8.1	6.6	59.8	61.6	60.8
10	3.7	5.9	4.9	62.2	64.1	63.1
11	4.6	8.2	6.4	62.3	60.8	61.6
12	4.4	5.2	4.8	62.7	64.7	63.7
Total	**4.5**	**6.9**	**5.7**	**61.6**	**62.8**	**62.3**

*Non-Hispanic.
Note: Vegetables defined as green salad, potatoes (excluding french fries, fried potatoes, or potato chips), carrots, or other vegetables.

SOURCE: Adapted from Danice K. Eaton et al., "Table 80. Percentage of High School Students Who Did Not Eat Vegetables and Who Ate Vegetables One or More Times/Day, by Sex, Race/Ethnicity, and Grade—United States, Youth Risk Behavior Survey, 2011," in "Youth Risk Behavior Surveillance—United States, 2011," *MMWR*, vol. 61, no. 4, June 8, 2012, http://www.cdc.gov/mmwr/pdf/ss/ss6104.pdf (accessed October 11, 2013)

TABLE 4.8

Percentages of high school students who ate vegetables 2 or 3 or more times/day, by sex, race/ethnicity, and grade, 2011

	Ate vegetables two or more times/day[a, b]			Ate vegetables three or more times/day[a, b]		
	Female	Male	Total	Female	Male	Total
Category	%	%	%	%	%	%
Race/ethnicity						
White[c]	27.2	30.9	29.1	13.3	15.5	14.4
Black[c]	23.2	26.7	24.9	14.2	17.3	15.8
Hispanic	23.8	29.7	26.8	13.7	18.1	16.0
Grade						
9	26.5	30.6	28.6	14.1	18.3	16.3
10	25.3	30.0	27.7	13.8	15.5	14.7
11	28.4	28.1	28.3	14.2	15.3	14.7
12	24.3	31.4	27.9	13.3	16.7	15.1
Total	**26.1**	**30.2**	**28.3**	**13.9**	**16.6**	**15.3**

[a]Green salad, potatoes (excluding French fries, fried potatoes, or potato chips), carrots, or other vegetables.
[b]During the 7 days before the survey.
[c]Non-Hispanic.

SOURCE: Adapted from Danice K. Eaton et al., "Table 82. Percentage of High School Students Who Ate Vegetables, by Sex, Race/Ethnicity, and Grade—United States, Youth Risk Behavior Survey, 2011," in "Youth Risk Behavior Surveillance—United States, 2011," *MMWR*, vol. 61, no. 4, June 8, 2012, http://www.cdc.gov/mmwr/pdf/ss/ss6104.pdf (accessed October 11, 2013)

increasing consumption of fast food is associated with excess weight gain and recommend that "regular consumption of fast food with large portion sizes and high energy density should be avoided."

Because high intake of sugar-sweetened beverages in childhood is linked to an increased risk of obesity, Gentry Lasater, Carmen Piernas, and Barry M. Popkin looked at beverage consumption patterns and trends among school-aged children in the United States between 1989–91 and 2007–08 and reported their findings in "Beverage Patterns and Trends among School-Aged Children in the U.S., 1989–2008" (*Nutrition Journal*, vol. 10, October 2, 2011). The researchers analyzed the dietary records of 3,583 children aged six to 11 years to determine the amounts of sugar-sweetened beverages (SSBs; e.g., soda, fruit drinks, sweetened coffee and tea, and sports drinks), caloric nutritional beverages (CNBs; e.g., 100% fruit and vegetable juice and high-fat low-sugar milk), and low-calorie beverages (LCBs; e.g., skim milk, unsweetened coffee and tea, and diet drinks) that were consumed per child. Over the course of the two-decade study period

TABLE 4.9

Percentage of students who drank 2 or 3 glasses of milk per day, by sex, race/ethnicity, and grade, 2011

	Drank two or more glasses/day of milk[a]			Drank three or more glasses/day of milk[a]		
	Female	Male	Total	Female	Male	Total
Category	%	%	%	%	%	%
Race/ethnicity						
White[b]	24.5	42.2	33.6	9.9	22.9	16.6
Black[b]	10.4	25.5	17.7	6.3	13.0	9.5
Hispanic	20.9	32.6	27.0	9.9	16.6	13.4
Grade						
9	24.6	41.1	32.9	11.8	22.5	17.2
10	24.5	39.5	32.3	11.0	21.0	16.2
11	18.8	35.7	27.4	7.4	17.2	12.4
12	17.8	33.4	25.8	6.5	18.4	12.6
Total	**21.6**	**37.6**	**29.9**	**9.3**	**20.0**	**14.9**

[a]During the 7 days before the survey.
[b]Non-Hispanic.

SOURCE: Adapted from Danice K. Eaton et al., "Table 85. Percentage of High School Students Who Drank Milk, by Sex, Race/Ethnicity, and Grade—United States, Youth Risk Behavior Survey, 2011," in "Youth Risk Behavior Surveillance—United States, 2011," *MMWR*, vol. 61, no. 4, June 8, 2012, http://www.cdc.gov/mmwr/pdf/ss/ss6104.pdf (accessed October 11, 2013)

the researchers find that the total caloric contribution from beverages remained constant, but that the types of beverages consumed changed. The consumption of SSBs increased and CNBs decreased in similar magnitude. A substantial increase in the consumption of certain SSBs, such as fruit drinks and soda, high-fat high-sugar milk, and sports drinks, coupled with a decrease in the consumption of high-fat low-sugar milk, was responsible for this shift. The percentage consuming SSBs as well as the amount per child (both portion size and the number of portions) increased significantly over time. Lasater, Piernas, and Popkin also observe that milk was displaced in children's diets by soda. The researchers applaud efforts to limit SSB consumption at schools made by the American Beverage Association with the support of the William J. Clinton Foundation and the American Heart Association, but believe that "further interventions to reduce SSB consumption within this age group should be considered."

The 2011 YRBSS confirmed that soda remains popular with high school students. More than one-quarter (27.8%) of students reported drinking at least one soda per day. (See Table 4.10.) More males (31.4%) than females (24%) drank one or more sodas per day, and female students (23.6%) were more likely than male students (18.4%) to report having had no soda or pop during the previous week. A greater proportion of white male students (34%) reported drinking soda than any other group in the survey, with white females having the lowest reported usage (23.2%). For both male and female students, ninth-graders were more likely to report drinking soda at least once per day than were students in any other grade.

Children's and Teens' Calorie Consumption Has Decreased

In *Trends in Intake of Energy and Macronutrients in Children and Adolescents from 1999–2000 through 2009–2010* (February 2013, http://www.cdc.gov/nchs/data/databriefs/db113.pdf), R. Bethene Ervin and Cynthia L. Ogden of the CDC National Center for Health Statistics report that average caloric intake for children and teens decreased between 1999–2000 and 2009–10. During this period, the average energy intake for boys decreased from 2,258 calories to approximately 2,100 calories, and the average energy intake for girls fell from 1,831 calories to 1,755 calories. (See Figure 4.4.)

In "Children in U.S. Are Eating Fewer Calories, Study Finds" (NYTimes.com, February 21, 2013), Sabrina Tavernise observes that while this decline, 7% for boys and 4% for girls, is not large enough to reverse the obesity epidemic, obesity rates for children have leveled off, and some cities have even reported modest declines. In a statement quoted by Tavernise, Marion Nestle, professor of nutrition, food studies, and public health at New York University, emphasizes that more dramatic changes are needed but acknowledges that the numbers are "trending in the right direction, and that's good news."

The Role of the Media

Despite television and print media antiobesity campaigns, many industry observers condemn corporate marketing efforts and media for continuing to assault children with unhealthy messages that encourage them to eat junk foods. The CDC defines junk foods as those that provide calories primarily through fats or added sugars and have minimal amounts of vitamins and minerals.

TABLE 4.10

Percentages of students who did not drink soda and drank soda at least once a day, 2011

[During the 7 days before the survey]

| | Did not drink soda or pop | | | Drank soda or pop one or more times/day | | |
| | Female | Male | Total | Female | Male | Total |
Category	%	%	%	%	%	%
Race/ethnicity						
White*	25.9	17.6	21.6	23.2	34.0	28.8
Black*	18.5	19.0	18.8	25.6	30.4	28.0
Hispanic	20.8	18.3	19.5	26.0	28.0	27.0
Grade						
9	19.3	16.0	17.6	26.4	32.8	29.7
10	22.9	17.9	20.3	24.7	29.6	27.3
11	26.9	20.0	23.4	21.2	31.7	26.6
12	26.2	20.5	23.3	22.7	31.2	27.0
Total	**23.6**	**18.4**	**20.9**	**24.0**	**31.4**	**27.8**

*Non-Hispanic.
Note: Soda defined as a can, bottle, or glass of soda or pop, not counting diet soda or diet pop.

SOURCE: Adapted from Danice K. Eaton et al., "Table 86. Percentage of High School Students Who Did Not Drink Soda or Pop and Who Drank Soda or Pop One or More Times/Day—United States, Youth Risk Behavior Survey, 2011," in "Youth Risk Behavior Surveillance—United States, 2011," *MMWR*, vol. 61, no. 4, June 8, 2012, http://www.cdc.gov/mmwr/pdf/ss/ss6104.pdf (accessed October 11, 2013)

FIGURE 4.4

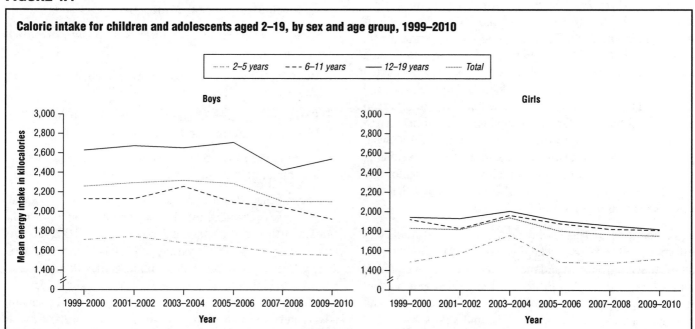

Caloric intake for children and adolescents aged 2–19, by sex and age group, 1999–2010

SOURCE: R. Bethene Ervin and Cynthia L. Ogden, "Figure 1. Mean Energy Intake for Children and Adolescents Aged 2–19 Years, by Sex and Age Group, 1999–2010," in "Trends in Intake of Energy and Macronutrients in Children and Adolescents from 1999–2000 through 2009–2010," *NCHS Data Brief*, no. 113, National Center for Health Statistics, February 2013, http://www.cdc.gov/nchs/data/databriefs/db113.pdf (accessed October 16, 2013)

The Interagency Working Group (IWG) on Food Marketed to Children, with representation from the CDC, the Federal Trade Commission, the U.S. Department of Agriculture (USDA), and the U.S. Food and Drug Administration (FDA), was formed in 2009 and tasked with recommending principles for the marketing of food to children to help the food industry self-regulate its marketing and advertising practices. In April 2011 the IWG released the fact sheet "Food for Thought: Interagency Working Group Proposal on Food Marketing to Children" (http://cspinet .org/new/pdf/FTC_foodmarket_factsheet110428%20.pdf) to discuss its principles for food marketing to children aged two to 16 years. The first principle is that the foods "make a meaningful contribution to a healthful diet" and contain fruit, vegetable, whole grain, fat-free or low-fat (1%) milk products, fish, extra lean meat or poultry, eggs, nuts and seeds, or beans. The second principle is that the foods should "contain limited amounts of nutrients that have a negative impact on health or weight," which is defined as a saturated fat content of 1 gram or less per serving or less than 15% of calories, 0 grams of trans-fat per serving, no more than 13 grams of added sugars per serving, and no more than 210 milligrams of sodium per serving. The principles are simply guidelines, and although they become effective in 2016, adherence to them is entirely voluntary.

According to the Robert Wood Johnson Foundation, in *F as in Fat: How Obesity Threatens America's Future* (2013, http://fasinfat.org/food-marketing/), in 2012 Congress asked the IWG to perform a cost-benefit analysis of the proposed voluntary guidelines. As of March 2014, that analysis had not been released, and the IWG proposal had not been implemented.

Many researchers and industry observers concur that the obesity epidemic cannot be effectively combated without dramatic changes in food marketing that is aimed at children. In "Protecting Children from Harmful Food Marketing: Options for Local Government to Make a Difference" (*Preventing Chronic Diseases*, vol. 8, no. 5, September 2011), Jennifer L. Harris and Samantha K. Graff note that although much of the marketing of calorie-dense, nutrient-poor foods to children is via nationwide media such as the Internet and television, it is also conducted using local venues such as billboards, restaurants, and schools. The researchers assert that "although the federal government has jurisdiction to regulate national media and the First Amendment to the U.S. Constitution limits what government at any level can do to restrict advertising, municipalities do have constitutionally viable options to protect children from the harmful food marketing that permeates their communities."

According to Harris and Graff, local food marketing efforts include product packaging, signs, and promotions in stores that are designed and placed at eye level for children, and school and local child-focused activities and product tie-ins that appeal to children by associating foods with popular movies, cartoon characters, and sports and entertainment celebrities. School-based promotions include food company incentives such as rewarding children for reading with coupons for free pizza; fund-raising programs that entail submitting proof of purchase of food items; branded food items that are served in school cafeterias, stores, and vending machines; corporate logos on scoreboards, book covers, and team jerseys; and sponsored books, workbooks, and materials with corporate logos and prominent mention of food products. Harris and Graff observe that logo placement, associations with celebrities, and video and Internet games are "designed to create lifelong customers by imprinting brand meaning into the minds of young children. Before children know better, they have learned to love the products they encounter most frequently and associate with positive experiences."

Harris and Graff suggest that local policies should restrict or limit the marketing of unhealthful food to children. For example, supermarkets and other retailers may opt to:

- Impose excise taxes or fees on sugar-sweetened beverages, and earmark a portion or all of the revenue to fund obesity prevention programs
- Limit sales of unhealthful food and beverages near schools before, during, and immediately after the school day
- Prohibit food sales in other retail venues that are frequented by children, such as toy stores

Restaurants and other food service providers may choose to:

- Eliminate use of trans fats
- Prohibit fast-food restaurants from opening near schools
- Establish nutritional standards for children's meals that include toys or other incentives

Schools can reduce children's exposure to food marketing by:

- Banning the sale and advertising of unhealthful foods on school property
- Requiring vendors to sharply restrict or eliminate the sale of unhealthful food and beverages
- Eliminating food company sponsorships, fund-raisers, and materials that are imprinted with corporate logos

According to Lorraine J. Weatherspoon et al., in "Consistency of Nutrition Recommendations for Foods Marketed to Children in the United States, 2009–2010" (*Preventing Chronic Diseases*, vol. 10, September 26, 2013), "advergames" are free online games that promote products to children. Weatherspoon et al. sought to identify whether foods marketed to children aged two to 11 years in advergames met nutrition recommendations of the Center for Science in the Public Interest, the FDA, the Institute of Medicine (IOM), and the USDA. They identified 143 websites that marketed 439 foods to children and analyzed the foods based on information including serving size and calories, from the food nutrient labels. Weatherspoon et al. conclude that a large number of foods with low nutritional value are marketed to children via advergames. Table 4.11 shows the proportion of meals and snacks marketed to children via advergames that met the nutritional recommendations of the four organizations. The researchers assert, "Companies that market foods to children should exercise social responsibility, and clear criteria and enforcement of food advertising guidelines

TABLE 4.11

Proportion of food marketed to children via "advergames" that met agency recommendations, by agency, 2009–10

Nutrient	USDA, n (%) Meets	Does not meet	FDA, n (%) Meets	Does not meet	CSPI, n (%) Meets	Does not meet	IOM, n (%) Meets	Does not meet	Meets standards of all organizations
Meals (sample size = 254)									
Total fat	**14 (5.5)**	**240 (94.5)**	**11 (4.3)**	**243 (95.7)**	**220 (86.6)**	**34 (13.4)**	**220 (86.6)**	**34 (13.4)**	**11 (4.3)**
Saturated fat	58 (22.8)	196 (77.2)	167 (65.7)	87 (34.3)	188 (74.0)	66 (26.0)	183 (72.0)	71 (28.0)	58 (22.8)
Added sugar	34 (13.4)	220 (86.6)	NA	NA	229 (90.2)	25 (9.8)	228 (89.8)	26 (10.2)	34 (13.4)[a]
Sodium	13 (5.1)	241 (94.9)	8 (3.1)	246 (96.9)	163 (64.2)	91 (35.8)	112 (44.1)	142 (55.9)	8 (3.1)
Cholesterol	230 (90.6)	24 (9.4)	253 (99.6)	1 (0.4)	NA	NA	NA	NA	230 (90.6)[b]
Snacks (sample size = 101)									
Total fat	**22 (21.8)**	**79 (78.2)**	**22 (21.8)**	**79 (78.2)**	**88 (87.1)**	**13 (12.9)**	**88 (87.1)**	**13 (12.9)**	**22 (21.8)**
Saturated fat	53 (52.5)	48 (47.5)	53 (52.5)	48 (47.5)	82 (81.2)	19 (18.8)	82 (81.2)	19 (18.8)	53 (52.5)
Added sugar	3 (3.0)	98 (97.0)	NA	NA	27 (26.7)	74 (73.3)	26 (25.7)	75 (74.3)	3 (3.0)[a]
Sodium	60 (59.4)	41 (40.6)	46 (45.5)	55 (54.5)	98 (97.0)	3 (3.0)	92 (91.1)	9 (8.9)	46 (45.5)
Cholesterol	101 (100)	0	101 (100)	0	NA	NA	NA	NA	101 (100)[b]

[a]Meets recommendations of USDA, CSPI, and IOM.
[b]Meets recommendations of USDA and FDA.
Notes: USDA = United States Department of Agriculture. FDA = US Food and Drug Administration. CSPI = Center for Science in the Public Interest. IOM = Institute of Medicine. NA = Not applicable.

SOURCE: Lorraine J. Weatherspoon et al., "Table 2. Proportion of Meals and Snacks Advertised through Advergames That Met Agency Recommendations, by Agency, United States, 2009–2010," in "Consistency of Nutrition Recommendations for Foods Marketed to Children in the United States, 2009–2010," *Preventing Chronic Diseases*, vol. 10, September 26, 2013, http://www.cdc.gov/pcd/issues/2013/pdf/13_0099.pdf (accessed October 21, 2013)

and regulations is warranted in the absence of consistent and enforceable voluntary standards."

The Role of Schools

In many parts of the country students are beginning to have some healthier beverage and food options in school. "Serving Healthy School Meals: Despite Challenges, Schools Meet USDA Nutrition Requirements" presents the results of a survey of school districts' ability to meet updated USDA nutrition standards for school meals conducted by The Kids' Safe and Healthful Foods Project, a joint effort of the Pew Charitable Trusts and the Robert Wood Johnson Foundation (September 2013, http://www .rwjf.org/en/research-publications/find-rwjf-research/2013/ 09/serving-healthy-school-meals.html). The survey, conducted in 2012, finds that the overwhelming majority (94%) of schools thought they would be able to implement the new standards, which call for more fruits, vegetables, and whole grains, and only fat-free and low-fat milk, by the end of the 2012–13 school year. Although schools were required to implement the new standards at the beginning of the 2012–13 school year, only 63% thought they would meet that deadline. Most schools (91%) cited obstacles to fully implementing the guidelines including lack of adequate equipment or training and problems with food costs and availability.

Not all schools, however, are ready to meet the new standards. In September 2013 the USDA reported that 524 schools (of about 100,000 nationwide) dropped out of the federally subsidized national school lunch program since the new standards were introduced in 2012. Some schools reported that so many students rejected the healthful lunches that their cafeterias were losing money. Schools that drop out of the program are no longer eligible for the federal funds that reimburse them for free and low-cost meals served to low-income students.

Many Schools Still Offer Unhealthful Food Choices

Food manufacturers and marketers know that schools are ideal sites to promote their products to children and teens. Nearly all youth attend school and spend many of their waking hours at school. Furthermore, the presence of foods in schools allows food companies to benefit from the implied endorsement of the schools and teachers. Many schools have vending machines, stores, or snack bars on campus that sell "competitive foods [which] are any foods or beverages sold or served at school separately from the USDA school meal programs." Competitive foods are usually low in nutrients and high in fat, sugar, and calories.

Until the 2014–15 school year the sale of competitive foods was essentially unregulated, and students often purchased these foods instead of, or in addition to, school meals. In December 2011 the USDA issued federal nutrition standards for competitive foods sold on school grounds and in June 2013 issued its "Smart Snacks in Schools" nutrition standards, which limit calories, fat, sugar, and sodium content of foods and beverages sold in school vending machines, cafeterias, and snack bars. Table 4.12 describes the new standards for competitive foods.

TABLE 4.12

U.S. Department of Agriculture competitive food standards for food sold in schools, 2013

Food/nutrient	Standard	Exemptions to the standard
General standard for competitive food	To be allowable, a competitive FOOD item must: (1) Meet all of the proposed competitive food nutrient standards; and (2) Be a grain product that contains 50% or more whole grains by weight or have whole grains as the first ingredient*; or (3) Have as the first ingredient* one of the non-grain main food groups: fruits, vegetables, dairy, or protein foods (meat, beans, poultry, seafood, eggs, nuts, seeds, etc.); or (4) Be a combination food that contains at least 1/4 cup fruit and/or vegetable; or (5) Contain 10% of the Daily Value (DV) of a nutrient of public health concern (i.e., calcium, potassium, vitamin D, or dietary fiber). Effective July 1, 2016 this criterion is obsolete and may not be used to qualify as a competitive food. *If water is the first ingredient, the second ingredient must be one of the above.	• Fresh and frozen fruits and vegetables with no added ingredients except water are exempt from all nutrient standards. • Canned fruits with no added ingredients except water, which are packed in 100% juice, extra light syrup, or light syrup are exempt from all nutrient standards. • Canned vegetables with no added ingredients except water or that contain a small amount of sugar for processing purposes to maintain the quality and structure of the vegetable are exempt from all nutrient standards.
NSLP/SBP Entrée items sold à la carte	Any entrée item offered as part of the lunch program or the breakfast program is exempt from all competitive food standards if it is served as a competitive food on the day of service or the day after service in the lunch or breakfast program	
Grain items	Acceptable grain items must include 50% or more whole grains by weight, or have whole grains as the first ingredient	
Total fats	Acceptable food items must have ≤35% calories from total fat as served	• Reduced fat cheese (including part-skim mozzarella) is exempt from the total fat standard. • Nuts and seeds and nut/seed butters are exempt from the total fat standard. • Products consisting of only dried fruit with nuts and/or seeds with no added nutritive sweeteners or fats are exempt from the total fat standard. • Seafood with no added fat is exempt from the total fat standard. Combination products are not exempt and must meet all the nutrient standards.
Saturated fats	Acceptable food items must have <10% calories from saturated fat as served	• Reduced fat cheese (including part-skim mozzarella) is exempt from the saturated fat standard. • Nuts and seeds and nut/seed butters are exempt from the saturated fat standard. • Products consisting of only dried fruit with nuts and/or seeds with no added nutritive sweeteners or fats are exempt from the saturated fat standard. Combination products are not exempt and must meet all the nutrient standards.
Trans fats	Zero grams of trans fat as served (≤0.5 g per portion).	
Sugar	Acceptable food items must have ≤35% of weight from total sugar as served.	• Dried whole fruits or vegetables; dried whole fruit or vegetable pieces; and dehydrated fruits or vegetables with no added nutritive sweeteners are exempt from the sugar standard. • Dried whole fruits, or pieces, with nutritive sweeteners that are required for processing and/or palatability purposes (i.e., cranberries, tart cherries, or blueberries) are exempt from the sugar standard. • Products consisting of only dried fruit with nuts and/or seeds with no added nutritive sweeteners or fats are exempt from the sugar standard.
Sodium	Snack items and side dishes sold à la carte: ≤230 mg sodium per item as served. Effective July 1, 2016 snack items and side dishes sold à la carte must be: ≤200 mg sodium per item as served, including any added accompaniments. Entrée items sold à la carte: ≤480 mg sodium per item as served, including any added accompaniments.	
Calories	Snack items and side dishes sold à la carte: ≤200 calories per item as served, including any added accompaniments. Entrée items sold à la carte: ≤350 calories per item as served including any added accompaniments.	
Accompaniments	Use of accompaniments is limited when competitive food is sold to students in school. The accompaniment must be included in the nutrient profile as part of the food item served and meet all proposed standards.	
Caffeine	Elementary and Middle School: foods and beverages must be caffeine-free with the exception of trace amounts of naturally occurring caffeine substances. High School: foods and beverages may contain caffeine.	

TABLE 4.12

U.S. Department of Agriculture competitive food standards for food sold in schools, 2013 [CONTINUED]

Food/nutrient	Standard	Exemptions to the standard
Beverages	Elementary School • Plain water or plain carbonated water (no size limit); • Low fat milk, unflavored (≤8 floz); • Non-fat milk, flavored or unflavored (≤8 floz), including nutritionally equivalent milk alternatives as permitted by the school meal requirements; • 100% fruit/vegetable juice (≤8 floz); and • 100% fruit/vegetable juice diluted with water (with or without carbonation), and no added sweeteners (≤8 floz).	
	Middle School • Plain water or plain carbonated water (no size limit); • Low-fat milk, unflavored (≤12 floz); • Non-fat milk, flavored or unflavored (≤12 floz), including nutritionally equivalent milk alternatives as permitted by the school meal requirements; • 100% fruit/vegetable juice (≤12 floz); and • 100% fruit/vegetable juice diluted with water (with or without carbonation), and no added sweeteners (≤12 floz).	
	High School • Plain water or plain carbonated water (no size limit); • Low-fat milk, unflavored (≤12 floz); • Non-fat milk, flavored or unflavored (≤12 floz), including nutritionally equivalent milk alternatives as permitted by the school meal requirements; • 100% fruit/vegetable juice (≤12 floz); • 100% fruit/vegetable juice diluted with water (with or without carbonation), and no added sweeteners (≤12 floz); • Other flavored and/or carbonated beverages (≤20 floz) that are labeled to contain ≤5 calories per 8 floz, or ≤10 calories per 20 floz; and • Other flavored and/or carbonated beverages (≤12 floz) that are labeled to contain ≤40 calories per 8 floz, or ≤60 calories per 12 fl oz.	
Sugar-free chewing gum	Sugar-free chewing gum is exempt from all of the competitive food standards and may be sold to students at the discretion of the local educational agency.	

Notes: NSLP = National School Lunch Program. SBP = School Breakfast Program.

SOURCE: "Summary of Interim Final Rule Competitive Food Standards," in "National School Lunch and School Breakfast Program: Nutrition Standards for All Foods Sold in School As Required by the Healthy, Hunger-Free Kids Act of 2010," *regulations.gov*, Food and Nutrition Service, June 28, 2013, http://www .regulations.gov/#!documentDetail;D=FNS-2011-0019-4718 (accessed October 23, 2013)

Besides selling food in schools, food manufacturers advertise on vending machines, posters, book covers, scoreboards, and banners and offer schools educational materials, contests in which children receive prizes or food rewards for achievement, and fund-raising opportunities. Some critics, including the Center for Science in the Public Interest, assert that the manufacturers are taking unfair advantage of cash-strapped school districts.

Food for Thought Has New Meaning at Many Schools

Some schools have taken novel approaches to improve students' diets. In 2013 the San Francisco Unified School District (SFUSD) began a program that would reinvent its school food system. Instead of focusing only on what students are eating, it focuses on how they are eating. The district hired a company to create healthful meals for its schools, and it is trying to change how students choose their lunches and the environments where they spend lunchtime. In "Improving School Lunch by Design" (NYTimes.com, October 16, 2013), Courtney E. Martin reports that in the SFUSD just 57% of students who qualify for free and reduced-cost lunches eat them. The district hopes to change this by involving students in the process in redesigned lunchrooms where elementary students sit at round tables and

eat family style—serving one another, with the healthiest foods offered first. Middle-schoolers can get lunch from mobile carts, and high school students can preorder lunches using mobile apps, which enable them to spend less time waiting in line and more time eating and socializing.

Another example of a school district working to improve nutrition, described by Gary D. Robertson in "N.C. Schools Better Than Most Going Local with Food" (Associated Press, October 23, 2013), is North Carolina's "Farm to School Census" programs, which involve purchasing food from local sources and planting edible gardens. The schools not only are better able to serve healthful meals and snacks using locally grown fruits and vegetables but also save money on food because local produce is less costly than products transported great distances.

The Media Can Deliver Powerful Nutrition and Health Education

Greater emphasis on children's diets has inspired the media to offer nutrition education. In 2013 *Sesame Street* (2013, http://www.sesamestreet.org/parents/topicsand activities/toolkits/food) produced programs aimed at families with children aged two to eight years on a wide range of nutrition topics: eating well on a budget, trying new foods, preparing and eating a healthful breakfast, healthful snacks, and how food arrives at the market and dinner table.

Children's television programming such as Disney's *Tasty Time with ZeFronk* offers easy-to-prepare recipes and aims to inspire young viewers to choose healthful meals and snacks in three-minute animated shorts. The Travel Channel's *Bizarre Foods America* exposes older children, teens, and adults to different cultures and foods. *Jamie Oliver's Food Revolution* follows English chef Jamie Oliver (1975–) as he tries to improve school lunch programs, teach students about healthy eating, and combat obesity.

Blending fitness and entertainment, video game makers have developed a genre of active rhythm games including *Dance Dance Revolution*, which features a workout mode that can track how many calories the user burns while playing. *In the Groove* and *Pump It Up: Exceed* are video games in which players try to match the onscreen action by stepping on different sections of a floor pad, and *Yourself!Fitness* and *Kinetic* offer teens exercise routines in video game formats. Nintendo's *Wii Fit* instructs and coaches users in yoga, balance games, strength training, aerobics, and simulated sports. *Just Dance 3* and its successor, *Just Dance 4*, are music video games that enable up to four players to dance to on-screen choreography. President Barack Obama (1961–) bought it for his daughters in December 2011.

FOOD AND BEVERAGE MARKETING PRACTICES IMPROVE. In 2005 the IOM published the report *Food Marketing to Children and Youth: Threat or Opportunity?* (http://www.iom.edu/Reports/2005/Food-Marketing-to-Children-and-Youth-Threat-or-Opportunity.aspx) to evaluate the influence of food marketing on the health of American children and teens. The IOM found that marketing practices, particularly television advertising, did not support a healthful diet and called on food and beverage companies and the media to promote programs and practices to support healthful eating. The IOM report offered 10 recommendations for promoting healthful diets to children and teens. The IOM Committee on Progress in Preventing Childhood Obesity followed up with the publications *Food Marketing and the Diets of Children and Youth* (2006, http://www.iom.edu/Activities/Children/KidsFoodMarketing .aspx), which included a framework to guide the development of marketing and advertising strategies to foster healthful food choices among children and teens, and *Progress in Preventing Childhood Obesity: How Do We Measure Up?* (2007, http://books.nap.edu/openbook.php?record_id= 11722), which addressed the competing interests of stakeholders and the challenges of balancing corporate goals with promoting children's health.

In November 2012 the IOM Standing Committee on Childhood Obesity Prevention held a workshop to assess progress made on food and beverage marketing aimed at children and youth and published presenters' findings in "Challenges and Opportunities for Change in Food Marketing to Children and Youth—Workshop Summary" (March 4, 2013, http://www.iom.edu/Reports/2013/Challenges-and-Opportunities-for-Change-in-Food-Marketing-to-Children-and-Youth.aspx). Presenters observed that limited to modest progress has been made toward implementing the recommendations in the IOM's 2006 report. They observed that integrated marketing communications, which use multiple media (videos on the Internet, ads on mobile phones, and advergames) to deliver and reinforce messages, is powerful. Marketing is often disguised as entertainment, and social networks provide additional marketing opportunities and despite progress in limiting food advertising to children, youth are still targeted by advertisers of unhealthful foods.

Presenters also described emerging policy initiatives and communication strategies. For example, companies such as The Walt Disney Company "can both offer and market healthier food to children and youth through self-regulation of the products they sell and advertise." They also observed that campaigns against tobacco advertising can serve as models for efforts to limit the marketing of unhealthful foods.

In "The Nation Needs to Do More to Address Food Marketing to Children" (*American Journal of Preventive Medicine*, vol. 42, no. 3, March 2012), Lori E. Dorfman and Margo G. Wootan assert that while schools have made progress by establishing nutrition standards for competitive foods, the food and beverage industry continues to bombard children with inducements to consume unhealthful foods. Dorfman and Wootan call on government to set nutrition standards for children's meals sold with toys or other incentives. They recommend that nonfat milk or water be served with meals rather than soda and urge the government to tax sugary drinks and use the resulting tax revenues to fund nutrition education and physical activity programs.

Physical Activity

School physical education (PE) programs, especially at the high school level, have been found lacking, and too few youth are physically active. Danice K. Eaton et al. of the CDC note in "Youth Risk Behavior Surveillance—United States, 2011" (*Morbidity and Mortality Weekly Report*, vol. 61, no. 4, June 8, 2012) that in 2011 fewer than one-third (28.7%) of high school students were physically active every day for at least 60 minutes, and just over half (55.6%) participated in muscle strengthening exercises on three or more days. (See Table 4.13.)

HEALTH RISKS AND CONSEQUENCES

The harmful health consequences of overweight and obesity can begin during childhood and adolescence.

TABLE 4.13

Percentages of high school students who met recommended levels of physical activity by sex, race/ethnicity, and grade, 2011

[WERE PHYSICALLY ACTIVE DOING ANY KIND OF PHYSICAL ACTIVITY (FOR EXAMPLE, PUSH-UPS, SIT-UPS, OR WEIGHT LIFTING) THAT INCREASED THEIR HEART RATE AND MADE THEM BREATHE HARD SOME OF THE TIME FOR A TOTAL OF AT LEAST 60 MINUTES/DAY ON 7 OF THE 7 DAYS BEFORE THE SURVEY]

	Physically active at least 60 minutes/day on all 7 days			Participated in muscle strengthening activities on 3 or more days		
	Female	Male	Total	Female	Male	Total
Category	%	%	%	%	%	%
Race/ethnicity						
White*	19.7	40.4	30.4	45.3	65.5	55.7
Black*	16.9	35.2	26.0	37.3	71.5	54.0
Hispanic	16.9	35.6	26.5	44.7	67.6	56.6
Grade						
9	22.2	38.8	30.7	49.8	68.6	59.3
10	18.1	42.6	30.8	43.3	68.8	56.5
11	18.0	36.2	27.3	41.3	64.9	53.4
12	14.9	34.9	25.1	39.8	63.8	52.2
Total	**18.5**	**38.3**	**28.7**	**43.8**	**66.7**	**55.6**

*Non-Hispanic.

Note: Because of changes in question context starting in 2011, national Youth Risk Behavior Survey (YRBS) prevalence estimates derived from the 60 minutes of physical activity question in 2011 are not comparable to those reported in 2009 or earlier. On the 2005–2009 national YRBS questionnaire, physical activity was assessed with three questions (in the following order) that asked the number of days students participated in: 1) at least 20 minutes of vigorous physical activity, 2) at least 30 minutes of moderate physical activity, and 3) at least 60 minutes of aerobic (moderate and vigorous) physical activity. On the 2011 national YRBS questionnaire, only the 60 minutes of aerobic physical activity question was included.

SOURCE: Danice K. Eaton et al., "Table 93. Percentage of High School Students Who Were Physically Active At Least 60 Minutes/Day on All 7 Days and Who Participated in Muscle Strengthening Activities on 3 or More Days, by Sex, Race/Ethnicity, and Grade—United States, Youth Risk Behavior Survey, 2011," in "Youth Risk Behavior Surveillance—United States, 2011," *MMWR*, vol. 61, no. 4, June 8, 2012, http://www.cdc.gov/mmwr/pdf/ss/ss6104.pdf (accessed October 11, 2013)

According to Gerald S. Berenson et al., in "Glycemic Status, Metabolic Syndrome, and Cardiovascular Risk in Children" (*Medical Clinics of North America*, vol. 95, no. 2, March 2011), approximately 40% of the U.S. population is overweight or obese by adolescence and "obesity in childhood is the most consistent predictor of adult heart disease." Berenson et al. also assert that the risk for cardiovascular disease increases at the 85th percentile of body weight, which is considerably below the 95th percentile considered to be dangerous by the CDC.

The most frequently occurring medical consequences of overweight among children and adolescents are:

• Elevated blood lipids—overweight children and adolescents display the same elevated levels of cholesterol, triglycerides (a fatty substance found in the blood), and/or low-density lipoproteins as overweight adults. These hyperlipidemias are linked to an increased risk for cardiovascular disease and premature mortality (death) in adulthood.

• Glucose intolerance and type 2 diabetes—glucose intolerance, a carbohydrate intolerance that varies in severity, is a forerunner of diabetes. The incidence of type 2 diabetes among adolescents is increasing in response to the national rise of overweight teens. A skin condition known as acanthosis nigricans (velvety thickening and darkening of skinfold areas at the neck, elbow, and behind the knee) often coexists with glucose intolerance in youth.

• Fatty liver disease—high concentrations of liver enzymes are associated with fatty degeneration of the liver (also called hepatic steatosis) and have been found in overweight children and adolescents. Excessively high blood insulin levels (hyperinsulinemia) may contribute to the genesis of this disease.

• Gallstones—although gallstones occur less frequently among children and adolescents who are overweight than in obese adults, nearly half of the cases of inflammation of the gallbladder (also called cholecystitis) in adolescents may be associated with overweight. Like adults, the risk for cholecystitis and gallstones in adolescents may decrease with weight reduction.

Another common health consequence of overweight is early maturation, a condition in which the skeletal age is more than three months greater than the chronological age. Early maturation is linked to overweight in adulthood and is also associated with the distribution of fat—it predicts that the fat will be predominantly located on the abdomen and trunk, which is in turn predictive of increased disease risk.

Less frequently occurring health consequences include hypertension, a condition that is nine times more frequent among children who are overweight, compared with children who have a healthy weight; obstructive sleep apnea (breathing becomes shallow or stops completely for short periods during sleep), a condition that afflicts an estimated 7% of overweight children; and orthopedic problems resulting from excessive stress on the feet, legs, and hips. Hypertension for children and adolescents aged one to 17 years is defined as average blood pressure readings at or above the 95th percentile (based on age, sex, and height) on at least three separate occasions. (See Table 4.14 and Table 4.15 for blood pressures by age and gender that are considered indicative of hypertension or at risk for hypertension; children and adolescents between the 90th and 95th percentiles for their age, sex, and height are at risk for developing hypertension.)

Metabolic Syndrome

The metabolic syndrome is a group of risk factors for atherosclerotic cardiovascular disease and type 2 diabetes mellitus in adults that include insulin resistance, obesity, hypertension, and hyperlipidemia. (Atherosclerosis is a hardening of the walls of the arteries caused by the buildup of fatty deposits on the inner walls of the arteries that interferes with blood flow.) Atherosclerotic cardiovascular disease is the leading cause of death among adults, but it rarely occurs in young people. Recently, however, the risk factors—high blood pressure, elevated triglycerides, obesity, and low levels of the "good" high-density lipoprotein (HDL) cholesterol—that are associated with the development of metabolic syndrome have been appearing during childhood. Berenson et al. indicate that in the United States more than 17% of children with a BMI greater than the 95th percentile are considered to have all the conditions that are associated with metabolic syndrome.

Mental Health Consequences

One of the most immediate, distressing, and widespread consequences of being overweight as described by children themselves is social discrimination and low self-esteem. Overweight and obese children and adolescents are at risk for psychological and social adjustment problems, such as considering themselves less competent than normal-weight youth in social, athletic, and appearance arenas, and for suffering from overall diminished self-worth.

In "Development of Mental Health Problems and Overweight between Ages 4 and 11 Years: A Population-Based Longitudinal Study of Australian Children" (*Academic Pediatrics*, vol. 13, no. 2, March–April 2013), Pauline W. Jansen et al. look at the relationship between mental health and overweight in children. The researchers find an association between overweight and mental health problems beginning at ages eight and nine and increasing among children ages 10 and 11. Overweight children had more problems with peers and emotional difficulties than did their healthy weight peers. Jansen et al. conclude that "in childhood, it appears that overweight precedes mental health problems, particularly peer problems."

SCREENING AND ASSESSMENT OF OVERWEIGHT CHILDREN AND ADOLESCENTS

In view of the rising prevalence of overweight youth, screening children and adolescents for overweight and risk for overweight has assumed a prominent place in pediatric practice (the medical specialty devoted to the diagnosis and treatment of children) and public health programs. The Recommendations for Preventive Pediatric Health Care by the American Academy of Pediatrics advise a frequent schedule of accurate weight and height measurements to determine whether children require further assessment or treatment for overweight. Screening distinguishes between youths who are not at risk of overweight, at risk of overweight, and overweight. Those deemed to be overweight receive an in-depth medical assessment; those considered at risk are assessed for changes in BMI, blood pressure, and cholesterol levels; and annual screening is advised for those who are not at risk of being overweight.

The comprehensive assessment that is performed on overweight children and adolescents generally includes obtaining a detailed medical history to identify any underlying medical conditions that may contribute to overweight and analyzing family history for the presence of familial risks for overweight or obesity. Relevant familial factors include the occurrence of obesity, eating disorders, type 2 diabetes, heart disease, high blood pressure, and abnormal lipid profiles such as high cholesterol among immediate family members. The assessment may also involve:

- A dietary evaluation to consider the quantity, quality, and timing of food consumed to identify foods and patterns of eating that may lead to excessive calorie intake. A food record or food diary may be used to assess eating habits.

- An evaluation of daily activities. This assessment involves an estimate of time that is devoted to exercise and activity as well as time spent on sedentary behaviors such as television, video games, and computer use.

- A physical examination to provide information about the extent of overweight and any complications of overweight, including high blood pressure. Children and adolescents with a BMI-for-age at or above the 95th percentile and who are athletic and muscular may be further assessed using the triceps skinfold measurement to assess body fat. A measurement of greater than the 95th percentile indicates that the child has excess fat rather than increased lean body mass or a large frame.

- Laboratory tests, such as cholesterol screening, that are dictated by the degree of overweight, family history, and the results of the physical examination. Table 4.16 shows the range of values for total blood cholesterol and low-density lipoprotein cho-

TABLE 4.14

Blood pressure levels for the 90th and 95th percentiles of blood pressure for boys ages 1 to 17 years

Age	BP percentile*	Systolic BP (mm Hg), by height percentile from standard growth curves							Diastolic BP (mm Hg), by height percentile from standard growth curves						
		5%	10%	25%	50%	75%	90%	95%	5%	10%	25%	50%	75%	90%	95%
1	90th	94	95	97	98	100	102	102	50	51	52	53	54	54	55
	95th	98	99	101	102	104	106	106	55	55	56	57	58	59	59
2	90th	98	99	100	102	104	105	106	55	55	56	57	58	59	59
	95th	101	102	104	106	108	109	110	59	59	60	61	62	63	63
3	90th	100	101	103	105	107	108	109	59	59	60	61	62	63	63
	95th	104	105	107	109	111	112	113	63	63	64	65	66	67	67
4	90th	102	103	105	107	109	110	111	62	62	63	64	65	66	66
	95th	106	107	109	111	113	114	115	66	67	67	68	69	70	71
5	90th	104	105	106	108	110	112	112	65	65	66	67	68	69	69
	95th	108	109	110	112	114	115	116	69	70	70	71	72	73	74
6	90th	105	106	108	110	111	113	114	67	68	69	70	70	71	72
	95th	109	110	112	114	115	117	117	72	72	73	74	75	76	76
7	90th	106	107	109	111	113	114	115	69	70	71	72	72	73	74
	95th	110	111	113	115	116	118	119	74	74	75	76	77	78	78
8	90th	107	108	110	112	114	115	116	71	71	72	73	74	75	75
	95th	111	112	114	116	118	119	120	75	76	76	77	78	79	80
9	90th	109	110	112	113	115	117	117	72	73	73	74	75	76	77
	95th	113	114	116	117	119	121	121	76	77	78	79	80	80	81
10	90th	110	112	113	115	117	118	119	73	73	74	75	76	77	78
	95th	114	115	117	119	121	122	123	77	78	79	80	80	81	82
11	90th	112	113	115	117	119	120	121	74	74	75	76	77	78	78
	95th	116	117	119	121	123	124	125	78	78	79	80	81	82	83
12	90th	115	116	117	119	121	123	123	75	75	76	77	78	78	79
	95th	119	120	121	123	125	126	127	79	79	80	81	82	83	83
13	90th	117	118	120	122	124	125	126	75	76	76	77	78	79	80
	95th	121	122	124	126	128	129	130	79	80	81	82	83	84	84
14	90th	120	121	123	125	126	128	128	76	76	77	78	79	80	80
	95th	124	125	127	128	130	132	132	80	81	81	82	83	84	85
15	90th	123	124	125	127	129	131	131	77	77	78	79	80	81	81
	95th	127	128	129	131	133	134	135	81	82	83	83	84	85	86
16	90th	125	126	128	130	132	133	134	79	79	80	81	82	82	83
	95th	129	130	132	134	136	137	138	83	83	84	85	86	87	87
17	90th	128	129	131	133	134	136	136	81	81	82	83	84	85	85
	95th	132	133	135	136	138	140	140	85	85	86	87	88	89	89

*Blood pressure percentile determined by a single measurement.

BP = blood pressure. mm Hg = millimeters of mercury.

SOURCE: "Table 16. Blood Pressure Levels for the 90th and 95th Percentiles of Blood Pressure for Boys Ages 1 to 17 Years," in *Overweight Children and Adolescents: Screen, Access, and Manage,* Centers for Disease Control and Prevention, National Center for Chronic Disease Prevention and Promotion, Division of Nutrition, Physical Activity and Obesity, May 2000, http://www.cdc.gov/nccdphp/dnpa/growthcharts/training/modules/module3/text/hypertension_tables.htm (accessed October 24, 2013)

TABLE 4.15

Blood pressure levels for the 90th and 95th percentiles of blood pressure for girls ages 1 to 17 years

Age	BP percentile*	Systolic BP (mm Hg), by height percentile from standard growth curves							Diastolic BP (mm Hg), by height percentile from standard growth curves						
		5%	10%	25%	50%	75%	90%	95%	5%	10%	25%	50%	75%	90%	95%
1	90th	97	98	99	100	102	103	104	53	53	53	54	55	56	56
	95th	101	102	103	104	105	107	107	57	57	57	58	59	60	60
2	90th	99	99	100	102	103	104	105	57	57	58	58	59	60	61
	95th	102	103	104	105	107	108	109	61	61	62	62	63	64	65
3	90th	100	100	102	103	104	105	106	61	61	61	62	63	63	64
	95th	104	104	105	107	108	109	110	65	65	65	66	67	67	68
4	90th	101	102	103	104	106	107	108	63	63	64	65	65	66	67
	95th	105	106	107	108	109	111	111	67	67	68	69	69	70	71
5	90th	103	103	104	106	107	108	109	65	66	66	67	68	68	69
	95th	107	107	108	110	111	112	113	69	70	70	71	72	72	73
6	90th	104	105	106	107	109	110	111	67	67	68	69	69	70	71
	95th	108	109	110	111	112	114	114	71	71	72	73	73	74	75
7	90th	106	107	108	109	110	112	112	69	69	69	70	71	72	72
	95th	110	110	112	113	114	115	116	73	73	73	74	75	76	76
8	90th	108	109	110	111	112	113	114	70	70	71	71	72	73	74
	95th	112	112	113	115	116	117	118	74	74	75	75	76	77	78
9	90th	110	110	112	113	114	115	116	71	72	72	73	74	74	75
	95th	114	114	115	117	118	119	120	75	76	76	77	78	78	79
10	90th	112	112	114	115	116	117	118	73	73	73	74	75	76	76
	95th	116	116	117	119	120	121	122	77	77	77	78	79	80	80
11	90th	114	116	116	117	118	119	120	74	74	75	75	76	77	77
	95th	118	118	119	121	122	123	124	78	78	79	79	80	81	81
12	90th	116	116	118	119	120	121	122	75	75	76	76	77	78	78
	95th	120	120	121	123	124	125	126	79	79	80	80	81	82	82
13	90th	118	118	119	121	122	123	124	76	76	77	78	78	79	80
	95th	121	122	123	125	126	127	128	80	80	81	82	82	83	84
14	90th	119	120	121	122	124	125	126	77	77	78	79	79	80	81
	95th	123	124	125	126	128	129	130	81	81	82	83	83	84	85
15	90th	121	121	122	124	125	126	127	78	78	79	79	80	81	82
	95th	124	125	126	128	129	130	131	82	82	83	83	84	85	86
16	90th	122	122	123	125	126	127	128	79	79	79	80	81	82	82
	95th	125	126	127	128	130	131	132	83	83	83	84	85	86	86
17	90th	122	123	124	125	126	128	128	79	79	79	80	81	82	82
	95th	126	126	127	129	130	131	132	83	83	83	84	85	86	86

*Blood pressure percentile determined by a single measurement.

BP = blood pressure. mm Hg = millimeters of mercury.

SOURCE: "Table 17. Blood Pressure Levels for the 90th and 95th Percentiles of Blood Pressure for Girls Ages 1 to 17 Years," in *Overweight Children and Adolescents: Screen, Access, and Manage,* Centers for Disease Control and Prevention, National Center for Chronic Disease Prevention and Promotion, Division of Nutrition, Physical Activity and Obesity, May 2000, http://www.cdc.gov/nccdphp/dnpa/growthcharts/training/modules/module3/text/hypertension_tables.htm (accessed October 248, 2013)

TABLE 4.16

Classification of cholesterol levels in high-risk children and adolescents

	Total cholesterol, ng/dL	LDL cholesterol, ng/dL
Acceptable	<170	<110
Borderline	170–199	110–129
High	Greater than or equal to 200	Greater than or equal to 130

Note: High-risk children are defined as those from families with hypercholesterolemia or premature cardiovascular disease.
LDL = low density lipoprotein. ng/dL = nanograms per deciliter.

SOURCE: "Table 15. Classification of Cholesterol Levels in High-Risk Children and Adolescents," in *Overweight Children and Adolescents: Screen, Assess, and Manage*, Centers for Disease Control and Prevention, National Center for Chronic Disease Prevention and Promotion, Division of Nutrition, Physical Activity and Obesity, 2000, http://www.cdc.gov/nccdphp/dnpa/growthcharts/training/modules/module3/text/cholesterol.htm (accessed October 24, 2013)

lesterol that are considered acceptable, borderline, and high.

- A mental health evaluation to determine the readiness of children and adolescents to change behaviors and to identify a history of eating disorders or depression that may require treatment. An assessment of the family's ability to support a child's weight-loss or weight-management efforts may also be performed.

INTERVENTION AND TREATMENT OF OVERWEIGHT AND OBESITY

In the absence of acute medical necessity, such as with children who are dangerously obese, most health professionals concur that drastic caloric restriction is an inappropriate weight-loss strategy for children who are still growing. Instead, they advise efforts to stabilize body weight with a healthful, balanced diet, increased physical activity, and education about nutrition, food choices, and preparation. This approach is especially effective for children who are just slightly overweight, because maintaining body weight often allows them to outgrow overweight and become normal-weight adults.

When active weight loss is indicated, it is generally for children with a BMI greater than the 95th percentile or those experiencing complications of overweight or obesity. Among children aged two to seven years, gradual weight loss of about 1 pound (0.5 kg) per month is advised. Older children with serious health risks who are severely overweight (BMI greater than 35) may be advised to lose between 1 and 2 pounds (0.5 and 0.9 kg) per week.

In "Pediatric Obesity: Etiology and Treatment" (*Pediatric Clinics of North America*, vol. 58, no. 5, October 2011), Melissa K. Crocker and Jack A. Yanovski of the NICHD observe that pediatric childhood obesity has been shown to have a tremendous impact on later health, even independent of adult weight. The researchers consider lifestyle modification and restricting energy intake to be the foundation of successful treatment of obesity in children. They explain that interventions for overweight and obese children range from basic diets and lifestyle interventions to more intensive very-low-energy diets, medications, and surgery. These methods achieve varying levels of success and all are optimally successful when the child and family are motivated and educated. Crocker and Yanovski assert that "the participation and cooperation of the entire family is critical regardless of the mode of therapy employed."

Crocker and Yanovski observe that dietary changes alone may benefit children who are overweight but are relatively ineffective for children and adolescents with severe obesity. Similarly, exercise without dietary intervention is relatively ineffective. Comprehensive approaches to weight loss that involve behavior modification to reduce screen time, increase physical activity, motivate children to improve their eating behavior, and engage the school system and family to support weight-loss goals appear to be more effective than diet alone.

Pharmacotherapy (drug treatment to support weight loss) has shown limited success when combined with diet and exercise. As of 2013, only one weight-loss drug, orlistat (a drug that induces weight loss by blocking the absorption of about one-third of the fat contained in a meal), was approved for use in children aged 16 years and younger. However, many physicians believe that in view of orlistat's limited effectiveness and potential side effects, it should be limited to children and adolescents with a BMI over the 95th percentile who also have significant obesity-related medical complications.

Some adolescents who are obese may be treated with weight-loss surgery. The National Institutes of Health criteria for adolescents aged 13 to 17 years are the same as those applied to adults: a BMI greater than or equal to 40 or a BMI greater than or equal to 35 with at least one coexisting serious medical condition such as type 2 diabetes, hypertension, or obstructive sleep apnea. In "Bariatric Surgery for Obese Children and Adolescents: A Review of the Moral Challenges" (*BMC Medical Ethics*, vol. 14, no. 18, April 2013), Bjørn Hofmann of the University College of Gjøvik, Norway, observes that the success of bariatric surgery in adults has fueled interest in the surgery for children and adolescents. Hofmann cautions, however, that although surgery may help obese youth avoid serious health problems, there is limited evidence of its safety and effectiveness in children and adolescents. Further, he writes, "exposing young people to potentially harmful treatment with uncertain outcomes is morally problematic" especially if there are less drastic or risky alternatives.

Meghan L. Butryn et al. of Drexel University examine in "Maintenance of Weight Loss in Adolescents: Current Status and Future Directions" (*Journal of Obesity*, January 2011) how different approaches (lifestyle modification, dietary and physical activity interventions, use of Internet, and medication) assist adolescents to maintain their weight loss. Butryn et al. find that lifestyle modification programs, especially those that involve parents, are likely to be more successful than other approaches because parents can exert a strong impact on the adolescent's behavior by supporting healthy eating and physical activity. Although definitive data are lacking, Internet-based interventions that maximize and prolong engagement and participation also appear promising, especially for adolescents without access to in-person treatment. Medication used as a component of a lifestyle modification program appears to offer some weight-maintenance benefits; however, adolescents must adhere to a low-fat diet when taking the medication.

Educating Parents

Researchers agree that primary prevention is the strategy with the greatest potential for reversing the alarming rise in overweight and obesity among children and teens. Public health educators recommend counseling parents and caregivers about healthy eating habits for children. They advise offering children a variety of healthful foods, in reasonable quantities, to assist children to make wise food choices. Children should be encouraged, but not forced, to sample new foods and should not be pressured to clean their plates. No foods or food groups should be entirely off-limits, or children may become fixated on obtaining the forbidden foods.

Although it is difficult to impress on children the future health risks that are associated with excess weight, parents should be informed that obese children are more likely to suffer from diabetes, heart, and joint diseases such as osteoarthritis, as well as breast and colon cancer. Adults should model healthy habits by consuming no more than 30% of calories from fat, exercising regularly, and limiting time spent in front of the television. Health educators are especially eager to reduce children's television viewing, with its destructive blend of junk-food advertising and enforced inactivity. Finally, health professionals caution that food should not be used to punish or reward behavior or as a way to comfort or console children. The undivided attention of a parent or caregiver or an expression of sympathy, reassurance, or encouragement may satisfy a child's need better than an ice cream cone or an order of french fries.

Multidisciplinary Treatment for Children and Teens

The Mass General Hospital for Children Weight Center in Boston, Massachusetts (August 23, 2013, http://www .massgeneral.org/digestive/news/newsarticle.aspx?id=3701)

recognizes that treating obesity in children requires a novel approach, one that addresses the many lifelong physical and mental health problems associated with it as well as family and social concerns. The Mass General program includes parents and other family members in the child's treatment and an array of practitioners deliver this family-centered care. The program uses a wide range of age-appropriate approaches to meet children's changing needs and has an established weight-loss surgery program for adolescents. It also collaborates with researchers investigating the genetics of obesity and the outcomes of weight-loss surgery.

Let's Move! National Program to Improve Children's Health

In February 2010 First Lady Michelle Obama (1964–) launched Let's Move! (http://www.letsmove.gov/), a comprehensive set of strategies aimed at combating childhood obesity. The antiobesity initiative involves private- and public-sector resources in alliances with states, local communities, athletic organizations, and schools. The ambitious program aims to:

- Inform parents to enable them to make healthy choices for their family

- Assist retailers and manufacturers to implement new nutritionally sound and user-friendly front-of-package labeling

- Educate health professionals about obesity to ensure they regularly monitor children's BMI, provide counseling for healthy eating, and write prescriptions for parents detailing the steps they can take to increase healthy eating and physical activity

- Use the media to enhance public awareness of the need to combat obesity through public service announcements, special programming, and marketing

- Promote use of the Food Environment Atlas, a USDA interactive database that helps identify communities with diet and obesity-related problems such as high incidences of diabetes; this information should prove useful for parents, educators, government, and businesses

- Improve food choices in schools by doubling the number of schools that participate in the Healthier U.S. School Challenge, which sets rigorous standards for schools' food quality, participation in meal programs, and physical activity and nutrition education

- Encourage food suppliers to decrease the amount of sugar, fat, and salt in school meals; increase whole grains; and double the amount of produce they serve within 10 years

- Improve Americans' access to healthful affordable foods by bringing grocery stores to underserved areas, helping places such as convenience stores and bodegas carry healthier food options, and investing in farmers' markets

- Increase physical activity by challenging children and adults to commit to physical activity five days per week for six weeks and supporting efforts to get children physically active in and outside of school

According to A. J. Pearlman, in "Let's Move! Active Schools Is Making Strides Nationwide" (October 24, 2013, http://www.letsmove.gov/blog/2013/10/24/let's-move-active-schools-making-strides-nationwide), since its launch more than 5,000 schools had joined Let's Move! as of October 2013. The campaign's website offers success stories involving children, chefs, faith-based and community organizations, mayors and municipal officials, parents, teachers, and schools. However, the program's emphasis on physical activity rather than eliminating junk food from children's diets has been criticized. For example, in "The Power of Ideas and the Ideas of Power: From Research to Policy in Global Health" (Lancet.com, July 1, 2013), Julio Frenk quotes Kevin Strong, a physician and founder of Dunk the Junk, who said, "Michelle Obama's Let's Move campaign has disregarded the science for fear of BIG-SODA backlash. Science clearly shows us that decreasing sugar intake, mainly in drinks, is the best way to reverse childhood obesity."

EATING DISORDERS

Overweight and obesity are among the most stigmatizing and least socially acceptable conditions in childhood and adolescence. Society, culture, and the media send children powerful messages about body weight and shape ideals. For girls these messages include the "thin ideal" and encouragement to diet and exercise. Messages to boys emphasize a muscular body and pressure to body build and even use potentially harmful dietary supplements and steroids. Sex has not been identified as a specific risk factor for obesity in children, but the pressure placed on girls to be thin may put them at a greater risk for developing eating-disordered behaviors. Although society presents boys with a wider range of acceptable body images, they are also at risk for developing disordered eating and body image disturbances.

Adolescence is a developmental period marked by great physical changes, and it is a time when many teens subject themselves to painful scrutiny. Uneven growth, puberty, and sexual maturation may make teens feel awkward and self-conscious about their bodies. Teenaged girls are especially susceptible to developing negative body images, ignoring other qualities and focusing exclusively on appearance to measure their self-worth. This single-minded, and often distorted, destructive focus can result in lowered self-esteem and increased risk for mental health problems, including eating disorders. The 2011 YRBSS found that 6% of female high school students engaged in dangerous dieting behaviors (vomiting or taking laxatives). (See Table 3.3 in Chapter 3.)

Who Is at Risk?

Although there are biological, genetic, and familial factors that predispose certain people to eating disorders such as anorexia nervosa (intense fear of becoming fat even when dangerously underweight) and bulimia nervosa (recurrent episodes of binge eating followed by purging to prevent weight gain), the emergence of these disorders is triggered by environmental factors. Chief among the environmental triggers is body image. Many researchers and health professionals believe that teenaged girls who identify with the idealized body images projected throughout U.S. culture are at an increased risk for eating disorders.

Other risk factors are peer group pressures and sociocultural forces such as the fashion and entertainment industries and the media. The National Eating Disorders Association identifies media definitions of attractiveness, beauty, and health as among the myriad factors that contribute to the rise of eating disorders.

Historically, most adolescents with eating disorders have been first- or second-born white females from middle- to upper-class families. Girls who suffer from anorexia are often academically successful, with athletic prowess or training in dance. They tend to be perfectionists, well behaved, emotionally dependent, socially anxious, and intent on receiving approval from others. Adolescent girls with bulimia are generally more extroverted and socially involved. According to the Eating Disorders Coalition for Research, Policy, and Action, in the fact sheet "Facts about Eating Disorders: What the Research Shows" (2009, http://www.eatingdisorderscoalition.org/documents/Talking pointsEatingDisordersFactSheetUpdated5-20-09.pdf), in the early 21st century the occurrence of eating disorders is increasing among younger children and throughout diverse ethnic and sociocultural groups.

Research reveals that the incidence of eating disorders in young children is relatively high. In "Eating Problems in Young Children—A Population-Based Study" (*Acta Paediatrica*, vol. 165, no. 10, October 2011), Monika Equit et al. of Saarland University questioned parents about the eating behavior of nearly 2,000 children. The researchers find that 34% of the children showed signs of restrictive eating disorders (intentional limitation or avoidance of nutrition), and 5% were worried about their weight.

Which Variables Are Associated with Dieting, Overweight, and Eating Disorders?

Dianne Neumark-Sztainer and Peter J. Hannan of the University of Minnesota analyzed a representative sample of 6,728 adolescents in grades five through 12 who completed Commonwealth Fund surveys about the health of adolescent girls and boys. The results of the research were detailed in the landmark study "Weight-Related Behaviors among Adolescent Girls and Boys: Results from a National Survey" (*Archives of Pediatrics and Adolescent Medicine*, vol. 154, no. 6, June 2000). The research aimed to assess the prevalence of dieting and disordered eating among adolescents; the sociodemographic, psychosocial, and behavioral variables that were associated with dieting and disordered eating; and whether adolescents report having discussed weight-related issues with their health care providers. (Neumark-Sztainer and Hannan defined disordered eating as weight-related behaviors such as anorexia and bulimia, self-induced vomiting, binge eating, inappropriate or extreme dieting, and obesity.)

Subjects were assessed by calculating their BMI and eliciting weight-related attitudes and behaviors. For example, dieting was assessed by asking such questions as "Have you ever been on a diet?" and "Why were you dieting?" Behaviors were assessed by posing a question such as "Have you ever binged and purged (which is when you eat a lot of food and then make yourself throw up, vomit, or take something that makes you have diarrhea) or not?" Subjects were also asked, "Right now, how would you describe yourself?" to gain an understanding of their perceptions of their weight. Psychosocial and behavioral variables including self-esteem, stress, depression, substance use (of tobacco, alcohol, or illegal drugs), and level of physical activity were also measured and scored using standardized questionnaires and inventories.

Alcohol and drug use were directly associated with dieting and disordered eating among girls and boys; however, the association between substance use and disordered eating was stronger than the association between substance use and dieting. Tobacco use was associated with dieting and disordered eating among girls, but not among boys.

In "Psychosocial Risk Factors for Eating Disorders" (*International Journal of Eating Disorders*, vol. 46, no. 5, July 2013), Pamela K. Keel and K. Jean Forney seek to identify risk factors for eating disorders in adolescents. Like other investigators, Keel and Forney find that an excessive drive for thinness, body dissatisfaction, negative self-evaluation, low self-esteem, and perfectionism are risk factors. These characteristics also influence the selection of peer groups, which in the case of adolescents at risk for eating disorders means choosing peers who share their traits and views, which in turn can magnify and reinforce insecurity about weight and body dissatisfaction.

In "Life Smart: A Pilot Study of a School-Based Program to Reduce the Risk of Both Eating Disorders and Obesity in Young Adolescent Girls and Boys" (*Journal of Pediatric Psychology*, vol. 38, no. 9, October 2013), Simon M. Wilksch and Tracey D. Wade describe the results of Life Smart, a school-based, eight-lesson interactive program aimed at reducing some of the known risk factors for eating disorders among male and female adolescents. Wilksch and Wade compared students' attitudes before and after the program to the attitudes of a control group of students who did not participate in the program. They find that among girls, program participation reduced shape and weight concern, one of the strongest risk factors, as well as body dissatisfaction and responses to peer teasing, and media messages. Although boys enjoyed the program, their perceptions and attitudes were not affected as much as those of the girls.

CHAPTER 5
DIETARY TREATMENT FOR OVERWEIGHT AND OBESITY

We rarely repent of having eaten too little.

—Thomas Jefferson

Americans have long been consumed with losing weight, seemingly willing to suffer deprivation and to embrace each new diet that debuts, even if the "new diet" is simply a twist on a previous weight-loss plan. The fixation with weight loss is so long-standing that even the word *diet* has assumed a new meaning. As a verb, diet means to eat and drink a prescribed selection of foods; however, since the latter part of the 20th century dieting became synonymous with an effort to lose weight.

During the 19th century fashionable body shapes and sizes varied from decade to decade, but most periods celebrated plumpness as a sign of health and prosperity and considered being thin a sign of poverty and ill health. At the start of the 20th century rising interest in dieting seemingly coincided with some of the social and cultural changes that would make it necessary: food became increasingly plentiful, and sedentary work and public transportation reduced Americans' level of physical activity. In *Fat History: Bodies and Beauty in the Modern West* (1997), Peter N. Stearns explains how fat became "a turn-of-the-century target" with anti-fat sentiments intensifying from the 1920s to the 21st century.

Stearns asserts that the contemporary obsession with fat arose in tandem with the dramatic growth in consumer culture, women's increasing equality, and changes in women's sexual and maternal roles. Dieting, with its emphasis on deprivation, self-control, and moral discipline, seemed the perfect antidote to the indulgence of consumer culture, and Stearns contends that "weight morality bore disproportionately on women precisely because of their growing independence, or seeming independence, from other standards."

Fashion trends fueled anti-fat sentiments as women shed the corsets that had created the illusion of narrow waists and aspired to duplicate the wasp-waisted silhouettes by becoming slimmer. The shorter, close-fitting "flapper" dresses of the 1920s revealed women's legs and rekindled their desire to be slender. The emergence of the first actuarial tables (data compiled to assess insurance risk and formulate life insurance premiums), which showed the relationship between overweight and premature mortality (death), reinforced the growing sentiment that thinness was the key to health and longevity. Capitalizing on the increasing interest in monitoring and reducing body weight, the new Detecto and Health-o-Meter bathroom scales enabled people to weigh themselves regularly in the privacy of their own home, as opposed to relying on periodic visits to the physician's office or the pharmacy to use the balance scale.

SELECTED MILESTONES IN THE HISTORY OF DIETING

Not unlike fashion trends, the history of dieting reveals the emergence and popularity of specific diets, which over time are cast aside in favor of different approaches but then are recycled and resurface as "new and miraculous." The first low-carbohydrate diet to earn popular acclaim was described by William Banting (1797–1878) during the 1860s. In *Letter on Corpulence, Addressed to the Public* (1863), Banting, then 66 years old, claimed that by adhering to his low-carbohydrate regimen he was never hungry and had lost 46 pounds (20.9 kg) of his initial 202 pounds (91.6 kg) in one year.

The Early to Mid-20th Century

The early 1900s marked the beginning of diets that restricted calories. *Diet and Health, with Key to the Calories* (1918) by Lulu Hunt Peters (1873–1930) advised readers to think in terms of consuming calories rather than food items and remained in print for 20 years. The 1920s saw the rise of very-low-calorie diets to promote weight loss. For example, the Hollywood 18-day diet advised just 585 calories per day, which required the dieter to eat mostly citrus fruit.

Throughout the 1920s and 1930s the low-calorie diet remained a popular weight-loss strategy. Other approaches, however, such as food-limiting plans that restricted dieters to just one or two foods (e.g., lamb chops, pineapples, grapefruits, or cabbage), were introduced, as were diets that prescribed combinations of certain foods and forbid others. For example, some diets prohibited eating protein and carbohydrates together; others were more specific, advising which vegetables could be served together. The 1930s also saw the first condemnations of carbohydrates as causes of overweight. A high-fat, low-fiber diet consisting primarily of milk and meat was thought to be protective against disease. The Italian poet Filippo Tommaso Marinetti (1876–1944) exhorted Italians to forgo their pasta because he claimed it made them sluggish, pessimistic, and fat.

In 1943 the U.S. Department of Agriculture (USDA) released the "Basic Seven" food guide in the *National Wartime Nutrition Guide*. It emphasized a patriotic wartime austerity diet that included between two and four servings of protein-rich meat and milk products, three servings of fruits or vegetables, and the rather vague recommendation of "bread, flour, and cereals every day and butter, fortified margarine—some daily."

In 1948 Esther Manz (1908–1996), a 208-pound (94.3-kg) homemaker, established Take Off Pounds Sensibly (TOPS; http://www.tops.org/), the first support-group program for weight loss. Manz was inspired to start the program after she attended childbirth preparation classes, where women benefited from mutual support and encouragement. As of March 2014, the annual membership of $28 supported the international nonprofit organization, which is based in Milwaukee, Wisconsin. Along with weekly meetings and private weigh-ins, TOPS participants are encouraged to adhere to a calorie-counting meal plan that is based on a program developed by the Academy of Nutrition and Dietetics. In "TOPS Quick Facts" (June 2013, http://www.tops.org/TOPS/Public Docs/Wellness/PI-009B-TOPSQuickFacts.pdf), TOPS indicates that in 2013 it had about 150,000 members in about 9,000 chapters worldwide. Members who achieve their weight goals become KOPS (Keep Off Pounds Sensibly) and often keep attending meetings to maintain their weight and serve as role models for others.

In 1950 the physician and biophysicist John W. Gofman (1918–2007) hypothesized that blood cholesterol was involved in the rise in coronary heart disease. Gofman found not only that heart attacks correlated with elevated levels of cholesterol but also that the cholesterol was contained in one lipoprotein particle: low-density lipoprotein (LDL). Early reports of the connection between overweight and elevated blood cholesterol intensified interest in weight loss, which was now promoted as a strategy for preventing heart disease. During the late 1950s injections of human chorionic gonadotropin, which was derived from the urine of pregnant women or animals, enjoyed fleeting popularity as a weight-loss agent; however, it was quickly proven entirely ineffective. Fad diets, such as a diet advocating the consumption of several bananas to satisfy sugar cravings and another that involved ingesting a blend of oils to boost metabolism, continued to lure Americans seeking quick weight loss. In 1959 the American Medical Association called dieting a "national neurosis."

In 1960 Metrecal, the first high-protein beverage, was widely advertised by the Mead Johnson Company as a weight-reducing aid. It was originally sold as a powder, which when mixed with 1 quart (0.9 L) of water yielded four 8-ounce (237-mL) glasses intended to serve as four meals per day, totaling 900 calories. The powder was made from milk, soy flour, starch, corn oil, yeast, vitamins, coconut oil, and vanilla, chocolate, or butterscotch flavoring. The low-calorie regimen enabled dieters to lose 10 pounds (4.5 kg) in a few weeks, without the trouble of meal preparation or counting calories. Later, Metrecal was sold in a premixed, liquid form that could be consumed right from the can. It was the forerunner of liquid diet products such as Slim-Fast.

Support Groups and Diet Books in the 1960s

The 1960s also witnessed the birth of Overeaters Anonymous (OA) and Weight Watchers. OA began as a support group modeled on the 12-step emotional, physical, and spiritual recovery program used by Alcoholics Anonymous. In *About OA* (2012, http://www .oa.org/pdfs/oafinalmediamaterials.pdf), the OA notes that about 7,000 OA groups meet each week in more than 80 countries. In 1961 Jean Nidetch (1923–), an overweight housewife in New York City, invited a few friends to her home to gain support for her efforts to diet and overcome an "obsession for cookies." From this first meeting, the friends gathered weekly, offering one another encouragement and sharing advice and ideas. The weekly support meetings proved successful, providing motivation and encouragement for long-term weight loss. In 1963 Nidetch incorporated Weight Watchers, and hundreds of people turned out for its first meeting. Weight Watchers grew in both size and popularity by developing nutritious and convenient eating plans and promoting exercise, cookbooks, healthful prepared food, and a magazine. The company became so successful that it was acquired by the H. J. Heinz Company in 1978. Weight Watchers states in "About Us: History and Philosophy" (2014, https:// www.weightwatchers.com/about/his/history.aspx) that approximately 1 million people attend Weight Watchers groups each week.

Two best-selling diet books also debuted during the 1960s. The first was Herman Taller's *Calories Don't Count* (1961), which told dieters to avoid carbohydrates and refined sugars and to eat a high-protein diet that included large quantities of unsaturated fat. The second was Irwin Maxwell Stillman and Samm Sinclair Baker's *The Doctor's Quick Weight Loss Diet* (1967), which instructed dieters to avoid carbohydrates altogether and to consume just meat, poultry, fish, cheese, eggs, and water. Although Taller and Stillman and Baker were not the first to tout low-carbohydrate diets, they introduced the first modern high-protein weight-loss diets. Taller's career as a diet guru ended abruptly in 1967, when he was convicted of mail fraud for the sale of safflower capsules as weight-loss aids. Stillman and Baker, however, followed up their wildly successful first book with several other additional weight-loss titles, including *The Doctor's Quick Teenage Diet* (1971), one of the first diet books to address the needs of overweight adolescents. High-protein, low-carbohydrate diets washed down by liberal amounts of alcohol were also advocated by other books from the 1960s, including Gardener Jameson's *The Drinking Man's Diet* (1965) and Sidney Petrie's *Martinis and Whipped Cream: The New Carbo-Cal Way to Lose Weight and Stay Slim* (1966) and *The Lazy Lady's Easy Diet: A Fast-Action Plan to Lose Weight Quickly for Sustained Slenderness and Youthful Attractiveness* (1969).

Development of Nonnutritive Sweeteners

During this same decade chemically processed, non-nutritive sweeteners were marketed as calorie- and guilt-free substitutes that enabled dieters to enjoy many of their favorite sweet treats. Saccharin, which is 300 times sweeter than sugar, was the first artificial sweetener to be widely used in diet foods and beverages. Other chemically processed, artificial, and nonnutritive sweeteners followed, including cyclamate, which was withdrawn from the U.S. market in 1969 because research findings in animals suggested that it might increase the risk of bladder cancer in humans. According to the National Cancer Institute, in "Artificial Sweeteners and Cancer" (August 5, 2009, http://www.cancer.gov/cancertopics/factsheet/Risk/artificial-sweeteners), animal studies have failed to demonstrate that cyclamate is a carcinogen (a substance known to cause cancer) or a cocarcinogen (a substance that enhances the effect of a cancer-causing substance); regardless, cyclamate is not approved for commercial use as a food additive in the United States.

Aspartame and acesulfame potassium were approved by the U.S. Food and Drug Administration (FDA) in 1981 and 1988, respectively. In 1999 the FDA approved the noncaloric sweetener sucralose for general use. Sucralose has gained popularity because it is derived from and tastes like sugar, has no aftertaste, does not promote tooth decay, and is deemed safe for use by pregnant women and diabetics, as well as by those in the general population who are trying to cut down on their sugar intake.

In 2002 the FDA approved neotame, another nonnutritive sweetener, for use as a general-purpose sweetener. Neotame is approximately 7,000 to 13,000 times sweeter than sugar and has been approved for use in food products including baked goods, nonalcoholic beverages (including soft drinks), chewing gum, confections and frostings, frozen desserts, gelatins and puddings, jams and jellies, processed fruits and fruit juices, toppings, and syrups.

In 2008 the FDA approved the sale of stevia, a naturally occurring, zero-calorie sweetener, as a sugar substitute. Stevia is sold in various forms: in combination with other naturally occurring flavors and sweeteners, such as the sugar alcohol erythritol, as well as on its own. Because it has a negligible effect on blood glucose, it is an attractive sugar alternative for people on low-carbohydrate diets.

However, some researchers think sugar substitutes may sabotage dieters by interfering with the body's own innate ability to monitor calorie consumption based on a food's flavor: sweet or savory. Susan E. Swithers of Purdue University reports in "Artificial Sweeteners Produce the Counterintuitive Effect of Inducing Metabolic Derangements" (*Trends in Endocrinology and Metabolism*, vol. 24, no. 9, September 2013) that research confirms that nonnutritive sweeteners promote weight gain, and increase risk for metabolic disorders. The researchers suggest that the consumption of nonnutritive sweeteners may result in sweet tastes no longer serving as consistent predictors of energy consumption and physiological consequences. This disconnect between the sweet taste cues and the caloric consequences may lead to a decrease in the ability of sweet tastes to stimulate the bodily responses that regulate energy balance.

The Atkins Diet, 1972

In 1972 the cardiologist Robert Atkins (1930–2003) published *Dr. Atkins' Diet Revolution: The High Calorie Way to Stay Thin Forever*, which provided a new explanation about how an extremely low-carbohydrate diet targets insulin to promote weight loss. Atkins called insulin, the hormone that regulates blood sugar levels, a "fat-producing hormone." He asserted that most overeaters are continually in a state of hyperinsulinism, in that they are primed and ever-ready to convert excess carbohydrates to fat. As a result, they have excess circulating insulin, which primes the body to store fat. Atkins contended that when people with hyperinsulinism dieted to lose weight—especially when they reduced their fat intake and increased carbohydrate consumption—their efforts were doomed to fail. He claimed that dieters could alter their metabolism and burn fat by inducing a state of ketosis (the accumulation of ketones from partly digested fats due to inadequate carbohydrate intake) that they monitored by testing their urine for the presence of ketones. Tired of limiting portion size, weighing and measuring their foods, counting calories, and assiduously avoiding fatty foods such as steak, bacon, butter, cheese, and heavy cream, dieters embraced the low-carbohydrate diet with religious fervor.

The high-protein, low-carbohydrate diet not only was satisfying but also produced the immediate benefit of weight loss through water loss because the body flushes the waste products of protein digestion in the form of urine. Especially during the early weeks of dieting this additional weight loss delivered a psychological boost to dieters and provided the motivation to continue. Many researchers and health professionals agreed with Atkins's premise that sharply limiting carbohydrate intake can help curb the appetite by maintaining even levels of insulin and preventing the insulin surges and blood sugar drops that may trigger hunger. For example, in "A High-Protein Diet Induces Sustained Reductions in Appetite, ad Libitum Caloric Intake, and Body Weight Despite Compensatory Changes in Diurnal Plasma Leptin and Ghrelin Concentrations" (*American Journal of Clinical Nutrition*, vol. 82, no. 1, July 2005), David S. Weigle et al. observe that there is considerable evidence that high-protein diets, such as the Atkins regimen, increase satiety (the feeling of fullness or satisfaction after eating). The researchers posit that the increased satiety produced by high-protein diets may help explain the weight loss produced by low-carbohydrate diets.

Critics of the low-carbohydrate regimen were concerned about the long-term health consequences of the high-fat diet and wondered if it might elevate cholesterol and triglyceride levels in people who by virtue of being overweight were already at increased risk for heart disease. There were also concerns that high-protein diets might cause kidney damage or bone loss over time. Rigorous research to compare the effectiveness and assess the health outcomes of low-carbohydrate and low-fat diets was not conducted until the late 1990s. Although Atkins enjoyed tremendous popularity, published a series of weight-loss books, and oversaw the sale of food products bearing his name, his contributions to the scientific understanding of nutrition and weight loss were not fully appreciated until the year preceding his death in 2003.

Pritikin and Other Diets of the 1970s

The 1970s also witnessed several fad diets. Robert Linn's *The Last Chance Diet—When Everything Else Has Failed* (1976) advised a protein-sparing fast, which was so dangerously deficient in essential nutrients that several deaths were attributed to it. In *The*

Complete Scarsdale Medical Diet Plus Dr. Tarnower's Lifetime Keep-Slim Program (1978), Herman Tarnower (1910–1980) advocated a fat-free, high-protein diet that allowed 700 calories per day.

At the close of the 1970s Nathan Pritikin's (1915–1985) *The Pritikin Program for Diet and Exercise* (1979) championed a nearly fat-free diet that consisted of fresh and cooked fruits and vegetables, whole grains, breads and pasta, and small amounts of lean meat, fish, and poultry, in concert with daily aerobic exercise. Advocating heart health and fitness, in 1975 Pritikin opened the Pritikin Longevity Center, where people could learn to modify not only their diet but also their lifestyle. Although Pritikin's plan, which essentially eliminated fat from the diet, was considered by many health professionals too extreme to gain long-term adherents, Pritikin enjoyed as loyal a following as did Atkins.

Jenny Craig, the Zone, and Other Diets of the Late 20th Century

During the 1980s Judy Mazel (1943–2007) resurrected the notion of specific food combinations as central to weight loss in *The Beverly Hills Diet* (1981). Mazel asserted that eating foods together, such as protein and carbohydrates, destroyed digestive enzymes and caused weight gain and poor digestion. Her diet featured an abundance of fruit, and some observers speculated that weight loss attributable to the diet resulted from the combined effects of caloric restriction and fluid loss resulting from diarrhea. Celebrity endorsements and Mazel's frequent media interviews stimulated interest in the diet.

In 1983 Jenny Craig (1932–) launched a weight-loss program that would become one of the world's two largest diet companies (the other being Weight Watchers). With over 725 centers in Australia, Guam, New Zealand, North America, and Puerto Rico, the company (2014, http://www.jennycraig.com/corporate/company-profile/) that bears her name sells prepared foods, along with other weight-loss materials. The company offers telephone and online support and home delivery of food and support materials. In 2002 the company founders Jenny Craig and Sid Craig (1932–2008) sold their majority stake in the company to ACI Capital Co. and MidOcean Capital Partners Inc., but retained 20% interest in the company.

The 1990s served up so-called new and revised versions of high-protein, high-fat, and low-carbohydrate diets and the low-fat diet. The cardiologist Dean Ornish (1953–) rekindled enthusiasm for low-fat eating with *Eat More, Weigh Less: Dr. Dean Ornish's Life Choice Program for Losing Weight Safely while Eating Abundantly* (1993). Atkins's 1999 update of *Dr. Atkins' New Diet Revolution*, which offered advice about how to achieve total wellness and weight loss, spent more than four years on the *New York Times* best-seller list and won over a new generation of dieters. Ornish's approach was directly opposed to Atkins's: he espoused the health benefits of vegetarianism and limiting dietary fat to just 10% of the total daily calories. However, both physicians encouraged readers to engage in moderate exercise, foster social support, and reconnect with themselves to support their physical and emotional well-being.

The diet that generated the most fanfare during the 1990s was by the biochemist Barry Sears (1947–), who published *The Zone: A Dietary Road Map* (1995). Sears's high-protein, low-carbohydrate plan promised that by eating the correct ratio of protein, fat, and carbohydrates dieters would lose weight permanently, avoid disease, enhance mental productivity, achieve maximum physical performance, balance and control insulin levels, and enter "that mysterious but very real state in which your body and mind work together at their ultimate best."

South Beach, the Glycemic Index, and Other Developments

Since the start of the 21st century the fiery debate about the merits of low-carbohydrate and low-fat diets has intensified, with both sides citing scientific evidence to support the supremacy of one diet as the healthier and more effective weight-loss strategy. The cardiologist Arthur Agatston (1947–) offered a kind of compromise between the two regimens in *The South Beach Diet: The Delicious, Doctor-Designed, Foolproof Plan for Fast and Healthy Weight Loss* (2003). Agatston condemned simple carbohydrates, such as white flour and white sugar, citing them as the source of the continuous cravings that sabotage dieters, but did not eliminate complex carbohydrates from the diet. (Carbohydrates are classified as simple or complex. The classification depends on the chemical structure of the particular food source and reflects how quickly the sugar is digested and absorbed. Simple carbohydrates have one or two sugars, whereas complex carbohydrates have three or more.) Agatston's diet recommended plenty of high-fiber foods, lean proteins, and healthful fats, while cutting back on, but not entirely banishing, bread, rice, pastas, and fruits.

Americans' enthusiasm for low-carbohydrate diets cooled during 2004, and Atkins Nutritionals Inc., the company that catapulted low-carbohydrate diets into a national obsession, filed for bankruptcy court protection in August 2005. Many dieters abandoned low-carbohydrate diets in favor of regimens that focused on the glycemic index—a ranking system for carbohydrates according to their immediate effect on blood glucose levels, in which a numerical value is assigned to a carbohydrate-rich food based on its average increase in blood glucose.

Diet books that extolled the virtues of the low glycemic index diet—including Michel Montignac's *Eat Yourself Slim* (1999), Rick Gallop's *The G.I. Diet: The Easy, Healthy Way to Permanent Weight Loss* (2002), and H. Leighton Steward et al.'s *The New Sugar Busters!: Cut Sugar to Trim Fat* (2003)—gained popularity. Proponents of low glycemic index diets observed that the regimen not only produced weight loss but also improved overall health by reducing the risk for both type 2 diabetes and cardiovascular disease.

In 2006 Stephen Lanzalotta offered *The Diet Code: Revolutionary Weight Loss Secrets from Da Vinci and the Golden Ratio*, which promotes Mediterranean-style eating and emphasizes bread, fish, cheese, vegetables, meat, nuts, and wine. In *Food Rules: An Eater's Manual* (2009) by Michael Pollan offers advice such as "eat mostly plants, especially leaves," "eat your colors," "limit your snacks to unprocessed plant food," "don't eat anything your great-grandmother wouldn't recognize as food," "avoid food products that contain more than five ingredients," and "avoid foods that contain high-fructose corn syrup." Some contemporary diets provide behavioral insights and strategies rather than food plans. For example, *The Eat This, Not That! No Diet! Diet: The World's Easiest Weight-Loss Plan* (2011) by David Zinczenko describes how to navigate the supermarket to select healthful foods, and *The Amen Solution: The Brain Healthy Way to Lose Weight and Keep It Off* (2011) by Daniel G. Amen describes how to determine an individual's type of overeating, such as compulsive overeater or emotional eater, and then tailor weight-loss and nutritional strategies for each type of overeater.

Weight-Loss Plans in 2014

Although diet industry observers cannot predict the next craze, they are certain that new diets will emerge. By 2014 a number of popular weight-loss plans stressed portion control and organic foods. Some of these programs had been around for many years. Nutrisystem, a diet delivery service, offered subscribers low-calorie, portion-controlled prepared meals, along with online and telephone access to weight management information and counselors. The program, in operation for more than 40 years, offered its customers convenience and simplicity by providing home delivery of a variety of shelf-stable foods that were low in fats and carbs and high in fiber. In its 2012 annual report (December 31, 2012, http://www.snl.com/IRWebLinkX/file.aspx?IID=4089088&FID=1500049935), the company indicated it had more than 7 million customers (although not all subscriptions were active) and that customers reported an average weight loss of 1 to 2 pounds (0.45 to 0.91 kg) per week and typically stayed on the program for 11 to 12 weeks.

Other diet plans that gained popularity in 2014 included juice fasts, raw-only plans, and the paleo diet, outlined by Loren Cordain in *The Paleo Diet Revised: Lose Weight and Get Healthy by Eating the Foods You Were Designed to Eat* (2010). Cordain suggests returning to the diet of hunter-gatherer times when humans consumed primarily animal products and plants. The high-protein, low glycemic index, and high fiber diet emphasizes lean meats and fish, fresh fruits, snacks, and non-starchy vegetables. Juice fasts aim to detox the body, improve health, and promote weight loss by restricting dieters to fruit and vegetable juices and water for periods ranging from two to 60 days. Raw food plans are often associated with veganism and comprise only foods such as fruits, vegetables, seeds, sprouts, nuts, and legumes that have not been cooked, processed, or heated above 115° F (46° C).

In "Three New Diets for Weight Loss: What Works and What Doesn't" (HuffingtonPost.com, June 6, 2013), Mark Hyman reviews three diets that debuted in 2012 or 2013. The Fast Diet recommends consuming just 600 calories per day for men and 550 for women two days per week and then eating anything desired the remaining five days. Hyman points out that while intermittent fasting may provide some health benefits and this diet could conceivably help reduce caloric intake, the lack of guidelines for the non-fasting days may result in unhealthful eating on those days. The Fast Metabolism Diet eliminates all processed foods, gluten, dairy, corn, soy, caffeine, and alcohol from the diet and recommends eating small meals and focusing on the quality of the food consumed. Hyman opines that this diet can effectively promote weight loss, but he observes that it is very restrictive—eliminating many familiar foods—and because it calls for weekly changes may be complicated to follow.

Hyman is most enthusiastic about Mark Bittman's VB6 diet, which advises no animal-derived foods before 6pm and then only whole, unprocessed foods after 6pm. This diet also aims to increase fruit and vegetable consumption. Bittman also counsels people to focus on health rather than weight.

AMERICANS' DIETS

Hazel A. B. Hiza and Lisa Bente of the Center for Nutrition Policy and Promotion offer in *Nutrient Content of the U.S. Food Supply: Developments between 2000 and 2006* (July 2011, http://www.cnpp.usda.gov/Publications/FoodSupply/Final_FoodSupplyReport_2006.pdf) historical data about the nutrients in the U.S. food supply and trends in Americans' diets. Trends include:

• An increase of 800 calories per day between 1960–69 and 2006

• An increase of 3.3 ounces (93 g) of carbohydrate per day between 1960–69 and 2006

• An increase of 1.3 ounces (38 g) of fat per day between 1960–69 and 2006

Americans' reduced their consumption of whole milk in favor of low-fat milk; increased consumption of cheese and legumes, nuts, and soy; and decreased consumption of grain products. Vegetable consumption declined, and there was a dramatic increase in consumption of salad, cooking, and other oils.

In September 2013 Bonnie Liebman of the Center for Science in the Public Interest published "The Changing American Diet" (http://cspinet.org/new/pdf/changing_american_diet_13.pdf), a "report card" rating Americans' food consumption patterns from 1970 to 2010. Liebman reports some modest improvements (decreased consumption of sugar, shortening, beef, whole milk, and white flour). She notes that Americans began eating more vegetables during the 1980s, but that vegetable and fruit consumption have stalled rather than increased and consumption of beef and pork continues to outpace that of chicken and fish. In 2010 Americans consumed about 500 calories more per day than they did in 1970. These calories come from more sweets, grains, and cheese. Americans also increased their fat intake, largely from increased consumption of pizza, burgers, fries and baked goods.

Dietary Guidelines for Americans

Every five years the *Dietary Guidelines for Americans* are updated and revised to translate the most current scientific knowledge about individual nutrients and food components into dietary recommendations that may be adopted by the public. The recommendations are based on the preponderance of scientific evidence for reducing the risk of chronic disease and promoting health.

According to the U.S. Department of Health and Human Services and the USDA, in *Dietary Guidelines for Americans, 2010* (December 2010, http://health.gov/dietaryguidelines/dga2010/DietaryGuidelines2010.pdf), a healthful diet includes plenty of fruits, vegetables, whole grains, and fat-free or low-fat milk and milk products, as well as lean meats, poultry, fish, beans, eggs, and nuts. A healthful diet is also low in saturated fats, trans fats (artificial fats created through the hydrogenation of oils, which solidifies the oil and limits the body's ability to regulate cholesterol), cholesterol, salt, and added sugars. Table 5.1 shows the recommended proportions of carbohydrate, protein, and fat for children, adolescents, and adults. Specific recommendations stipulate that fewer than 10% of calories should come from saturated fatty acids, and trans fatty acids, which are considered to be the most harmful to health, should be avoided. Cholesterol intake should be less than 300 milligrams per day. Total fat intake should not exceed 20% to 35% of calories. Preferred fat sources are fish, nuts, and vegetable oils containing polyunsaturated and monounsaturated fatty acids. Lean, low-fat, or fat-free meats, poultry, dry beans, and milk or milk products are preferable to full-fat foods. Daily sodium intake should be 2,300 milligrams or less for people to age 51 and 1,500 milligrams or less for older adults, African Americans, and people with diabetes, hypertension, or chronic kidney disease.

In general, the guidelines encourage most Americans to eat fewer calories, increase their physical activity, and choose nutrient-dense foods. They advocate increased consumption of fruits, vegetables, whole grains, and fat-free or low-fat milk and milk products. For example, two cups of fruit and two and a half cups of vegetables per day are recommended for a 2,000-calorie diet, along with three or more servings of whole-grain products per day and three cups per day of fat-free or low-fat milk or equivalent milk

TABLE 5.1

Recommended proportions of carbohydrate, protein, and fat, by age group, 2010

	Carbohydrate	Protein	Fat
Young children (1–3 years)	45–65%	5–20%	30–40%
Older children and adolescents (4–18 years)	45–65%	10–30%	25–35%
Adults (19 years and older)	45–65%	10–35%	20–35%

SOURCE: "Table 2-4. Recommended Macronutrient Proportions by Age," in *Dietary Guidelines for Americans, 2010*, 7th ed., U.S. Department of Health and Human Services and U.S. Department of Agriculture, December 2010, http://health.gov/dietaryguidelines/dga2010/dietaryguidelines2010.pdf (accessed October 25, 2013)

products. The guidelines also advise consuming at least half of all grains as whole grains and increasing seafood consumption by replacing some meat and poultry with seafood. Figure 5.1 shows three ways to ensure that at least half of all grains consumed are whole grains.

Table 5.2 compares four eating patterns: the typical American adult diet, the Mediterranean diet, the Dietary Approaches to Stop Hypertension (DASH) eating plan, and the USDA-recommended food pattern. Compared with the typical American adult diet, the other eating patterns contain greater quantities of vegetables, fruits, beans and peas, whole grains, fat-free and low-fat milk and milk products, and oils and smaller amounts of solid fats, added sugars, and sodium. The other eating patterns also emphasize less red and processed meat and more seafood than the typical American adult diet. Table 5.3 shows the amounts of various food groups that are recommended each day or each week at calorie levels ranging from 1,000 to 3,200.

The guidelines specifically address weight management by advising Americans to "maintain calorie balance over time to achieve and sustain a healthy weight" and to "focus on consuming nutrient-dense foods and beverages." For people who are overweight, the guidelines advise gradual, steady weight loss by decreasing caloric consumption while maintaining sufficient nutrients and increasing physical activity. Parents of overweight children are counseled to

FIGURE 5.1

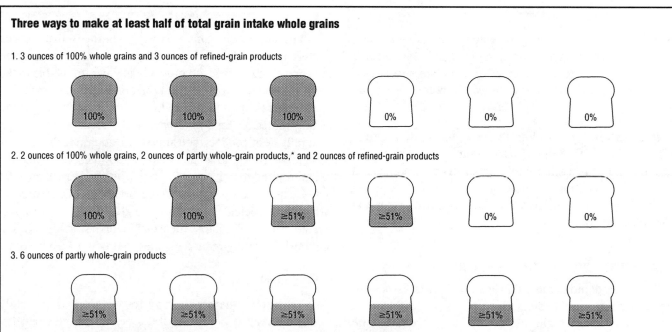

Three ways to make at least half of total grain intake whole grains

1. 3 ounces of 100% whole grains and 3 ounces of refined-grain products

2. 2 ounces of 100% whole grains, 2 ounces of partly whole-grain products,* and 2 ounces of refined-grain products

3. 6 ounces of partly whole-grain products

Notes: Each one-ounce slice of bread represents a 1 ounce-equivalent of grains: 1 one-ounce slice bread; 1 ounce uncooked pasta or rice; 1/2 cup cooked rice, pasta, or cereal; 1 tortilla (6" diameter); 1 pancake (5" diameter); 1 ounce ready-to-eat cereal (about 1 cup cereal flakes). The figure uses an example for a person whose recommendation is 6 ounces of total grains with at least 3 ounces from whole grains per day.
*Partly whole-grain products depicted are those that contribute substantially to whole-grain intake. For example, products that contain at least 51% of total weight as whole grains or those that provide at least 8 grams of whole grains per ounce-equivalent.

SOURCE: "Figure 4-1. Three Ways to Make At Least Half of Total Grains Whole Grains," in *Dietary Guidelines for Americans, 2010*, 7th ed., U.S. Department of Health and Human Services and U.S. Department of Agriculture, December 2010, http://health.gov/dietaryguidelines/dga2010/dietaryguidelines2010.pdf (accessed October 25, 2013)

TABLE 5.2

Comparison of typical U.S. intake, Mediterranean diet, DASH diet, and U.S. Department of Agriculture (USDA) recommended food intake

Pattern	Usual U.S. intake adults[a]	Mediterranean patterns Greece (G) Spain (S)	DASH	USDA food pattern
Food groups				
Vegetables: total (c)	1.6	1.2 (S)–4.1 (G)	2.1	2.5
Dark-green (c)	0.1	nd[b]	nd	0.2
Beans and peas (c)	0.1	<0.1 (G)–0.4 (S)	See protein foods	0.2
Red and orange (c)	0.4	nd	nd	0.8
Other (c)	0.5	nd	nd	0.6
Starchy (c)	0.5	nd–0.6 (G)	nd	0.7
Fruit and juices (c)	1.0	1.4 (S)–2.5 (G) (including nuts)	2.5	2.0
Grains: total (oz)	6.4	2.0 (S)–5.4 (G)	7.3	6.0
Whole grains (oz)	0.6	nd	3.9	≥3.0
Milk and milk products (Dairy products) (c)	1.5	1.0 (G)–2.1 (S)	2.6	3.0
Protein foods:				
Meat (oz)	2.5	3.5 (G)–3.6 (S) (including poultry)	1.4	1.8
Poultry (oz)	1.2	nd	1.7	1.5
Eggs (oz)	0.4	nd–1.9 (S)	nd	0.4
Fish/seafood (oz)	0.5	0.8 (G)–2.4 (S)	1.4	1.2
Beans and peas (oz)	See vegetables	See vegetables	0.4 (0.1 c)	See vegetables
Nuts, seeds, and soy products (oz)	0.5	See fruits	0.9	0.6
Oils (g)	18.0	19 (S)–40 (G)	25	27
Solid fats (g)	43.0	nd	nd	16[c]
Added sugars (g)	79.0	nd–24 (G)	12	32[c]
Alcohol (g)	9.9	7.1 (S)–7.9 (G)	nd	nd[d]

[a]1 day mean intakes for adult males and females, adjusted to 2,000 calories and averaged.
[b]nd = Not determined.
[c]Amounts of solid fats and added sugars are examples only of how calories from solid fats and added sugars in the USDA Food Patterns could be divided.
[d]In the USDA Food Patterns, some of the calories assigned to limits for solid fats and added sugars may be used for alcohol consumption instead.
DASH = Dietary Approaches to Stop Hypertension. USDA = United States Department of Agriculture.

SOURCE: "Table 5-1. Eating Pattern Comparison: Usual U.S.. Intake, Mediterranean, DASH, and USDA Food Patterns, Average Daily Intake at or Adjusted to a 2,000 Calorie Level," in *Dietary Guidelines for Americans, 2010*, 7th ed., U.S. Department of Health and Human Services and U.S. Department of Agriculture, December 2010, http://health.gov/dietaryguidelines/dga2010/dietaryguidelines2010.pdf (accessed October 21, 2011)

reduce the rate of weight gain while children grow and develop and to consult a health care provider before placing children on weight-reduction diets. Women are encouraged to achieve and maintain a healthy weight before becoming pregnant.

In an effort to expand on the guidelines and improve their utility, in 2011 the USDA debuted a new, simple graphic food icon called MyPlate to offer Americans a simple representation of how to construct a healthful meal and diet. (See Figure 5.2.) There is a full discussion of MyPlate in Chapter 10.

HOW WEIGHT-LOSS DIETS WORK

Research demonstrates that weight loss is associated with the length of the diet, the pre-diet weight (people who are more overweight tend to lose more weight, more quickly than those who are only mildly overweight), and the number of calories consumed. Any diet that restricts caloric intake such that calories consumed are less than those expended will promote short-term weight loss. The key to weight loss through diet is adherence—if people do not stick to their diet, then they will not lose weight.

The successes achieved using regimens that restrict dieters to a single food or food group such as grapefruit, pineapple, or cabbage are probably in part attributable to the human hankering for variety. When limited to just one food, most dieters experience boredom: there is just no appeal to eating the same food at every meal, for days on end, so naturally less food is consumed. In addition, these diets generally rely on low-calorie foods, so that even if dieters were inspired to consume 15 grapefruits per day, their total daily caloric consumption would be about 1,200 calories, which is sufficient to produce weight loss for most overweight people. Similarly, diets that involve stringent portion control effectively reduce calories to produce weight loss.

Low-Calorie Diets

Traditional dietary therapy for weight loss generally seeks to create a deficit of 500 to 1,000 calories per day with the intent of promoting weight loss of between 1 to 2 pounds (0.5 to 0.9 kg) per week. Low-calorie diets for men usually range from 1,200 to 1,600 calories per day; for women, low-calorie diets contain between 1,000 and 1,200 calories per day. (See Table 5.3 for examples of the recommended percentages of nutrients in low-calorie diets.)

TABLE 5.3

Recommended intake amounts at various calorie levels

For each food group or subgroup[a], recommended average daily intake amounts[b] at all calorie levels. Recommended intakes from vegetable and protein foods subgroups are per week.

Calorie level of pattern[c]	1,000	1,200	1,400	1,600	1,800	2,000	2,200	2,400	2,600	2,800	3,000	3,200
Fruits	1 c	1 c	1 1/2 c	1 1/2 c	1 1/2 c	2 c	2 c	2 c	2 c	2 1/2 c	2 1/2 c	2 1/2 c
Vegetables[d]	1 c	1 1/2 c	1 1/2 c	2 c	2 1/2 c	2 1/2 c	3 c	3 c	3 1/2 c	3 1/2 c	4 c	4 c
Dark-green vegetables	1/2 c/wk	1 c/wk	1 c/wk	1 1/2 c/wk	1 1/2 c/wk	1 1/2 c/wk	2 c/wk	2 c/wk	2 1/2 c/wk	2 1/2 c/wk	2 1/2 c/wk	2 1/2 c/wk
Red and orange vegetables	2 1/2 c/wk	3 c/wk	3 c/wk	4 c/wk	5 1/2 c/wk	5 1/2 c/wk	6 c/wk	6 c/wk	7 c/wk	7 c/wk	7 1/2 c/wk	7 1/2 c/wk
Beans and peas (legumes)	1/2 c/wk	1/2 c/wk	1/2 c/wk	1 c/wk	1 1/2 c/wk	1 1/2 c/wk	2 c/wk	2 c/wk	2 1/2 c/wk	2 1/2 c/wk	3 c/wk	3 c/wk
Starchy vegetables	2 c/wk	3 1/2 c/wk	3 1/2 c/wk	4 c/wk	5 c/wk	5 c/wk	6 c/wk	6 c/wk	7 c/wk	7 c/wk	8 c/wk	8 c/wk
Other vegetables	1 1/2 c/wk	2 1/2 c/wk	2 1/2 c/wk	3 1/2 c/wk	4 c/wk	4 c/wk	5 c/wk	5 c/wk	5 1/2 c/wk	5 1/2 c/wk	7 c/wk	7 c/wk
Grains[e]	3 oz-eq	4 oz-eq	5 oz-eq	5 oz-eq	6 oz-eq	6 oz-eq	7 oz-eq	8 oz-eq	9 oz-eq	10 oz-eq	10 oz-eq	10 oz-eq
Whole grains	1 1/2 oz-eq	2 oz-eq	2 1/2 oz-eq	3 oz-eq	3 oz-eq	3 oz-eq	3 1/2 oz-eq	4 oz-eq	4 1/2 oz-eq	5 oz-eq	5 oz-eq	5 oz-eq
Enriched grains	1 1/2 oz-eq	2 oz-eq	2 1/2 oz-eq	2 oz-eq	3 oz-eq	3 oz-eq	3 1/2 oz-eq	4 oz-eq	4 1/2 oz-eq	5 oz-eq	5 oz-eq	5 oz-eq
Protein foods[d]	2 oz-eq	3 oz-eq	4 oz-eq	5 oz-eq	5 oz-eq	5 1/2 oz-eq	6 oz-eq	6 1/2 oz-eq	6 1/2 oz-eq	7 oz-eq	7 oz-eq	7 oz-eq
Seafood	3 oz/wk	5 oz/wk	6 oz/wk	8 oz/wk	8 oz/wk	8 oz/wk	9 oz/wk	10 oz/wk	10 oz/wk	11 oz/wk	11 oz/wk	11 oz/wk
Meat, poultry, eggs	10 oz/wk	14 oz/wk	19 oz/wk	24 oz/wk	24 oz/wk	26 oz/wk	29 oz/wk	31 oz/wk	31 oz/wk	34 oz/wk	34 oz/wk	34 oz/wk
Nuts, seeds, soy products	1 oz/wk	2 oz/wk	3 oz/wk	4 oz/wk	4 oz/wk	4 oz/wk	4 oz/wk	5 oz/wk	5 oz/wk	5 oz/wk	5 oz/wk	5 oz/wk
Dairy[f]	2 c	2 1/2 c	2 1/2 c	3 c	3 c	3 c	3 c	3 c	3 c	3 c	3 c	3 c
Oils[g]	15 g	17 g	17 g	22 g	24 g	27 g	29 g	31 g	34 g	36 g	44 g	51 g
Maximum SoFAS[h] limit, Calories (% of calories)	137 (14%)	121 (10%)	121 (9%)	121 (8%)	161 (9%)	258 (13%)	266 (12%)	330 (14%)	362 (14%)	395 (14%)	459 (15%)	596 (19%)

[a] All foods are assumed to be in nutrient-dense forms, lean or low-fat and prepared without added fats, sugars, or salt. Solid fats and added sugars may be included up to the daily maximum limit identified in the table. Food items in each group and subgroup are:

Fruits — All fresh, frozen, canned, and dried fruits and fruit juices: for example, oranges and orange juice, apples and apple juice, bananas, grapes, melons, berries, raisins.

Vegetables

- Dark-green vegetables — All fresh, frozen, and canned dark-green leafy vegetables and broccoli, cooked or raw: for example, broccoli; spinach; romaine; collard, turnip, and mustard greens.
- Red and orange vegetables — All fresh, frozen, and canned red and orange vegetables, cooked or raw: for example, tomatoes, red peppers, carrots, sweet potatoes, winter squash, and pumpkin.
- Beans and peas (legumes) — All cooked beans and peas: for example, kidney beans, lentils, chickpeas, and pinto beans. Does not include green beans or green peas. (See additional comment under protein foods group.)
- Starchy vegetables — All fresh, frozen, and canned starchy vegetables: for example, white potatoes, corn, green peas.
- Other vegetables — All fresh, frozen, and canned other vegetables, cooked or raw: for example, iceberg lettuce, green beans, and onions.

Grains

- Whole grains — All whole-grain products and whole grains used as ingredients: for example, whole-wheat bread, whole-grain cereals and crackers, oatmeal, and brown rice.
- Enriched grains — All enriched refined-grain products and enriched refined grains used as ingredients: for example, white breads, enriched grain cereals and crackers, enriched pasta, white rice.

Protein foods — All meat, poultry, seafood, eggs, nuts, seeds, and processed soy products. Meat and poultry should be lean or low-fat and nuts should be unsalted. Beans and peas are considered part of this group as well as the vegetable group, but should be counted in one group only.

Dairy — All milks, including lactose-free and lactose-reduced products and fortified soy beverages, yogurts, frozen yogurts, dairy desserts, and cheeses. Most choices should be fat-free or low-fat. Cream, sour cream, and cream cheese are not included due to their low calcium content.

[b] Food group amounts are shown in cup (c) or ounce-equivalents (oz-eq). Oils are shown in grams (g). Quantity equivalents for each food group are:
- Grains, 1 ounce-equivalent is: 1 one-ounce slice bread; 1 ounce uncooked pasta or rice 1/2 cup cooked rice, pasta, or cereal; 1 tortilla (6" diameter); 1 pancake (5" diameter); 1 ounce ready-to-eat cereal (about 1 cup cereal flakes).
- Vegetables and fruits, 1 cup equivalent is: 1 cup raw or cooked vegetable or fruit 1/2 cup dried vegetable or fruit; 1 cup vegetable or fruit juice; 2 cups leafy salad greens.
- Protein foods, 1 ounce-equivalent is: 1 ounce lean meat, poultry, seafood; 1 egg; 1 Tbsp peanut butter 1/2 ounce nuts or seeds. Also, 1/4 cup cooked beans or peas may also be counted as 1 ounce-equivalent
- Dairy, 1 cup equivalent is: 1 cup milk, fortified soy beverage, or yogurt; 1/2 ounces natural cheese (e.g., cheddar); 2 ounces of processed cheese (e.g., American).

[c] Food intake patterns at 1,000, 1,200, and 1,400 calories meet the nutritional needs of children ages 2 to 8 years. Patterns from 1,600 to 3,200 calories meet the nutritional needs of children ages 9 years and older and adults. If a child ages 4 to 8 years needs more calories and, therefore, is following a pattern at 1,600 calories or more, the recommended amount from the dairy group can be 2 1/2 cups per day. Children ages 9 years and older and adults should not use the 1,000, 1,200, or 1,400 calorie patterns.

[d] Vegetable and protein foods subgroup amounts are shown in this table as weekly amounts, because it would be difficult for consumers to select foods from all subgroups daily.

[e] Whole-grain subgroup amounts shown in this table are minimums. More whole grains up to all of the grains recommended may be selected, with offsetting decreases in the amounts of enriched refined grains.

[f] The amount of dairy foods in the 1,200 and 1,400 calorie patterns have increased to relect new RDAs for calcium that are higher than previous recommendations for children ages 4 to 8 years.

[g] Oils and soft margarines include vegetable, nut, and fish oils and soft vegetable oil table spreads that have notrans fats.

[h] SoFAS are calories from solid fats and added sugars. The limit for SoFAS is the remaining amount of calories in each food pattern after selecting the specified amounts in each food group in nutrient-dense forms (forms that are fat-free or low-fat and with no added sugars). The number of SoFAS is lower in the 1,200, 1,400, and 1,600 calorie patterns than in the 1,000 calorie pattern. The nutrient goals for the 1,200 to 1,600 calorie patterns are higher and require that more calories be used for nutrient-dense foods from the food groups.

SOURCE: "Appendix 7. USDA Food Patterns," in *Dietary Guidelines for Americans, 2010*, 7th ed., U.S. Department of Health and Human Services and U.S. Department of Agriculture, December 2010, http://health.gov/dietaryguidelines/dga2010/dietaryguidelines2010.pdf (accessed October 25, 2013)

FIGURE 5.2

MyPlate aims to help consumers plan healthful meals

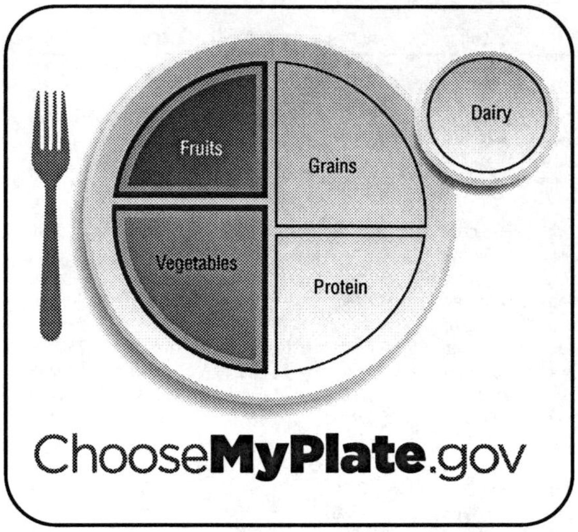

ChooseMyPlate.gov

SOURCE: "MyPlate," in *News and Media* U.S. Department of Agriculture, September 19, 2011, http://www.choosemyplate.gov/images/MyPlateImages/halfplate/PDF/myplate_grayscale_half.pdf (accessed October 25, 2013)

The most successful low-calorie diets take individual food preferences into account to custom-tailor the diet. Table 5.4 and Table 5.5 show examples of how traditional American cuisine may be used to create a low-calorie diet containing 1,200 and 1,600 calories per day, respectively. Table 5.6 incorporates regional southern cuisine into a reduced-calorie diet. Table 5.7 illustrates how Asian American cuisine may be adapted to 1,200- and 1,600-calorie-per-day diets, and Table 5.8 shows how Mexican American cuisine may be adapted for low-calorie diets. Table 5.9 is a sample of a reduced-calorie diet that vegetarians who eat milk and eggs but no meat or fish can use to lose weight. Food exchanges, such as those shown in Table 5.10, enable dieters to enjoy a variety of foods in their reduced-calorie meals, which can prevent boredom and the tendency to abandon the diet.

Research reveals that reducing fat in the diet is an effective way to reduce calories and that when low-calorie diets are combined with low-fat diets, better weight loss is achieved than through calorie reduction alone. Furthermore, although very-low-calorie diets that provide about 500 calories per day have been demonstrated to produce greater initial weight loss than low-calorie diets, the long-term weight loss is not different between the two regimens.

Low-Carbohydrate Diets

During the first decade of the 21st century several rigorous research studies reported that low-carbohydrate diets were as effective, or even more effective, in producing short-term weight loss than low-fat diets. The low-carbohydrate diets owed much of their success to adherence—dieters were better able to stick with their diets, and as a result achieved better results. Another hypothesis about the success of low-carbohydrate regimens is that dieters do not feel as hungry as they do on other diets because protein is the most satisfying of the three macronutrients: carbohydrates, fats, and proteins.

The scientific premise of low-carbohydrate diets is that consuming certain carbohydrates can cause surges in blood sugar and insulin that not only stimulate appetite and weight gain but may also increase the risk for diabetes and heart disease. At first, low-carbohydrate diets viewed all carbohydrates as equally harmful. Increasingly, however, low-carbohydrate diets distinguished between simple and complex carbohydrates, which contain simple (single or double) or complex (three or more) sugars.

Examples of single sugars from foods include fructose, which is found in fruits, and galactose, which is found in milk products. Double sugars include lactose in dairy products; maltose, which is found in certain vegetables and in beer; and sucrose (table sugar). Examples of complex carbohydrates, which are often referred to as starches, include breads, cereals, legumes, brown rice, and pastas. Simple carbohydrates occur naturally in fruits, milk products, and vegetables and, like complex carbohydrates, contain vitamins and minerals, which distinguishes them from the refined simple sugars many nutritionists advise against (or at least recommend limiting in the diet). The simple carbohydrates most nutritionists call "empty calories" are the processed and refined sugars found in candy, table sugar, and sodas, as well as in foods such as white flour and polished white rice.

Besides distinguishing between simple and complex carbohydrates, low-carbohydrate regimens rely on a measure known as the glycemic index (GI), which ranks foods based on how rapidly their consumption raises blood glucose levels. The GI measures how much blood sugar increases over a period of two or three hours after a meal. Carbohydrate foods that break down quickly during digestion have the highest GI. The GI may be used to determine if a particular food will trigger the problematical "carbohydrate–blood sugar–insulin cascade." High-GI foods are those that are rapidly digested and absorbed or transformed metabolically into glucose.

Examples of foods with GI scores of 70 or above are cake, cookies, doughnuts, honey, french fries, rice, baked potato, and white bread. In contrast, lentils have a GI of 29, whereas broccoli, peanuts, and spinach have GIs of less than 15. Carbohydrates that break down slowly, such as whole-grain breads and cereals, beans, leafy greens, or

TABLE 5.4

Sample reduced calorie menus, traditional American cuisine—1,200 calories

	Calories	Fat (grams)	% Fat	Exchange for
Breakfast				
• Whole wheat bread, 1 medium slice	70	1.2	15	(1 bread/starch)
• Jelly, regular, 2 tsp	30	0	0	(1/2 fruit)
• Cereal, shredded wheat, 1/2 cup	104	1	4	(1 bread/starch)
• Milk, 1%, 1 cup	102	3	23	(1 milk)
• Orange juice, 3/4 cup	78	0	0	(1 1/2 fruit)
• Coffee, regular, 1 cup	5	0	0	(free)
Breakfast total	**389**	**5.2**	**10**	
Lunch				
• Roast beef sandwich:				
Whole wheat bread, 2 medium slices	139	2.4	15	(2 bread/starch)
Lean roast beef, unseasoned, 2 oz	60	1.5	23	(2 lean protein)
Lettuce, 1 leaf	1	0	0	(1 vegetable)
Tomato, 3 medium slices	10	0	0	
Mayonnaise, low calorie, 1 tsp	15	1.7	96	(1/3 fat)
• Apple, 1 medium	80	0	0	(1 fruit)
• Water, 1 cup	0	0	0	(free)
Lunch total	**305**	**5.6**	**16**	
Dinner				
• Salmon, 2 ounces edible	103	5	44	(2 lean protein)
• Vegetable oil, 1 1/2 tsp	60	7	100	(1 1/2 fat)
• Baked potato, 3/4 medium	100	0	0	(1 bread/starch)
• Margarine, 1 tsp	34	4	100	(1 fat)
• Green beans, seasoned, with margarine, 1/2 cup	52	2	4	(1 vegetable) (1/2 fat)
• Carrots, seasoned	35	0	0	(1 vegetable)
• White dinner roll, 1 small	70	2	28	(1 bread/starch)
• Iced tea, unsweetened, 1 cup	0	0	0	(free)
• Water, 2 cups	0	0	0	(free)
Dinner total	**454**	**20**	**39**	
Snack				
• Popcorn, 2 1/2 cups	69	0	0	(1 bread/starch)
• Margarine, 3/4 tsp	30	3	100	(3/4 fat)
Total	**1,247**	**34–36**	**24–26**	

Calories	1,247	Saturated fat, % kcals	7	
Total carbohydrate, % kcals	58	Cholesterol, mg	96	
Total fat, % kcals	26	Protein, % kcals	19	
*Sodium, mg	1,043			

Note: Calories have been rounded. Kcal = kilo calorie.
1,200: 100% RDA met for all nutrients except vitamin E 80%, vitamin B$_2$ 96%, vitamin B$_6$ 94%, calcium 68%, iron 63%, and zinc 73%.
*No salt added in recipe preparation or as seasoning. Consume at least 32 ounces of water.

SOURCE: "Appendix D. Traditional American Cuisine—1,200 Calories," in *The Practical Guide: Identification, Evaluation, and Treatment of Overweight and Obesity in Adults*, National Institutes of Health, National Heart, Lung, and Blood Institute, North American Association for the Study of Obesity, October 2000, http://www.nhlbi.nih.gov/guidelines/obesity/prctgd_b.pdf (accessed October 25, 2013)

cruciferous vegetables (which include mustard greens, cabbage, broccoli, cauliflower, kale, and brussels sprouts), generate slower glucose release into the bloodstream and lower GI scores—50 or less. Eating low-GI foods supports weight loss by enhancing satiety and thereby decreasing total food consumption.

The measurement of GI began during the 1990s, following the discovery that specific carbohydrates such as potatoes and cornflakes raised blood sugar faster than others such as brown rice and oatmeal. Harvard University School of Public Health researchers used GI to calculate glycemic load—a measure that considers the food's GI and the amount of carbohydrates contained in a single serving. For example, many whole fruits, vegetables, and grains have low glycemic loads, which when consumed prompt a moderate rise in blood glucose and insulin. When the same fruits, vegetables, and grains are squeezed or pulverized into juice or flour, their glycemic load increases—effectively rendering them with the same high glycemic load of sugar water.

After consuming a meal with a high glycemic load, blood sugar rises higher and faster than it does after eating a meal with a low glycemic load. In an effort to recover from the resulting peaks and plummets, the brain transmits a hunger signal long before the next meal is due. Wildly fluctuating blood sugar and insulin may result in overeating, which in turn causes overweight. For people who are overweight or physically inactive,

TABLE 5.5

Sample reduced calorie menus, traditional American cuisine—1,600 calories

	Calories	Fat (grams)	% Fat	Exchange for
Breakfast				
• Whole wheat bread, 1 medium slice	70	1.2	15.4	(1 bread/starch)
• Jelly, regular, 2 tsp	30	0	0	(1/2 fruit)
• Cereal, shredded wheat, 1 cup	207	2	8	(2 bread/starch)
• Milk, 1%, 1 cup	102	3	23	(1 milk)
• Orange juice, 3/4 cup	18	0	0	(1 1/2 fruit)
• Coffee, regular, 1 cup	5	0	0	(free)
• Milk, 1%, 1 oz	10	0.3	27	(1/8 milk)
Breakfast total	**502**	**6.5**	**10**	
Lunch				
• Roast beef sandwich:				
Whole wheat bread, 2 medium slices	139	2.4	15	(2 bread/starch)
Lean roast beef, unseasoned, 2 oz	60	1.5	23	(2 lean protein)
American cheese, low fat and low sodium, 1 slice, 3/4 oz	46	1.8	36	(1 lean protein)
Lettuce, 1 leaf	1	1	0	
Tomato, 3 medium slices	10	0	0	(1 vegetable)
Mayonnaise, low calorie, 2 tsp	30	3.3	99	(2/3 fat)
• Apple, 1 medium	8	0	0	(1 fruit)
• Water, 1 cup	0	0	0	(free)
Lunch total	**366**	**9**	**22**	
Dinner				
• Salmon, 3 ounces edible	155	7	40	(3 lean protein)
• Vegetable oil, 1 1/2 tsp	60	7	100	(1 1/2 fat)
• Baked potato, 3/4 medium	100	0	0	(1 bread/starch)
• Margarine, 1 tsp	34	4	100	(1 fat)
• Green beans, seasoned, with margarine, 1/2 cup	52	2	4	(1 vegetable) (1/2 fat)
• Carrots, seasoned, with margarine, 1/2 cup	52	2	4	(1 vegetable) (1/2 fat)
• White dinner roll, 1 medium	80	3	33	(1 bread/starch)
• Ice milk, 1/2 cup	92	3	28	(1 bread/starch) (1/2 fat)
• Iced tea, unsweetened, 1 cup	0	0	0	(free)
• Water, 2 cups	0	0	0	(free)
Dinner total	**625**	**28**	**38**	
Snack				
• Popcorn, 2 1/2 cups	69	0	0	(1 bread/starch)
• Margarine, 1/2 tsp	58	6.5	100	(1 1/2 fat)
Total	**1,613**	**50**	**28**	

Calories	1,613	Saturated fat, % kcals	8	
Total carbohydrate, % kcals	55	Cholesterol, mg	142	
Total fat, % kcals	29	Protein, % kcals	19	
*Sodium, mg	1,341			

Note: Calories have been rounded. Kcal = kilo calorie.
1,600: 100% RDA met for all nutrients except vitamin E 99%, iron 73%, and zinc 91%.
No salt added in recipe preparation or as seasoning. Consume at least 32 ounces of water.

SOURCE: "Appendix D. Traditional American Cuisine—1,600 Calories," in *The Practical Guide: Identification, Evaluation, and Treatment of Overweight and Obesity in Adults*, National Institutes of Health, National Heart, Lung, and Blood Institute, North American Association for the Study of Obesity, October 2000, http://www.nhlbi.nih.gov/guidelines/obesity/prctgd_b.pdf (accessed October 25, 2013)

another potential danger of consuming foods with high glycemic loads is that they may already be insulin resistant, and the overexertion of insulin-producing cells in the pancreas that is required to metabolize the high glycemic loads may ultimately exhaust their insulin-producing cells, leading to diabetes.

Weight-loss diets based on the GI sharply restrict high-index foods in favor of low-index foods. Proponents of low-carbohydrate, low-GI food diets observe that consuming foods with low glycemic loads stabilizes blood sugar and insulin to prevent the fluctuations that can cause overeating and may increase the risk for diabetes.

They also assert that reliance on low-fat diets inadvertently led to diets that were high in simple carbohydrates and indirectly promoted overweight and diabetes in the United States.

Low-Fat Diets

Low-fat diets reduce caloric intake by reducing fat consumption. Fat has 9 calories per gram, whereas protein and carbohydrates have 4 calories per gram. These diets rely on the high-fiber content of complex carbohydrates to satisfy dieters. High-fiber foods also slow the absorption of carbohydrates, so they do not provoke a rapid rise in blood sugar and insulin.

TABLE 5.6

Sample reduced calorie menus, southern cuisine

	1,600 calories	1,200 calories
Breakfast		
• Oatmeal, prepared with 1% milk, low fat	1/2 cup	1/2 cup
• Milk, 1%, low fat	1/2 cup	1/2 cup
• English muffin	1 medium	—
• Cream cheese, light, 18% fat	1 T	—
• Orange juice	3/4 cup	1/2 cup
• Coffee	1 cup	1 cup
• Milk, 1%, low fat	1 oz	1 oz
Lunch		
• Baked chicken, without skin	2 oz	2 oz
• Vegetable oil	1 tsp	1/2 tsp
• Salad:		
Lettuce	1/2 cup	1/2 cup
Tomato	1/2 cup	1/2 cup
Cucumber	1/2 cup	1/2 cup
• Oil and vinegar dressing	2 tsp	1 tsp
• White rice	1/2 cup	1/4 cup
• Margarine, diet	1/2 tsp	1/2 tsp
• Baking powder biscuit, prepared with vegetable oil	1 small	1/2 small
• Margarine	1 tsp	1 tsp
• Water	1 cup	1 cup
Dinner		
• Lean roast beef	3 oz	2 oz
• Onion	1/4 cup	1/4 cup
• Beef gravy, water-based	1 T	1 T
• Turnip greens	1/2 cup	1/2 cup
• Margarine, diet	1/2 tsp	1/2 tsp
• Sweet potato, baked	1 small	1 small
• Margarine, diet	1/2 tsp	1/4 tsp
• Ground cinnamon	1 tsp	1 tsp
• Brown sugar	1 tsp	1 tsp
• Corn bread prepared with margarine, diet	1/2 medium slice	1/2 medium slice
• Honeydew melon	1/4 medium	1/8 medium
• Iced tea, sweetened with sugar	1 cup	1 cup
Snack		
• Saltine crackers, unsalted tops	4 crackers	4 crackers
• Mozzarella cheese, part skim, low sodium	1 oz	1 oz

Calories	1,653	Calories	1,225
Total carbohydrate, % kcals	53	Total carbohydrate, % kcals	50
Total fat, % kcals	28	Total fat, % kcals	31
*Sodium, mg	1,231	*Sodium, mg	867
Saturated fat, % kcals	8	Saturated fat, % kcals	9
Cholesterol, mg	172	Cholesterol, mg	142
Protein, % kcals	20	Protein, % kcals	21

1,600: 100% RDA met for all nutrients except vitamin E 97%, magnesium 98%, iron 78%, and zinc 90%.
1,200: 100% RDA met for all nutrients except vitamin E 82%, vitamin B$_1$ & B$_2$ 95%, vitamin B$_3$ 99%, vitamin B$_6$ 88%, magnesium 83%, iron 56%, and zinc 70%.
*No salt added in recipe preparation or as seasoning. Consume at least 32 ounces of water.
Kcal = kilo calorie.

SOURCE: "Appendix D. Southern Cuisine—Reduced Calorie," in *The Practical Guide: Identification, Evaluation, and Treatment of Overweight and Obesity in Adults*, National Institutes of Health, National Heart, Lung, and Blood Institute, North American Association for the Study of Obesity, October 2000, http://www.nhlbi.nih.gov/guidelines/obesity/prctgd_b.pdf (accessed October 25, 2013)

TABLE 5.7

Sample reduced calorie menus, Asian American cuisine

	1,600 calories	1,200 calories
Breakfast		
• Banana	1 small	1 small
• Whole wheat bread	2 slices	1 slice
• Margarine	1 tsp	1 tsp
• Orange juice	3/4 tsp	3/4 tsp
• Milk 1%, low fat	3/4 cup	3/4 cup
Lunch		
• Beef noodle soup, canned, low sodium	1/2 cup	1/2 cup
• Chinese noodle and beef salad:		
Roast beef	3 oz	2 oz
Peanut oil	1 1/2 tsp	1 tsp
Soya sauce, low sodium	tsp	1 tsp
Carrots	1/2 cup	1/2 cup
Zucchini	1/2 cup	1/2 cup
Onion	1/4 cup	1/4 cup
Chinese noodles, soft type	1/4 cup	1/4 cup
• Apple	1 medium	1 medium
• Tea, unsweetened	1 cup	1 cup
Dinner		
• Pork stir-fry with vegetables:		
Pork cutlet	2 oz	2 oz
Peanut oil	1 tsp	1 tsp
Soya sauce, low sodium	1 tsp	1 tsp
Broccoli	1/2 cup	1/2 cup
Carrots	1 cup	1 cup
Mushrooms	1/4 cup	1/2 cup
• Steamed white rice	1 cup	1/2 cup
• Tea, unsweetened	1 cup	1 cup
Snack		
• Almond, cookies	2 cookies	—
• Milk 1%, low fat	1/2 cup	1/2 cup

Calories	1,609	Calories	1,220
Total carbohydrate, % kcals	56	Total carbohydrate, % kcals	55
Total fat, % kcals	27	Total fat, % kcals	27
*Sodium, mg	1,296	*Sodium, mg	1,043
Saturated fat, % kcals	8	Saturated fat, % kcals	8
Cholesterol, mg	148	Cholesterol, mg	117
Protein, % kcals	20	Protein, % kcals	21

1,600: 100% RDA net for all nutrients except zinc 95%, iron 87%, and calcium 93%
1,200: 100% RDA net for all nutrients except vitamin E 75%, calcium 84%, magnesium 98%, iron 66%, and zinc 77%
*No salt added in recipe preparation or as seasoning. Consume at least 32 ounces of water.
Kcal = kilo calorie.

SOURCE: "Appendix D. Asian American Cuisine—Reduced Calorie," in *The Practical Guide: Identification, Evaluation, and Treatment of Overweight and Obesity in Adults*, National Institutes of Health, National Heart, Lung, and Blood Institute, North American Association for the Study of Obesity, October 2000, http://www.nhlbi.nih.gov/guidelines/obesity/prctgd_b.pdf (accessed October 25, 2013)

Table 5.11 shows some food substitutions that may be made to reduce the dietary fat content. Besides making substitutions, many fat-free or low-fat food products are available—from fat-free frozen desserts to reduced-fat peanut butter. Dieters, however, are often cautioned that fat-free or reduced-fat foods are not calorie-free and that their consumption will not result in weight loss when more of the reduced-fat foods are consumed than would be eaten of the full-fat versions. For example, eating twice as many baked tortilla chips would actually result in higher caloric intake than a single serving of regular tortilla chips. (See Table 5.12.)

Low-Fat versus Low-Carbohydrate Diets

In the absence of rigorous scientific research and studies demonstrating the long-term safety and effectiveness of low-carbohydrate and low-fat diets,

TABLE 5.8

Sample reduced calorie menus, Mexican American cuisine

	1,600 calories	1,200 calories
Breakfast		
• Cantaloupe	1 cup	1/2 cup
• Farina, prepared with 1% low fat milk	1/2 cup	1/2 cup
• White bread	1 slice	1 slice
• Margarine	1 tsp	1 tsp
• Jelly	1 tsp	1 tsp
• Orange juice	1 1/2 cup	3/4 cup
• Milk, 1%, low fat	1/2 cup	1/2 cup
Lunch		
• Beef enchilada:		
Tortilla, corn	2 tortillas	2 tortillas
Lean roast beef	2 1/2 oz	2 oz
Vegetable oil	2/3 tsp	2/3 tsp
Onion	1 T	1 T
Tomato	4 T	4 T
Lettuce	1/2 cup	1/2 cup
Chili peppers	2 tsp	2 tsp
Refried beans, prepared with vegetable oil	1/4 cup	1/4 cup
• Carrots	5 sticks	5 sticks
• Celery	6 sticks	6 sticks
• Milk, 1%, low fat	1/2 cup	—
• Water	—	1 cup
Dinner		
• Chicken taco:		
Tortilla, corn	1 tortilla	1 tortilla
Chicken breast, without skin	2 oz	1 oz
Vegetable oil	2/3 tsp	2/3 tsp
Cheddar cheese, low fat and low sodium	1 oz	1/2 oz
Guacamole	2 T	2 T
Salsa	1 T	1 T
• Corn, seasoned with	1/2 cup	1/2 cup
margarine	1/2 tsp	—
• Spanish rice without meat	1/2 cup	1/2 cup
• Banana	1 large	1/2 large
• Coffee	1 cup	1/2 cup
• Milk, 1%	1 oz	1 oz

Calories	1,638	Calories	1,239
Total carbohydrate, % kcals	56	Total carbohydrate, % kcals	58
Total fat, % kcals	27	Total fat, % kcals	26
*Sodium, mg	1,616	*Sodium, mg	1,364
Saturated fat, % kcals	9	Protein, % kcals	8
Cholesterol, mg	153	Cholesterol, mg	91
Protein, % kcals	20	Protein, % kcals	19

1,600: 100% RDA met for all nutrients except vitamin in E 97% and zinc 84%.
1,200: 100% RDNA met for all nutrients except vitamin E 71%, vitamin B₁ & B₃ 91%, vitamin B₂ & iron 90%, and calcium 92%.
*No salt in recipe preparation or as seasoning. Consume at least 32 ounces of water.
Kcal = kilo calorie.

SOURCE: "Appendix D. Mexican American Cuisine—Reduced Calorie," in *The Practical Guide: Identification, Evaluation, and Treatment of Overweight and Obesity in Adults*, National Institutes of Health, National Heart, Lung, and Blood Institute, North American Association for the Study of Obesity, October 2000, http://www.nhlbi.nih.gov/guidelines/obesity/prctgd_b.pdf (accessed October 25, 2013)

TABLE 5.9

Sample reduced calorie menus, lacto-ovo vegetarian cuisine

	1,600 calories	1,200 calories
Breakfast		
• Orange	1 medium	1 medium
• Pancakes, made with 1% lowfat milk and egg whites	3 4" circles	2 4" circles
• Pancake syrup	2 T	1 T
• Margarine, diet	1 1/2 tsp	1 1/2 tsp
• Milk, 1%, lowfat	1 cup	1/2 cup
• Coffee	1 cup	1 cup
• Milk, 1%, lowfat	1 oz	1 oz
Lunch		
• Vegetable soup, canned, low sodium	1 cup	1/2 cup
• Bagel	1 medium	1/2 medium
• Processed American cheese, lowfat	3/4 oz	—
• Spinach salad:		
Spinach	1 cup	1 cup
Mushrooms	1/2 cup	1/2 cup
• Salad dressing, regular calorie	2 tsp	2 tsp
• Apple	1 medium	1 medium
• Iced tea, unsweetened	1 cup	1 cup
Dinner		
• Omelette:		
Egg whites	4 large eggs	4 large eggs
Green pepper	2 T	2T
Onion	2 T	2T
Mozzarella cheese, made from part skim milk, low sodium	1 oz	1/2 oz
Vegetable oil	1 T	1/2 T
• Brown rice, seasoned with	1/2 cup	1/2 cup
margarine, diet	1/2 tsp	1/2 tsp
• Carrots, seasoned with	1/2 cup	1/2 cup
Margarine, diet	1/2 tsp	1/2 tsp
• Whole wheat bread	1 slice	1 slice
• Margarine, diet	1 tsp	1 tsp
• Fig bar cookie	1 bar	1 bar
• Tea	1 cup	1 cup
• Honey	1 tsp	1 tsp
• Milk, 1%, lowfat	3/4 cup	3/4 cup

Calories	1,650	Calories	1,205
Total carbohydrate, % kcals	56	Total carbohydrate, % kcals	60
Total fat, % kcals	27	Total fat, % kcals	25
*Sodium, mg	1,829	*Sodium, mg	1,335
Saturated fat, % kcals	8	Saturated fat, % kcals	7
Cholesterol, mg	82	Cholesterol, mg	44
Protein, % kcals	19	Protein, % kcals	18

1,600: 100% RDA met for all nutrients except vitamin E 92%, vitamin B₃ 97%, vitamin B₆ 67%, iron 73%, and zinc 68%.
1,200: 100% RDA met for all nutrients except vitamin E 75%, vitamin B₁ 92%, vitamin B₃ 69%, vitamin B₆ 59%, iron 54%, and zinc 46%.
*No salt added in recipe preparation or as seasoning. Consume at least 32 ounces of water.
Kcal = kilo calorie.

SOURCE: "Appendix D. Lacto-Ovo Vegetarian Cuisine—Reduced Calorie," in *The Practical Guide: Identification, Evaluation, and Treatment of Overweight and Obesity in Adults*, National Institutes of Health, National Heart, Lung, and Blood Institute, North American Association for the Study of Obesity, June 1998, http://www.nhlbi.nih.gov/guidelines/obesity/practgde.htm (accessed October 25, 2013)

many investigators and health professionals hesitate to proclaim one diet's superiority over all others. Nevertheless, there is consensus that although some diets may produce greater initial weight loss, most perform similarly over time, and that the best predictor of successful weight loss is adherence to a diet.

In "A Randomized Trial of Energy-Restricted High-Protein versus High-Carbohydrate, Low-Fat Diet in Morbid Obesity" (*Obesity*, vol. 21, no. 9, September 2013), Riccardo Dalle Grave et al. compared the long-term effects of high-protein versus high-carbohydrate diet combined with cognitive behavior therapy in 88 study participants. The researchers compared the percentage of weight lost at one year, the attrition rate (how many subjects failed to adhere to the diet), and changes in

TABLE 5.10

Food exchange list

Within each group, these foods can be exchanged for each other. You can use this list to give yourself more choices.

Vegetables contain 25 calories and 5 grams of carbohydrate. One serving equals:
- 1/2 cup   Cooked vegetables (carrots, broccoli, zucchini, cabbage, etc.)
- 1 cup   Raw vegetables or salad greens
- 1/2 cup   Vegetable juice

If you're hungry, eat more fresh or steamed vegetables.

Fat free and very low fat milk contains 90 calories and 12 grams of carbohydrate per serving. One serving equals:
- 8 oz   Milk, fat free or 1% fat
- 1/4 cup   Yogurt, plain nonfat or low fat
- 1 cup   Yogurt, artificially sweetened

Very lean protein choices have 35 calories and 1 gram of fat per serving. One serving equals:
- 1 oz   Turkey breast or chicken breast, skin removed
- 1 oz   Fish fillet (flounder, sole, scrod, cod, haddock, halibut)
- 1 oz   Canned tuna in water
- 1 oz   Shellfish (clams, lobster, scallop, shrimp)
- 3/4 cup   Cottage cheese, nonfat or lowfat
- 2 each   Egg whites
- 1/4 cup   Egg substitute
- 1 oz   Fat free cheese
- 1/2 cup   Beans—cooked (black beans, kidney, chickpeas, or lentils): count as 1 starch/bread and 1 very lean protein

Medium fat proteins have 75 calories and 5 grams of fat per serving. One serving equals:
- 1 oz   Beef (any prime cut), corned beef, ground beef**
- 1 oz   Pork chop
- 1 each   Whole egg (medium)**
- 1 oz   Mozzarella cheese
- 1/4 cup   Ricotta cheese
- 4 oz   Tofu (note that this is a heart-healthy choice)

****Choose these very infrequently.**

Fats contain 45 calories and 5 grams of fat per serving. One serving equals:
- 1 tsp   Oil (vegetable, corn, canola, olive, etc.)
- 1 tsp   Butter
- 1 tsp   Stick margarine
- 1 tsp   Mayonnaise
- 1 T   Reduced fat margarine or mayonnaise
- 1 T   Salad dressing
- 1 T   Cream cheese
- 2 T   Lite cream cheese
- 1/8   Avocado
- 8 large   Black olives
- 10 large   Stuffed green olives
- 1 slice   Bacon

Fruits contain 15 grams of carbohydrates and 60 calories. One serving equals:
- 1 small   Apple, banana, orange, nectarine
- 1 medium   Fresh peach
- 1   Kiwi
- 1/2   Grapefruit
- 1/2   Mango
- 1 cup   Fresh berries (strawberries, raspberries, or blueberries)
- 1 cup   Fresh melon cubes
- 1/8   Honeydew melon
- 4 oz   Unsweetened juice
- 4 tsp   Jelly or jam

Lean protein choices have 55 calories and 2 to 3 grams of fat per serving. One serving equals:
- 1 oz   Chicken—dark meat, skin removed
- 1 oz   Turkey—dark meat, skin removed
- 1 oz   Salmon, swordfish, herring, catfish, trout
- 1 oz   Lean beef (flank steak, London broil, tenderloin, roast beef)*
- 1 oz   Veal, roast, or lean chop*
- 1 oz   Lamb, roast, or lean chop*
- 1 oz   Pork, tenderloin, or fresh ham*
- 1 oz   Lowfat luncheon meats (with 3 grams or less of fat per ounce)
- 1/4 cup   4.5% cottage cheese
- 2 medium   Sardines

***Limit to 1 to 2 times per week.**

Starches contain 15 grams of carbohydrate and 80 calories per serving. One serving equals:
- 1 slice   Bread (white, pumpernickel, whole wheat, rye)
- 2 slice   Reduced calorie or "lite" bread
- 1/4 (1 oz)   Bagel (varies)
- 1/2   English muffin
- 1/2   Hamburger bun
- 3/4 cup   Cold cereal
- 1/3 cup   Rice, brown or white—cooked
- 1/3 cup   Barley or couscous—cooked
- 1/3 cup   Legumes (dried beans, peas, or lentils)—cooked
- 1/2 cup   Pasta—cooked
- 1/2 cup   Bulgur—cooked
- 1/2 cup   Corn, sweet potato, or green peas
- 3 oz   Baked sweet or white potato
- 3/4 oz   Pretzels
- 3 cups   Popcorn, hot-air popped or microwave (80-percent light)

SOURCE: "Appendix E. Food Exchange List," in *The Practical Guide: Identification, Evaluation, and Treatment of Overweight and Obesity in Adults*, National Institutes of Health, National Heart, Lung, and Blood Institute, North American Association for the Study of Obesity, October 2000, http://www.nhlbi.nih.gov/guidelines/obesity/prctgd_b.pdf (accessed October 25, 2013)

cardiovascular risk factors and find that there were no significant differences between the two diets.

Although there is no single winner in the diet wars, research has dispelled some of the fears about the safety and effectiveness of low-carbohydrate diets. Low-carbohydrate diets appear to be safe and effective in the short term, but long-term outcomes are still unclear. Some results suggest that higher protein and fat intakes lead to lower total caloric intake by producing earlier satiety, but these diets have not been shown to alter fundamental eating behaviors, nor have they demonstrated, as many of their proponents argue, the ability to modify caloric balance such that weight loss persists when more calories are consumed than expended.

TABLE 5.11

Low calorie, lower fat food alternatives

Instead of...		Replace with...
• Evaporated whole milk		• Evaporated fat free (skim) or reduced fat (2%) milk
• Whole milk		• Low fat (1%), reduced fat (2%), or fat free (skim) milk
• Ice cream		• Sorbet, sherbet, lowfat or fat free frozen yogurt, or ice milk (check label for calorie content)
• Whipping cream		• Imitation whipped cream (made with fat free [skim] milk) or lowfat vanilla yogurt
• Sour cream		• Plain lowfat yogurt
• Cream cheese	**Dairy**	• Neufchatel or "light" cream cheese or fat free cream cheese
• Cheese (cheddar, Swiss, jack)	**Products**	• Reduced calorie cheese, low calorie processed cheese, etc.
		• Fat free cheese
• American cheese		• Fat free American cheese or other types of fat free cheeses
• Regular (4%) cottage cheese		• Lowfat (1%) or reduced fat (2%) cottage cheese
• Whole milk mozzarella cheese		• Part skim low-moisture mozzarella cheese
• Whole milk ricotta cheese		• Part skim milk ricotta cheese
• Coffee cream (half and half) or nondairy creamer (liquid, power)		• Low fat (1%) or reduced fat (2%) milk or nonfat dry milk power
• Ramen noodles		• Rice or noodles (spaghetti, macaroni, etc.)
• Pasta with white sauce (alfredo)	**Cereals, grains**	• Pasta with red sauce (marinara)
• Pasta with cheese sauce	**and pasta**	• Pasta with vegetables (primavera)
• Granola		• Bran flakes, crispy rice, etc.
		• Cooked grits or oatmeal
		• Whole grains (e.g., couscous, barley, bulgur, etc.)
		• Reduced fat granola
• Cold cuts or lunch meats (bologna, salami, liverwurst, etc.)		• Lowfat cold cuts (95% to 97% fat free lunch meats, lowfat pressed meats)
• Hot dogs (regular)		• Lower fat hot dogs
• Bacon or sausage		• Canadian bacon or lean ham
• Regular ground beef		• Extra lean ground beef such as ground round or ground turkey (read labels)
• Chicken or turkey with skin, duck, or goose		• Chicken or turkey without skin (white meat)
• Oil-packed tuna		• Water-packed tuna (rinse to reduce sodium content)
• Beef (chuck, rib, brisket)	**Meat, fish,**	• Beef (round, loin) (trimmed of external fat) (choose select grades)
• Pork (spareribs, untrimmed loin)	**and poultry**	• Pork tenderloin or trimmed, lean smoked ham
• Frozen breaded fish or fried fish (homemade or commercial)		• Fish or shellfish, unbreaded (fresh, frozen, canned in water)
• Whole eggs		• Egg whites or egg substitutes
• Frozen TV dinners (containing more than 13 gram of fat per serving)		• Frozen TV dinners (containing less than 13 grams of fat per serving and lower in sodium)
• Chorizo sausage		• Turkey sausage, drained well (read label)
		• Vegetarian sausage (made with tofu)
• Croissants, brioches, etc.		• Hard French rolls or soft "brown 'n serve" rolls
• Donuts, sweet rolls, muffins, scones, or pastries		• English muffins, bagels, reduced fat or fat free muffins or scones
• Party crackers		• Lowfat crackers (choose lower in sodium)
• Saltine or soda crackers (choose lower in sodium)	**Baked goods**	
• Cake (pound, chocolate, yellow)		• Cake (angel food, white, gingerbread)
• Cookies		• Reduced fat or fat free cookies (graham crackers, ginger snaps, fig bars) (compare calorie level)
• Nuts	**Snacks and**	• Popcorn (air-popped or light microwave), fruits, vegetables
• Ice cream, e.g., cones or bars	**sweets**	• Frozen yogurt, frozen fruit, or chocolate pudding bars
• Custards or puddings (made with whole milk)		• Puddings (made with skim milk)
• Regular margarine or butter		• Light-spread margarines, diet margarine, or whipped butter, tub or squeeze bottle
• Regular mayonnaise		• Light or diet mayonnaise or mustard
• Regular salad dressings	**Fats, oils, and**	• Reduced calorie or fat free salad dressings, lemon juice, or plain, herb-flavored, or wine vinegar
	salad dressings	
• Butter or margarine on toast or bread		• Jelly, jam, or honey on bread or toast
• Oils, shortening, or lard		• Nonstick cooking spray for stir-frying or sautéing
		• As a substitute for oil or butter, use applesauce or prune puree in baked goods
• Canned cream soups		• Canned broth-based soups
• Canned beans and franks	**Miscellaneous**	• Canned baked beans in tomato sauce
• Gravy (home made with fat and/or milk)		• Gravy mixes made with water or homemade with the fat skimmed off and fat free milk included
• Fudge sauce		• Chocolate syrup
• Avocado on sandwiches		• Cucumber slices or lettuce leaves
• Guacamole dip or refried beans with lard		• Salsa

SOURCE: "Appendix C. Instead of...Replace with...," in *The Practical Guide: Identification, Evaluation, and Treatment of Overweight and Obesity in Adults*, National Institutes of Health, National Heart, Lung, and Blood Institute, North American Association for the Study of Obesity, October 2000, http://www.nhlbi.nih.gov/guidelines/obesity/prctgd_b.pdf (accessed October 25, 2013)

TABLE 5.12

Calories in fat-free or reduced-fat and regular food

Fat free or reduced fat	Calories	Regular	Calories
Reduced fat peanut butter, 2 T	187	Regular peanut butter, 2 T	191
Cookies		Cookies	
Reduced fat chocolate chip cookies, 3 cookies (30 g)	118	Regular chocolate chip cookies, 3 cookies (30 g)	142
Fat free fig cookies, 2 cookies (30 g)	102	Regular fig cookies, 2 cookies (30 g)	111
Ice cream		Ice cream	
Nonfat vanilla frozen yogurt (1% fat), 1/2 cup	100	Regular whole milk vanilla frozen yogurt (3–4% fat), 1/2 cup	104
Light vanilla ice cream (7% fat), 1/2 cup	111	Regular vanilla ice cream (11% fat), 1/2 cup	133
Fat free caramel topping, 2 T	103	Caramel topping, homemade with butter, 2 T	103
Low fat granola cereal, approx. 1/2 cup (55 g)	213	Regular granola cereal, approx 1/2 cup (55 g)	257
Low fat blueberry muffin, 1 small (2 1/2 inch)	131	Regular blueberry muffin, 1 small (2 1/2 inch)	138
Baked tortilla chips, 1 oz.	113	Regular tortilla chips, 1 oz.	143
Low fat cereal bar, 1 bar (1.3 oz.)	130	Regular cereal bar, 1 bar (1.3 oz.)	140

SOURCE: "Fat Free or Reduced Fat [versus] Regular," in *The Practical Guide: Identification, Evaluation, and Treatment of Overweight and Obesity in Adults*, National Institutes of Health, National Heart, Lung, and Blood Institute, North American Association for the Study of Obesity, October 2000, http://www.nhlbi .nih.gov/guidelines/obesity/prctgd_b.pdf (accessed October 25, 2013)

CHAPTER 6
PHYSICAL ACTIVITY, DRUGS, SURGERY, AND OTHER TREATMENTS FOR OVERWEIGHT AND OBESITY

Lack of activity destroys the good condition of every human being, while movement and methodical physical exercise save it and preserve it.

—Plato

One credible hypothesis about the cause of the epidemic of overweight and obesity in the United States is the progressive decrease in physical activity expended in daily life—for work, transportation, and household chores. Some researchers contend that by reducing daily physical activity, the caloric imbalance between calories consumed and expended has shifted to favor weight gain. Although no data conclusively prove this hypothesis, there is some evidence to support it.

Among the studies that support the premise that Americans' sedentary lifestyle has precipitated the obesity epidemic is a landmark study that examined the diets of an Amish community in Ontario, Canada. In "Physical Activity in an Old Order Amish Community" (*Medicine and Science in Sports and Exercise*, vol. 36, no. 1, January 2004), David R. Bassett, Patrick L. Schneider, and Gertrude E. Huntington describe the "Amish paradox"—that despite a diet that is high in fat, calories, and refined sugar, the Amish community had a scant 4% obesity rate, compared with 31% in the general U.S. population. The researchers chose this particular Amish population because it has rejected technological advances such as automobiles and electricity, and its physically demanding lifestyle is comparable to the way Americans lived 150 years ago. (Other Amish communities that have assumed occupations less physically active than farming have obesity rates that are similar to those found in the general U.S. population.) Bassett, Schneider, and Huntington analyzed the daily routines of 98 Amish people and found that the men averaged 18,425 steps per day and the women 14,196 steps per day, compared with the recommended 10,000 steps per day that most Americans struggle to achieve. The Amish men performed about 10 hours per week of vigorous

exercise and the women spent 3.4 hours engaged in heavy lifting, shoveling, digging, shoeing horses, or tossing straw bales. The men devoted an additional 42.8 hours per week and the women an average of 39.2 hours to moderate physical activities such as gardening, performing farm-related chores, or doing laundry.

PHYSICAL ACTIVITY

In sharp contrast to the Amish farmers, many Americans are not physically active. In "How Much Physical Activity Do Adults Need?" (December 1, 2011, http://www.cdc.gov/physicalactivity/everyone/guidelines/adults.html), the U.S. Centers for Disease Control and Prevention (CDC) defines the minimum recommended physical activity level for adults as: moderate-intensity aerobic physical activity for 150 minutes every week and muscle-strengthening activities on at least two days per week, or vigorous-intensity physical activity for 75 minutes or more every week and muscle-strengthening activities on at least two days per week. Table 6.1 shows that the percentage of men and women who met the federal guidelines for aerobic and muscle-strengthening exercise increased between 1999 and 2011; however, in 2011 just 21% of Americans obtained the physical activity prescribed by the guidelines. That year only 11.2% of men and 5.3% of women aged 75 years and older met the guidelines for leisure-time physical activity, compared with about 32% of men and 20% of women aged 18 to 44 years. Across all age groups, a lower percentage of women met the guidelines than men.

Table 6.1 shows that the overall percentage of adults considered to be inactive (meeting neither the aerobic nor the muscle-strengthening activity guidelines) decreased from 56.6% in 1998 to 47.6% in 2011; however, inactivity was higher among specific groups. For example, the percentage of inactive adults was higher among non-Hispanic African Americans (55%) and Hispanics (56.3%) than among non-Hispanic whites (46.2%). Inactivity declined

TABLE 6.1

Participation in leisure-time physical activities that meet federal guidelines for adults, by selected characteristics, selected years 1998–2011

[Data are based on household interviews of a sample of the civilian noninstitutionalized population]

| | 2008 Physical Activity Guidelines for Americans[a] | | | | | | | |
| | Met both aerobic activity and muscle-strengthening guidelines | | | | Met neither aerobic activity nor muscle-strengthening guideline | | | |
Characteristic	1998	2000	2010	2011	1998	2000	2010	2011
				Percent				
18 years and over, age-adjusted[b, c]	14.3	15.0	20.7	21.0	56.6	54.7	49.1	47.6
18 years and over, crude[c]	14.5	15.1	20.4	20.6	56.3	54.6	49.5	48.1
Age								
18–44 years	18.9	18.9	25.7	26.0	50.7	49.1	43.1	41.4
18–24 years	23.8	23.8	29.6	30.3	46.5	44.5	39.4	36.2
25–44 years	17.4	17.3	24.3	24.5	51.9	50.6	44.4	43.3
45–64 years	11.4	12.8	17.7	17.5	58.8	57.6	51.0	51.5
45–54 years	13.2	14.5	19.2	18.8	56.9	55.4	48.9	49.9
55–64 years	8.6	10.1	15.9	16.1	61.8	61.0	53.7	53.3
65 years and over	5.5	6.8	10.4	11.3	71.0	67.0	64.6	60.3
65–74 years	7.0	8.4	13.6	14.3	65.6	60.3	59.9	54.3
75 years and over	3.5	4.9	6.4	7.7	77.8	75.0	70.3	67.7
Sex[b]								
Male	17.5	17.9	25.1	25.0	50.8	49.6	43.8	43.5
Female	11.4	12.3	16.5	17.2	61.9	59.4	54.0	51.5
Sex and age								
Male:								
18–44 years	23.0	23.0	31.8	31.9	44.3	43.0	37.1	36.7
45–54 years	16.1	16.0	20.9	19.6	52.9	52.7	45.2	48.4
55–64 years	9.4	11.3	19.1	17.6	58.2	58.7	50.1	50.5
65–74 years	9.5	9.4	16.6	16.8	58.9	55.3	55.6	50.8
75 years and over	4.9	7.1	9.1	11.2	69.5	66.7	62.8	59.0
Female:								
18–44 years	14.9	15.0	19.6	20.2	56.9	55.0	49.0	46.1
45–54 years	10.5	13.1	17.5	17.9	60.8	57.9	52.4	51.4
55–64 years	7.8	9.0	13.1	14.7	65.0	63.1	57.0	56.0
65–74 years	5.1	7.7	11.0	12.1	70.9	64.3	63.6	57.2
75 years and over	2.6	3.6	4.6	5.3	83.0	80.0	75.3	73.8
Race[b, d]								
White only	14.8	15.7	21.4	21.7	55.2	53.1	47.6	46.2
Black or African American only	11.7	12.2	17.2	17.9	65.7	64.6	58.5	55.0
American Indian or Alaska Native only	16.0	10.6*	12.7*	17.0	57.6	67.1	54.0	51.4
Asian only	13.5	14.1	17.8	16.8	59.1	55.0	51.7	52.6
Native Hawaiian or other Pacific Islander only	—	*	*	*	—	*	*	*
2 or more races	—	19.0	25.9	24.1	—	52.8	45.0	45.6
Hispanic origin and race[b, d]								
Hispanic or Latino	9.4	9.2	14.4	15.4	67.7	66.5	60.2	56.3
Mexican	8.7	8.1	13.2	14.0	69.5	67.0	60.7	56.7
Not Hispanic or Latino	14.9	15.8	21.9	22.0	55.3	53.2	47.2	46.1
White only	15.5	16.5	22.9	23.1	53.6	51.4	45.0	44.0
Black or African American only	11.7	12.2	17.4	18.1	65.8	64.6	58.4	55.1
Education[e, f]								
No high school diploma or GED	4.6	4.3	7.7	7.4	76.3	74.0	69.8	68.3
High school diploma or GED	8.6	9.5	12.7	12.2	64.6	61.7	59.0	59.0
Some college or more	18.2	18.9	25.0	25.4	48.0	47.1	42.1	40.8
Percent of poverty level[b, g]								
Below 100%	8.0	9.3	12.0	11.7	71.3	68.0	63.9	61.5
100%–199%	9.0	9.0	12.7	13.9	67.1	65.5	60.6	58.7
200%–399%	12.6	13.2	19.2	19.5	58.0	56.8	50.6	48.6
400% or more	20.2	20.5	29.1	29.5	46.2	45.0	36.9	36.4
Hispanic origin and race and percent of poverty level[b, d, g]								
Hispanic or Latino:								
Below 100%	4.6	4.4	8.9	8.4	78.0	75.2	68.6	66.1
100%–199%	7.0	5.0	9.3	11.7	71.2	72.2	66.7	61.8
200%–399%	11.1	10.2	15.7	17.5	63.8	63.1	57.6	52.6
400% or more	17.4	19.6	28.1	27.9	55.6	52.8	42.5	40.0

TABLE 6.1

Participation in leisure-time physical activities that meet federal guidelines for adults, by selected characteristics, selected years 1998–2011 [CONTINUED]

[Data are based on household interviews of a sample of the civilian noninstitutionalized population]

	2008 Physical Activity Guidelines for Americans[a]							
	Met both aerobic activity and muscle-strengthening guidelines				Met neither aerobic activity nor muscle-strengthening guideline			
Characteristic	1998	2000	2010	2011	1998	2000	2010	2011
				Percent				
Not Hispanic or Latino:								
White only:								
Below 100%	9.9	11.7	13.7	14.4	66.9	63.5	60.5	58.7
100%–199%	9.6	10.3	14.1	14.9	65.1	62.6	56.4	56.3
200%–399%	13.1	13.9	20.0	19.5	56.1	54.7	48.6	46.9
400% or more	20.2	21.0	29.9	30.4	45.2	43.7	35.2	34.6
Black or African American only:								
Below 100%	7.1	9.5	11.3	11.0	74.6	72.1	66.9	63.4
100%–199%	8.8	9.5	11.7	13.6	69.8	69.2	67.0	61.7
200%–399%	10.6	11.8	20.8	22.8	64.5	64.3	53.3	51.4
400% or more	21.2	17.6	26.1	25.1	54.2	54.9	47.7	44.8
Disability measure[b, h]								
Any basic actions difficulty or complex activity limitation	10.2	10.3	13.6	13.2	64.4	62.2	59.1	58.7
Any basic actions difficulty	9.8	10.3	13.8	12.7	64.8	62.1	59.2	59.2
Any complex activity limitation	7.7	7.2	8.9	9.7	71.9	71.2	67.2	66.7
No disability	16.0	17.0	24.2	24.7	52.5	50.6	43.3	41.3
Geographic region[b]								
Northeast	14.2	17.0	20.2	19.5	57.0	51.8	49.1	50.9
Midwest	15.0	16.4	20.7	22.0	54.9	53.4	49.7	47.7
South	11.8	12.1	18.8	18.3	61.4	59.7	51.8	50.8
West	18.5	16.7	24.0	25.3	49.5	50.1	44.5	40.3
Location of residence[b]								
Within MSA[i]	14.9	15.7	21.8	22.1	55.8	54.1	47.8	46.2
Outside MSA[i]	12.2	12.3	14.5	14.9	59.7	56.9	56.9	55.3

*Estimates are considered unreliable.

[a]Starting with *Health, United States, 2010,* measures of physical activity shown in this table changed to reflect the federal 2008 Physical Activity Guidelines for Americans. This table presents four measures of physical activity that are of interest to the public health community: the percentage of adults who met the federal 2008 guidelines for both aerobic activity and muscle strengthening; the percentage who met neither the aerobic activity guideline nor the muscle-strengthening guideline; the percentage who met the aerobic activity guideline; and the percentage who met the muscle-strengthening guideline. Persons who met neither the aerobic activity nor the muscle-strengthening guideline were unable to be active, were completely inactive, or had some aerobic or muscle-strengthening activities but amounts were insufficient to meet the guidelines. The percentage of persons who met the aerobic activity guideline includes those who may or may not have also met the muscle-strengthening guideline. Similarly, the percentage of persons who met the muscle-strengthening guideline includes those who may or may not have also met the aerobic activity guideline. The federal 2008 guidelines recommend that for substantial health benefits adults perform at least 150 minutes (2 hours and 30 minutes) a week of moderate-intensity, or 75 minutes (1 hour and 15 minutes) a week of vigorous-intensity aerobic physical activity, or an equivalent combination of moderate- and vigorous-intensity aerobic activity. Aerobic activity should be performed in episodes of at least 10 minutes, and preferably, should be spread throughout the week. The 2008 guidelines also recommend that adults perform muscle-strengthening activities that are moderate or high intensity and involve all major muscle groups on 2 or more days a week, because these activities provide additional health benefits.
[b]Estimates are age-adjusted to the year 2000 standard population using five age groups: 18–44 years, 45–54 years, 55–64 years, 65–74 years, and 75 years and over. Age-adjusted estimates in this table may differ from other age-adjusted estimates based on the same data and presented elsewhere if different age groups are used in the adjustment procedure.
[c]Includes all other races not shown separately, unknown education level, and unknown disability status.
[d]The race groups, white, black, American Indian or Alaska Native, Asian, Native Hawaiian or Other Pacific Islander, and 2 or more races, include persons of Hispanic and non-Hispanic origin. Persons of Hispanic origin may be of any race. Starting with 1999 data, race-specific estimates are tabulated according to the 1997 Revisions to the Standards for the Classification of Federal Data on Race and Ethnicity and are not strictly comparable with estimates for earlier years. The five single-race categories plus multiple-race categories shown in the table conform to the 1997 Standards. Starting with 1999 data, race-specific estimates are for persons who reported only one racial group; the category 2 or more races includes persons who reported more than one racial group. Prior to 1999, data were tabulated according to the 1977 Standards with four racial groups, and the Asian only category included Native Hawaiian or Other Pacific Islander. Estimates for single-race categories prior to 1999 included persons who reported one race or, if they reported more than one race, identified one race as best representing their race. Starting with 2003 data, race responses of other race and unspecified multiple race were treated as missing, and then race was imputed if these were the only race responses. Almost all persons with a race response of other race were of Hispanic origin.
[e]Estimates are for persons aged 25 and over and are age-adjusted to the year 2000 standard population using five age groups: 25–44 years, 45–54 years, 55–64 years, 65–74 years, and 75 years and over.
[f]GED is General Educational Development high school equivalency diploma.
[g]Percent of poverty level is based on family income and family size and composition using U.S. Census Bureau poverty thresholds. Missing family income data were imputed for 1997 and beyond.
[h]Any basic actions difficulty or complex activity limitation is defined as having one or more of the following limitations or difficulties: movement difficulty, emotional difficulty, sensory (seeing or hearing) difficulty, cognitive difficulty, self-care (activities of daily living or instrumental activities of daily living) limitation, social limitation, or work limitation. Starting with 2007 data, the hearing question, a component of the basic actions difficulty measure, was revised. Consequently, data prior to 2007 are not comparable with data for 2007 and beyond.
[i]MSA is metropolitan statistical area. Starting with 2006 data, MSA status is determined using 2000 census data and the 2000 standards for defining MSAs.

SOURCE: Adapted from "Table 67. Participation in Leisure-Time Aerobic and Muscle-Strengthening Activities That Meet the 2008 Federal Physical Activity Guidelines for Americans among Adults Aged 18 Years and over, by Selected Characteristics: United States, 1998–2011," in *Health, United States, 2012: With Special Feature on Emergency Care,* Centers for Disease Control and Prevention, National Center for Health Statistics, 2013, http://www.cdc.gov/nchs/data/hus/hus12.pdf (accessed October 8, 2013)

with increasing education, from 68.3% of people with no high school diploma to 40.8% of those with at least some college. Similarly, inactivity declined with increasing income: 61.5% of people at or below poverty level income were inactive, compared with 36.4% of people whose incomes were 400% or more above the poverty level.

Figure 6.1 reveals that while men were more likely than women to report regularly engaging in leisure-time physical activity across all age groups in early 2013, the difference was relatively small among people aged 25 to 64 years. Figure 6.2 shows that in early 2013 non-Hispanic white adults (51.9%) were more likely than non-Hispanic African American adults (41.1%) or Hispanic adults (38.8%) to report having participated in sufficient leisure-time physical activity to meet the federal guidelines.

Physical Activity and Weight Loss

Increasing physical activity and exercise is an important element of weight-loss regimens, although the addition of exercise to a diet program generally does not produce substantially greater weight loss—most of the weight that is lost is attributable to decreased caloric intake. By favorably affecting blood lipids, increased and sustained physical activity does offer many direct and indirect health benefits, including reducing risks for cardiovascular heart disease and type 2 diabetes beyond the risk reduction possible through diet alone. Physical activity lowers low-density lipoprotein (LDL) cholesterol ("bad cholesterol") and triglycerides, increases high-density lipoprotein (HDL) cholesterol ("good cholesterol"), reduces abdominal fat, and may protect against a decrease in muscle mass during weight loss.

Like those who have been inactive or sedentary, overweight people are advised to initiate physical activity slowly and gradually. Walking and swimming at a slow pace are ideal activities because they are enjoyable, easy to schedule, and less likely to produce injuries than many competitive sports. Table 6.2 is an example of a walking program that progressively increases physical activity. Furthermore, because the amounts of activity and the resulting health benefits are functions of the duration, intensity, and frequency of the activity, the same health benefits can be obtained through long sessions of moderately intense activity, such as brisk walking, as in shorter sessions of more strenuous activity, such as running. Table 6.3 shows how a moderate amount of activity, physical activity that uses about 150 calories of energy per day for a total of about 1,000 calories per week, can

FIGURE 6.1

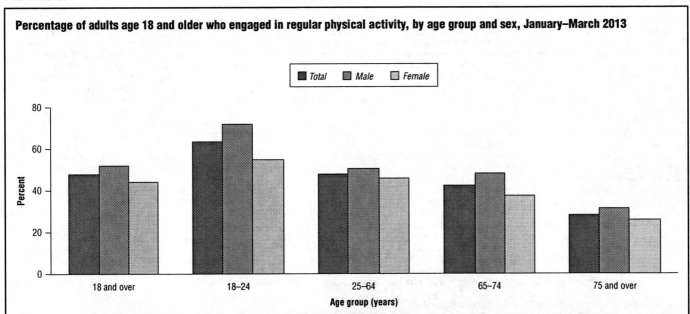

Percentage of adults age 18 and older who engaged in regular physical activity, by age group and sex, January–March 2013

Notes: Data are based on household interviews of a sample of the civilian noninstitutionalized population. Estimates in this figure are limited to leisure-time physical activity only. This measure reflects an estimate of leisure-time aerobic activity motivated by the 2008 federal *Physical Activity Guidelines for Americans,* which are being used for Healthy People 2020 Objectives (3). The 2008 guidelines refer to any kind of aerobic activity, not just leisure-time aerobic activity, so the leisure-time aerobic activity estimates in this figure may underestimate the percentage of adults who met the 2008 guidelines for aerobic activity. This figure presents the percentage of adults who met the 2008 federal guidelines for aerobic activity. The 2008 federal guidelines recommend that for substantial health benefits, adults perform at least 150 minutes a week of moderate-intensity aerobic physical activity, or 75 minutes a week of vigorous-intensity aerobic physical activity, or an equivalent combination of moderate- and vigorous-intensity aerobic activity. The 2008 guidelines state that aerobic activity should be performed in episodes of at least 10 minutes, and preferably it should be spread throughout the week. The analyses excluded the 1.4% of persons with unknown physical activity participation.

SOURCE: Brian W. Ward, Jeannine S. Schiller, and Gulnur Freeman, "Figure 7.2. Percentage of Adults Aged 18 Years and over Who Met the 2008 Federal Physical Activity Guidelines for Aerobic Activity through Leisure-Time Aerobic Activity, by Age Group and Sex: United States, January–March 2013," in *Early Release of Selected Estimates Based on Data from the January–March 2013 National Health Interview Survey,* Centers for Disease Control and Prevention, National Center for Health Statistics, September 2013, http://www.cdc.gov/nchs/data/nhis/earlyrelease/earlyrelease201309_07.pdf (accessed October 7, 2013)

FIGURE 6.2

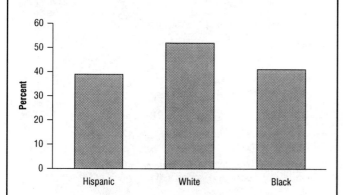

Percentage of adults aged 18 and older who engaged in regular physical activity, by race/ethnicity, January–March 2013

Notes: Data are based on household interviews of a sample of the civilian noninstitutionalized population. Estimates in this figure are limited to leisure-time physical activity only. This measure reflects an estimate of leisure-time aerobic activity motivated by the 2008 federal *Physical Activity Guidelines for Americans*, which are being used for Healthy People 2020 Objectives (3). The 2008 guidelines refer to any kind of aerobic activity, not just leisure-time aerobic activity, so the leisure-time aerobic activity estimates in this figure may underestimate the percentage of adults who met the 2008 guidelines for aerobic activity. This figure presents the percentage of adults who met the 2008 federal guidelines for aerobic activity. The 2008 federal guidelines recommend that for substantial health benefits, adults perform at least 150 minutes a week of moderate-intensity aerobic physical activity, or 75 minutes a week of vigorous-intensity aerobic physical activity, or an equivalent combination of moderate-and vigorous-intensity aerobic activity. The 2008 guidelines state that aerobic activity should be performed in episodes of at least 10 minutes, and preferably it should be spread throughout the week. The analyses excluded the 1.4% of persons with unknown physical activity participation. Estimates are age-sex adjusted using the projected 2000 U.S. population as the standard population and using five age groups: 18–24, 25–34, 35–44, 45–64, and 65 and over.

SOURCE: Brian W. Ward, Jeannine S. Schiller, and Gulnur Freeman, "Figure 7.3. Age-Sex-Adjusted Percentage of Adults Aged 18 Years and over Who Met the 2008 Federal Physical Activity Guidelines for Aerobic Activity through Leisure-Time Aerobic Activity, by Race/ Ethnicity: United States, January–March 2013," in *Early Release of Selected Estimates Based on Data from the January–March 2013 National Health Interview Survey*, Centers for Disease Control and Prevention, National Center for Health Statistics, September 2013, http://www.cdc.gov/nchs/data/nhis/earlyrelease/earlyrelease201309_07 .pdf (accessed October 7, 2013)

be obtained in a variety of ways. The table also indicates how performing common household chores, and even self-care activities such as using a wheelchair, may be used to fulfill requirements for moderate amounts of physical activity. Changing routines to include walking up stairs rather than taking an elevator or parking farther than usual from work or school are ways to increase physical activity incrementally. Even reducing sedentary time, such as hours spent in front of the television or computer, can serve to increase energy expenditure.

Table 6.3 also shows the relationship between the intensity and duration of physical activities by comparing the amount of time an adult must spend performing each activity to expend 150 calories. It is interesting to note that just five additional minutes of walking at a moderate pace expends the same number of calories as walking at a brisk pace.

TABLE 6.2

A sample walking program

	Warm up	Exercising	Cool down	Total time
Week 1				
Session A	Walk 5 min.	Then walk briskly 5 min.	Then walk more slowly 5 min.	15 min.
Session B	Repeat above pattern			
Session C	Repeat above pattern			

Continue with at least three exercise sessions during each week of the program.

	Warm up	Exercising	Cool down	Total time
Week 2	Walk 5 min.	Walk briskly 7 min.	Walk 5 min.	17 min.
Week 3	Walk 5 min.	Walk briskly 9 min.	Walk 5 min.	19 min.
Week 4	Walk 5 min.	Walk briskly 11 min.	Walk 5 min.	21 min.
Week 5	Walk 5 min.	Walk briskly 13 min.	Walk 5 min.	23 min.
Week 6	Walk 5 min.	Walk briskly 15 min.	Walk 5 min.	25 min.
Week 7	Walk 5 min.	Walk briskly 18 min.	Walk 5 min.	28 min.
Week 8	Walk 5 min.	Walk briskly 20 min.	Walk 5 min.	30 min.
Week 9	Walk 5 min.	Walk briskly 23 min.	Walk 5 min.	33 min.
Week 10	Walk 5 min.	Walk briskly 26 min.	Walk 5 min.	36 min.
Week 11	Walk 5 min.	Walk briskly 28 min.	Walk 5 min.	38 min.
Week 12	Walk 5 min.	Walk briskly 30 min.	Walk 5 min.	40 min.

Week 13 on: Gradually increase your brisk walking time to 30 to 60 minutes, three or four times a week. Remember that your goal is to get the benefits you are seeking and enjoy your activity.

SOURCE: "A Sample Walking Program," in *The Practical Guide: Identification, Evaluation, and Treatment of Overweight and Obesity in Adults*, National Institutes of Health, National Heart, Lung, and Blood Institute, North American Association for the Study of Obesity, October 2000, http://www.nhlbi.nih.gov/guidelines/obesity/prctgd_b.pdf (accessed October 25, 2013)

In "Weight Loss, Exercise or Both and Cardiometabolic Risk Factors in Obese Older Adults: Results of a Randomized Controlled Trial" (*International Journal of Obesity*, vol. 38, no. 3, March 2014), Matthew F. Bouchonville et al. examine the effects of exercise on weight loss and cardiovascular risk factors. The researchers assigned 107 obese subjects to one of three regimes: diet only, diet and exercise, or a control group. Bouchonville et al. find that body weight decreased similarly in the diet and exercise and the diet alone groups. However, subjects in the diet and exercise group had improved insulin sensitivity and the presence of metabolic syndrome decreased 40% in the diet and exercise group compared with 15% in the diet alone group.

Donal J. O'Gorman and Anna Krook observe in "Exercise and the Treatment of Diabetes and Obesity" (*Medical Clinics of North America*, vol. 95, no. 5, September 2011) that there is a significant dose-response to the effect of exercise and that recommendations such as the minimum amount of physical activity needed to maintain or improve cardiovascular health are not sufficient to prevent weight gain or promote weight loss. The researchers suggest that exercise recommendations for people seeking to lose weight may have to be revised upward to achieve these objectives. O'Gorman and Krook also reiterate that "exercise by itself exerts clinically beneficial effects in both lean

TABLE 6.3

Examples of moderate amounts of physical activity

Common chores	Sporting activities	
Washing and waxing a car for 45–60 minutes	Playing volleyball for 45–60 minutes	**Less vigorous**
Washing windows or floors for 45–60 minutes	Playing touch football for 45 minutes	**more time***
Gardening for 30–45 minutes	Walking 1 3/4 miles in 35 minutes (20 min/mile)	
Wheeling self in wheelchair for 30–40 minutes	Basketball (shooting baskets) for 30 minutes	
Pushing a stroller 1 1/2 miles in 30 minutes	Bicycling 5 miles in 30 minutes	
Raking leaves for 30 minutes	Dancing fast (social) for 30 minutes	
Walking 2 miles in 30 minutes (15 min/mile)	Water aerobics for 30 minutes	
Shoveling snow for 15 minutes	Swimming laps for 20 minutes	
Stairwalking for 15 minutes	Basketball (playing a game) for 15–20 minutes	
	Jumping rope for 15 minutes	**More vigorous,**
	Running 1 1/2 miles in 15 minutes	**less time**

Note: A moderate amount of physical activity is roughly equivalent to physical activity that uses approximately 150 calories of energy per day, or 1,000 calories per week.
*Some activities can be performed at various intensities; the suggested durations correspond to expected intensity of effort.

SOURCE: "Appendix H. Examples of Moderate Amounts of Physical Activity," in *The Practical Guide: Identification, Evaluation, and Treatment of Overweight and Obesity in Adults*, National Institutes of Health, National Heart, Lung, and Blood Institute, North American Association for the Study of Obesity, October 2000, http://www.nhlbi.nih.gov/guidelines/obesity/prctgd_b.pdf (accessed October 25, 2013)

and obese subjects, even in the absence of effects on weight—it exerts an effect on metabolism and changes in gene expression (regulation of the process by which the heritable effects of a gene are displayed)."

O'Gorman and Krook assert that there has been relatively little rigorous research to evaluate the effect of exercise on weight loss. Many studies call for about 150 minutes of exercise per week, or 30 minutes of physical activity on all or most days of the week. O'Gorman and Krook observe that this amount of exercise is only equivalent to a 150- to 200-calorie energy expenditure per day or about 700 to 1,000 calories per week. As such, it is not surprising that this level of exercise does not compare favorably in terms of weight loss with diets that result in a 500-calorie-per-day reduction, or about 3,500 calories per week. O'Gorman and Krook report that there have been just two studies that matched the energy expenditure of exercise with that of a calorie-restricted diet. When exercise and diet both resulted in a deficit of 500 or 700 calories per day, both regimens produced comparable weight loss. O'Gorman and Krook conclude that "exercise is an effective weight-loss strategy but the accumulated energy expenditure required for weight reduction may be greater than the general recommendations."

EXERCISE MAY COUNTER GENES THAT INCREASE THE RISK OF OBESITY. A gene variant known as FTO (fat mass and obesity associated) is known to increase the risk of obesity by 20% to 30%. In "Physical Activity Attenuates the Influence of FTO Variants on Obesity Risk: A Meta-analysis of 218,166 Adults and 19,268 Children" (*PLoS Medicine*, vol. 8, no. 11, November 2011), Tuomas O. Kilpeläinen et al. analyze the results of 45 research studies of adults and nine studies conducted with children and adolescents to determine whether physical activity modifies or reduces the risk that is associated with the FTO gene. The researchers

find that moderate physical activity—about an hour per day, five days per week—moderated the influence of the gene. Among physically active adults with the FTO gene variant, the risk of obesity was reduced by about 30%. Kilpeläinen et al. conclude that physical activity "is a particularly effective way of controlling body weight in individuals with a genetic predisposition towards obesity and thus contrast with the determinist view held by many that genetic influences are unmodifiable."

MEDICATION

Pharmacotherapy for weight loss involves the use of drugs as one of several strategies including diet, physical activity, behavioral therapy, counseling, and participation in group-support programs that in combination can work to achieve weight loss. Adding weight-loss medications to a comprehensive treatment program consisting of diet, physical activity, and counseling can increase weight loss by 5 to 20 pounds (2.3 to 9.1 kg) during the first six months of treatment. While this is only a modest improvement, demand for weight-loss drugs is high.

The decision to add prescription drugs to a treatment program takes into account the individual's body mass index (BMI; body weight in kilograms divided by height in meters squared), other medical problems, and coexisting risk factors. Table 6.4 shows the therapies that are appropriate for people with differing BMIs and takes into account the presence of comorbidities (the coexistence of two or more diseases) such as diabetes, severe obstructive sleep apnea, or heart disease.

Most drugs used for weight loss are anorexiants (appetite suppressants), which act on neurotransmitters (natural chemical substances that convey impulses from one nerve cell to another) in the brain. Anorexiant drugs vary depending on which neurotransmitters they affect: some affect

TABLE 6.4

A guide to selecting weight loss treatment by body mass index (BMI)

Treatment	BMI category				
	25–26.9	27–29.9	30–34.9	35–39.9	≥40
Diet, physical activity, and behavior therapy	With comorbidities	With comorbidities	+	+	+
Pharmacotherapy		With comorbidities	+	+	+
Surgery				With comorbidities	

- Prevention of weight gain with lifestyle therapy is indicated in any patient with a BMI ≥25 kg/m², even without comorbidities, while weight loss is not necessarily recommended for those with a BMI of 25–29.9 kg/m² or a high waist circumference, unless they have two or more comorbidities.
- Combined therapy with a low-calorie diet (LCD), increased physical activity, and behavior therapy provide the most successful intervention for weight loss and weight maintenance.
- Consider pharmacotherapy only if a patient has not lost 1 pound per week after 6 months of combined lifestyle therapy.

The + represents the use of indicated treatment regardless of comorbidities.

SOURCE: "Table 3. A Guide to Selecting Treatment," in *The Practical Guide: Identification, Evaluation, and Treatment of Overweight and Obesity in Adults*, National Institutes of Health, National Heart, Lung, and Blood Institute, North American Association for the Study of Obesity, October 2000, http://www.nhlbi.nih.gov/guidelines/obesity/prctgd_b.pdf (accessed October 25, 2013)

catecholamines such as dopamine and norepinephrine; others affect serotonin; and a third class of drugs acts on more than one neurotransmitter. The drugs, which include phentermine, diethylpropion, and phendimetrazine, act by increasing the secretion of dopamine, norepinephrine, or serotonin, by inhibiting reuptake of neurotransmitters (causing their effects to last longer), or by inducing a combination of both mechanisms.

Another class of weight-loss drugs blocks the absorption of fat. Orlistat, which was approved by the U.S. Food and Drug Administration (FDA) in 1999, decreases fat absorption in the digestive tract by about one-third. Because it also inhibits absorption of water and vitamins, some users suffer from cramping and diarrhea.

Table 6.5 describes the drugs that may be prescribed for weight loss. The determination of which type of drug to prescribe is based on individual patient characteristics: anorexiant drugs work best for people who are preoccupied with food and feel constantly hungry, orlistat may be effective for those who are unwilling to reduce fat from their diet, and phentermine may help reduce food cravings.

Several weight-loss drugs that appeared effective and were popular among consumers have been withdrawn from the U.S. market due to the number and severity of adverse side effects associated with their use. During the 1990s a combination of two drugs—phentermine and fenfluramine, commonly known as "phen-fen"—was prescribed for long-term use (more than three months). However, rare but unacceptable side effects, including serious damage to the heart valves, prompted the withdrawal of fenfluramine and a similar drug, dexfenfluramine, in September 1997. Phentermine is still approved for short-term use.

In June 2012 the FDA approved the first new prescription weight-management drug in over a decade: Belviq. As reported by the FDA, in "FDA Approves Belviq to Treat Some Overweight or Obese Adults" (June 27, 2012, http://www.fda.gov/NewsEvents/Newsroom/PressAnnouncements/ucm309993.htm), clinical trials had shown that obese and overweight individuals who combined Belviq with a program of exercise and a reduced-calorie diet were more likely to lose weight than those who engaged in the same program without using Belviq. After up to a year using Belviq, those in the study had an average weight loss of 3% to 3.7%. Belviq activates serotonin 2C receptors in the brain, which is thought to help people feel full after eating smaller amounts of food.

Less than a month later the FDA also approved Qsymia for prescription as a weight-management drug. Qsymia is a combination of a low does of phentermine and topiramate (a drug used to prevent seizures and migraine headaches). As reported by the FDA in "FDA Approves Weight-Management Drug Qsymia" (July 17, 2012, http://www.fda.gov/NewsEvents/Newsroom/PressAnnouncements/ucm312468.htm), when used in combination with a reduced-calorie diet and regular physical activity Qsymia helped obese and overweight adults lose weight. After one year of treatment with Qsymia, nearly two-thirds of patients in the clinical trials had lost 5% or more of their body weight.

Over-the-Counter Use of Orlistat

In February 2007 the FDA approved the over-the-counter (nonprescription) sale of orlistat, at doses lower than it had previously approved for prescription sale. In 2008 consumers began buying 60-milligram capsules sold under the brand names Alli and Xenical. The FDA recommended it be used in combination with a reduced-calorie, low-fat diet and an exercise program. The introduction of orlistat as an over-the-counter product made it the only nonprescription FDA-approved product for weight loss, since the FDA had withdrawn phenylpropanolamine in

TABLE 6.5

Prescription drugs approved for obesity treatment, 2013

Weight-loss drug	Approved for	How it works	Common side effects
Orlistat Sold as Xenical by prescription Over-the-counter version sold as Alli	Xenical: adults and children ages 12 and older Alli: adults only	Blocks some of the fat that you eat, keeping it from being absorbed by your body.	Stomach pain, gas, diarrhea, and leakage of oily stools. Note: Rare cases of severe liver injury reported. Should not be taken with cyclosporine.
Lorcaserin Sold as Belviq	Adults	Acts on the serotonin receptors in the brain. This may help you eat less and feel full after eating smaller amounts of food.	Headaches, dizziness, feeling tired, nausea, dry mouth, cough, and constipation. Should not be taken with selective serotonin reuptake inhibitors (SSRIs) and monoamine oxidase inhibitor (MAOI) medications.
Phentermine-topiramate Sold as Qsymia	Adults	A mix of two drugs: phentermine (suppresses your appetite and curbs your desire to eat) and topiramate (used to treat seizures or migraine headaches). May make you feel full and make foods taste less appealing.	Tingling of hands and feet, dizziness, taste alterations (particularly with carbonated beverages), trouble sleeping, constipation, and dry mouth. Note: Sold only through certified pharmacies. MAY LEAD TO BIRTH DEFECTS. DO NOT TAKE QSYMIA IF YOU ARE PREGNANT OR PLANNING A PREGNANCY.
Other appetite suppressant drugs (drugs that curb your desire to eat), which include • phentermine • benzphetamine • diethylpropion • phendimetrazine Sold under many names	Adults	Increase chemicals in the brain that affect appetite. Make you feel that you are not hungry or that you are full. Note: Only FDA approved for a short period of time (up to 12 weeks).	Dry mouth, difficulty sleeping, dizziness, headache, feeling nervous, feeling restless, upset stomach, diarrhea, and constipation.

SOURCE: "Table 1. Prescription Drugs Approved for Obesity Treatment," in *Prescription Medications for the Treatment of Obesity*, Weight-control Information Network, National Institute of Diabetes and Digestive and Kidney Diseases, National Institutes of Health, July 5, 2013, http://win.niddk.nih.gov/publications/PDFs/Prescription_Medications.pdf (accessed October 25, 2013)

2005. The FDA notes in "FDA Drug Safety Communication: Completed Safety Review of Xenical/Alli (Orlistat) and Severe Liver Injury" (May 26, 2010, http://www.fda.gov/Drugs/DrugSafety) that in rare cases orlistat can cause severe liver damage. Those taking the drug are advised to be watchful for signs of liver problems, such as itching, yellow eyes or skin, and dark urine.

Research Focuses on New Weight-Loss Drugs

Research is underway to test new drugs and drug combinations to help achieve weight loss. In "Prescription Medications for the Treatment of Obesity" (October 25, 2013, http://win.niddk.nih.gov/publications/prescription.htm), the Weight-Control Information Network (an information service of the National Institute of Diabetes and Digestive and Kidney Diseases, one of the National Institutes of Health) describes the following drug-development strategies:

• combining drugs that suppress appetite with drugs that treat addiction or reduce cravings

• stimulating hormones such as leptin that reduce appetite or increase satiety

• shrinking the blood vessels that supply fat cells to prevent the fat cells from growing

• targeting genes that affect body weight

• altering bacteria in the gut to control weight

Beloranib, an injected drug that was undergoing clinical trials in 2013, aims to help the body produce less fat and burn off excess fat as fuel. Zafgan, the company developing the drug, hopes it will produce weight loss comparable to that produced by baratric surgery. In "New Entrant in Obesity Drug Race Targets Body, Not the Mind" (Reuters.com, August 23, 2013), Esha Dey reports that Beloranib is not expected to be available until at least mid-2018.

According to Roger A. H. Adan, in "Mechanisms Underlying Current and Future Anti-obesity Drugs" (*Trends in Neuroscience*, vol. 36, no. 2, February 2013), effective drug therapy may have to target multiple pathways involved in the regulation of energy balance including the circuits and endocrine signals in the brain that govern hunger and satiety. Adan observes that because people respond differently to weight-loss drugs, optimal treatment entails a personalized approach in which the right drug is used in combination with lifestyle changes.

SURGERY

Bariatric (weight-loss) surgery is considered a good treatment option only for people for whom all other treatment methods have failed and who have a BMI of 30 or greater in the presence of comorbidities, or a BMI of 40 or higher regardless of comorbidities. Two types of surgical procedures have been demonstrated to be effective in producing weight loss maintained for five years: restrictive techniques, which reduce gastric volume, and malabsorptive procedures, which not only limit food intake but also alter digestion. An example of the first type is banded gastroplasty, in which an inflatable band that can be adjusted to different diameters is placed around the stomach, reducing its size and thus the amount of food that it can digest. (See Figure 6.3.) Another restrictive technique is sleeve gastrectomy, in which the stomach is reduced to about 25% of its original size. The Roux-en-Y gastric bypass is an example of the second technique. On average, patients maintain a weight loss of 25% to 40% of their preoperative body weight after these procedures.

Bariatric surgeries generally improve patients' quality of life by causing weight loss and the resolution of many weight-related conditions, such as sleep apnea, joint pain, and diabetes. Furthermore, in "Bariatric Surgery Is Associated with a Reduced Risk of Mortality in Morbidly Obese Patients with a History of Major Cardiovascular Events" (*American Surgeon*, vol. 78, no. 6, June 2012), Rebecca J. Johnson et al. report that bariatric surgery patients had a lower death rate than a comparable group of clinically severe obese individuals (people with BMIs of 40 or higher) who had not had surgery.

Bariatric surgical procedures are generally performed laparoscopically—via a tube inserted through a small incision in the abdomen, as opposed to open surgery. This reduces, but does not eliminate, the risk of complications, which can include death. According to Muhammad Asad Khan et al., in "Perioperative Risk Factors for 30-Day Mortality after Bariatric Surgery: Is Functional Status Important?" (*Surgical Endoscopy*, vol. 27, no. 5, May 2013), people without comorbidities and a BMI equal to or less than 50 have the lowest reported mortality rates and the fewest postsurgical complications. Not unexpectedly, those with a BMI equal to or greater than 60 with one or more comorbidities have higher mortality rates. The possibility of death or other complications due to bariatric surgery is why it is generally only recommended in cases where other obesity treatments have failed and the risks from the obesity itself are high.

People who undergo weight-loss surgeries require lifelong medical monitoring. After surgery, they are no longer able to eat in the way to which they were accustomed. Those who have undergone gastric bypass experience "dumping syndrome" when they ingest significant amounts of calorie-dense food, with symptoms such as sweating, palpitations, lightheadedness, and nausea. Over time most become conditioned not to eat such foods. Patients who have had gastric restriction surgery can only eat a limited amount of food during a single sitting without vomiting, so they must eat several small meals per day to maintain adequate nutrition. Those who do not adhere to a prescribed regimen of vitamins and minerals may develop vitamin and iron deficiencies. There are also potential postoperative and long-term complications following surgery, such as wound infections, hernias at the incision site, and gallstones. Generally, however, patients fare extremely well, experiencing dramatic improvement and even complete resolution of diabetes, hypertension (high blood pressure), and infertility, as well as improved mobility, self-esteem, and overall quality of life.

Robin Schroeder, Jordan M. Garrison Jr., and Mark S. Johnson explain in "Treatment of Adult Obesity with Bariatric Surgery" (*American Family Physician*, vol. 84, no. 7, October 1, 2011) that although there have been no long-term randomized controlled trials (studies that randomly assign some people to have the surgery and others to forgo it), currently available research shows that bariatric surgery significantly improves and frequently eliminates many obesity-related conditions (e.g., diabetes, hypertension, hyperlipidemia [elevated blood lipids]) and has a beneficial effect on mortality. More than 90% of bariatric surgeries are performed laparoscopically (using a

FIGURE 6.3

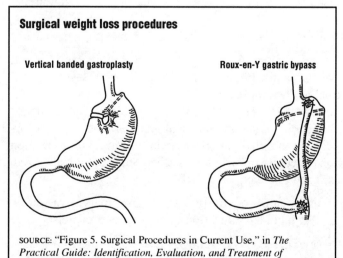

Surgical weight loss procedures

Vertical banded gastroplasty

Roux-en-Y gastric bypass

SOURCE: "Figure 5. Surgical Procedures in Current Use," in *The Practical Guide: Identification, Evaluation, and Treatment of Overweight and Obesity in Adults*, National Institutes of Health, National Heart, Lung, and Blood Institute, North American Association for the Study of Obesity, October 2000, http://www.nhlbi.nih.gov/guidelines/obesity/prctgd_b.pdf (accessed October 28, 2013)

thin tube that is inserted in a small incision to insert instruments and perform the procedure), which results in fewer wound complications, shorter hospital stays, and more rapid recovery than open surgery.

The Number of Weight-Loss Surgeries

Schroeder, Garrison, and Johnson report that the number of bariatric surgical procedures performed in the United States rose from 13,365 in 1998 to more than 200,000 in 2008. The American Society for Metabolic and Bariatric Surgery (an organization that advocates for the study and practice of bariatric surgery) reports in the fact sheet "Metabolic and Bariatric Surgery" (May 2013, http://s3 .amazonaws.com/publicASMBS/Resources/Fact-Sheets/ Metabolic-Bariatric-Surgery-Fact-Sheet-ASMBS2012.pdf) that approximately 160,000 people had bariatric surgery in 2010, just 1% of the population of people who met the guidelines for bariatric surgery.

Bariatric Surgery Can Benefit the Whole Family

In "Halo Effect for Bariatric Surgery" (*Archives of Surgery*, vol. 146, no. 10, October 2011), Gavitt A. Woodard et al. of the Stanford University School of Medicine discuss changes in weight and health behaviors of 35 patients who underwent bariatric surgery and their families for one year. The researchers find that one year after surgery the families (spouses, children, and other relatives of the surgical patients) lost significant amounts of weight, increased their activity levels, and adopted other healthy behaviors. They drank less alcohol, watched less television, and reported fewer instances of emotional eating. Woodard et al. conclude that "this study demonstrates that performing a gastric bypass operation on 1 patient has a halo of positive effect on the weight, eating habits, activity levels, and health behaviors of the entire family."

COUNSELING AND BEHAVIORAL THERAPY

Weight-loss counseling and behavioral therapy aim to assist people to develop the skills needed to identify and modify behaviors and patterns of thinking that undermine weight-control efforts. Behavioral strategies include self-monitoring of weight, food intake, and physical activity; identifying and controlling stimuli that provoke overeating; identifying and solving problems; and using family and social support systems to reinforce weight-control efforts. Counseling and behavioral therapy are often perceived as necessary components of comprehensive weight-loss treatment, but are also viewed as labor intensive because educating and supporting people seeking to lose weight is time consuming. The effort also requires the active participation of everyone who may be involved in treatment: the affected individuals, their families, physicians, nurses, nutritionists, dieticians, exercise instructors, and mental health professionals. In view of the considerable resources

that must be allocated to deliver counseling and behavioral therapy, it is important to know if these approaches promote weight loss effectively.

Erin S. LeBlanc et al. considered the evidence supporting the efficacy of counseling and behavioral therapy as well as other treatment methods and present their findings in "Effectiveness of Primary Care–Relevant Treatments for Obesity in Adults: A Systematic Evidence Review for the U.S. Preventive Services Task Force" (*Annals of Internal Medicine*, vol. 155, no. 7, October 4, 2011). The researchers report that counseling to promote change in diet, exercise, or both, and behavioral therapy to help patients acquire the skills, motivations, and support to change diet and exercise patterns enabled obese patients to achieve modest but clinically significant and sustained (one to two years) weight loss. Furthermore, LeBlanc et al. observe that because control groups also frequently received some form of counseling, education, or support, they might have underestimated the effectiveness of counseling.

Not unexpectedly, more intensive programs, with higher numbers of treatment sessions and/or more frequent contact, were generally more successful and produced greater weight loss, as were those that incorporated behavioral therapy. Behavioral therapy–based treatments resulted in 6.6 pounds (3 kg) greater weight loss, compared with control groups, after 12 to 18 months. LeBlanc et al. also indicate that weight-loss treatment reduced diabetes incidence among people with prediabetes.

Pharmacotherapy also improved weight loss. People who received drug treatment (orlistat) along with behavioral intervention had greater weight loss, compared with those who were given a placebo. LeBlanc et al. conclude that behavioral weight-loss interventions, with or without pharmacotherapy, produce clinically meaningful weight loss.

A Study of Three Weight-Loss Counseling Approaches

In "Changes in Eating, Physical Activity, and Related Behaviors in a Primary-Care-Based Weight Loss Intervention" (*International Journal of Obesity* [London], vol. 37, no. S12–S18, August 2013), Sheri Volger et al. analyzed changes in eating and physical activity in adults who participated in a two-year behavioral weight-loss intervention conducted in a primary care setting. Study participants were assigned to either:

- usual care—quarterly visits to a primary care setting that included education about diet and exercise

- brief lifestyle counseling—quarterly primary care visits plus monthly counseling sessions about weight control

- enhanced brief lifestyle counseling—quarterly primary care visits, monthly lifestyle counseling, and a choice of meal replacements or weight-loss medication

After two years, participants in the two groups that included lifestyle counseling had significantly more improvement in self-reported measures of appetite control, dietary intake, and physical activity than did the participants receiving only usual care. At month 24, participants in the brief lifestyle counseling had lost an average of 6.4 pounds (2.9 kg), and those in enhanced brief lifestyle counseling had lost average of 10.1 pounds (4.6 kg). By comparison, those receiving usual care had lost 3.7 pounds (1.7 kg) on average. Volger et al. conclude, "a primary care-based lifestyle intervention delivered by primary care providers, with the assistance of auxiliary health care workers, can result in clinically meaningful weight loss in some patients."

Comparing Weight-Loss Using a Clinic-Based Program and a Commercial Program

Steven Fox reports in "Advantages Seen with Clinic-Based Weight-Loss Programs" (Medscape.com, October 19, 2011) that Adam Tsai et al. conducted a pilot study in Denver, Colorado, and presented their findings at the Obesity Society 29th Annual Scientific Meeting in Orlando, Florida, in 2011. The researchers indicated that some clinic-based weight-loss programs may produce better outcomes than commercial weight-loss programs.

Tsai et al. compared the efficacy of two programs: Weight Watchers and a clinic-based individualized treatment approach. Study subjects were randomly assigned to attend Weight Watchers for 17 weeks or to receive 12 individual counseling sessions lasting from 20 to 30 minutes with a nurse nutritionist. Subjects assigned to the clinic program were offered the option of using meal replacements or using the weight-loss medication phentermine. Four months after completing the programs, the subjects were evaluated for weight loss, blood pressure, waist circumference, and health-related quality of life.

Tsai et al. find that the subjects in the clinic-based group lost significantly more weight than those in the commercial weight-loss program. However, no significant differences in blood pressure, waist circumference, or health-related quality of life were found between the two groups of subjects.

Comparing Weight-Loss Counseling from a Primary Care Physician and a Commercial Program

Interestingly, the results of a study comparing people receiving weight-loss guidance from a primary care physician and those participating in Weight Watchers indicate that the commercial program yields better results. Susan A. Jebb et al. find in "Primary Care Referral to a Commercial Provider for Weight Loss Treatment versus Standard Care: A Randomised Controlled Trial" (*Lancet*, vol. 378, no. 9801, October 22, 2011) that after 12 months subjects attending Weight Watchers lost twice as much weight as those who received only physician guidance (15 pounds

[6.8 kg] versus 7 pounds [3.2 kg]). Participants in the Weight Watchers group also had greater reductions in waist circumference and fat mass. Jebb et al. conclude that "referral by a primary health care professional to a commercial weight loss programme that provides regular weighing, advice about diet and physical activity, motivation, and group support can offer a clinically useful early intervention for weight management in overweight and obese people that can be delivered at large scale."

New Approaches

Comprehensive and holistic weight-loss programs that address diet, nutrition, physical activity, stress and an array of emotional and behavioral issues promise to help people seeking lasting weight loss and better health. Working with individuals, groups, and corporations many of these programs combine high-tech and high-touch approaches. For example, Retrofit, started by Mark Hyman in March 2011, promises to help people lose weight and become healthier over the course of 12 months using team support from a registered dietician, exercise physiologist, behavior coach, and program manager. Clients meet via weekly Skype meetings and their activity and weight are monitored using wireless activity trackers and scales. As of March 2014 the Retrofit program cost roughly $125 a month.

Weight-Loss Counseling Online

An expanding array of diet, counseling, and support group programs are available on the Internet; however, there is little comparative research available on these programs, including any studies to determine their efficacy. In the landmark study "A Randomized Trial Comparing Human E-Mail Counseling, Computer-Automated Tailored Counseling, and No Counseling in an Internet Weight Loss Program" (*Archives of Internal Medicine*, vol. 166, no. 15, August 2006), Deborah F. Tate, Elizabeth H. Jackvony, and Rena R. Wing sought to determine whether computer-generated feedback, delivered via the Internet, would prove to be a viable alternative to human counseling via e-mail. They compared the effects of custom-tailored computer-automated interactions with an Internet program that provided weight-loss counseling from a human via e-mail.

Participants were randomly selected to be in one of three treatment groups: human e-mail counseling, computer-automated feedback, or no counseling. All the subjects received one weight-loss group session, coupons for meal replacements, and access to an interactive website, but the human e-mail counseling and computer-automated feedback groups also had access to an e-diary and a message board. The human e-mail counseling group received weekly e-mail feedback from a counselor, the computer-automated feedback group received automated, custom-tailored messages, and the control group did not receive any counseling. Recommendations included calorie-restricted diets of between 1,200 and 1,500 calories per day, daily exercise equivalent to walking for 30 minutes, and instructions about how to use meal replacement products. All the participants were encouraged to self-monitor their diet and exercise using diaries and calorie books. Both groups accessed the same website, which featured weekly reporting and graphs of weight, weekly e-mail prompts to report weight, weekly weight-loss tips via e-mail, recipes, and a weight-loss e-buddy network system that enabled users to interact with other dieters with similar characteristics via e-mail.

The primary outcome measure used to compare the groups was change in body weight from baseline at three and six months. Both the human and automated e-counseling groups had greater reductions in weight than the control group at each weigh-in. Tate, Jackvony, and Wing conclude that automated computer feedback was as effective as human e-mail counseling.

Kevin O. Hwang et al. describe in "Website Usage and Weight Loss in a Free Commercial Online Weight Loss Program: Retrospective Cohort Study" (*Journal of Medical Internet Research*, vol. 15, no. 1, January 2013) the association between use of SparkPeople, a free commercial online weight-loss program, and weight loss. Hwang et al. find that active participation—logging-in, entering weight, or entering food at least four times per 30 days—was associated with greater weight loss. The researchers posit that in addition to engagement with the program, "weight self-monitoring leads to frequent modification of diet and exercise behavior in response to weights," which in turn spurs weight-loss efforts.

Mobile Apps for Weight-Loss

Smartphones offer dieters a wide range of mobile apps to help motivate them and track diet and exercise. In "Evidence-Based Strategies in Weight-Loss Mobile Apps" (*American Journal of Preventive Medicine*, vol. 45, no. 5, November 2013), Sherry Pagoto et al. look at 31 weight-loss apps to determine whether they contain any of 20 behavioral strategies that have proven effective. The researchers report that the apps include an average of less than 20% of the strategies proven to be effective. The top two apps—MyNetDiary PRO and MyNetDiary—included 65% of the strategies. Out of the 20 strategies, seven were not included in any app. Pagoto et al. feel that many of the strategies that were included in the apps, such as barcode scanners to instantly obtain products' nutritional information, social networks where users can support one another, email and text reminders, and diaries for tracking exercise and food intake, are helpful, but hope that the next generation of apps will incorporate additional strategies.

COMPLEMENTARY AND ALTERNATIVE THERAPIES

Many complementary and alternative medicine practices such as yoga, Dahn (a holistic mind-body training method), and mindful eating (which teaches greater awareness of bodily sensations such as hunger and satiety [the feeling of fullness or satisfaction after eating] and helps people to identify "emotional eating") have been used to promote weight loss. However, acupuncture (the Chinese practice of inserting extremely thin, sterile needles into any of 360 specific points on the body) and hypnosis are the only alternative medical practices that have been studied as potential treatments for obesity. Several studies report that acupuncture does not appear to have any benefit greater than a placebo.

Hypnosis is an altered state of consciousness. It is a state of heightened awareness and suggestibility and enables focused concentration that may be used to alter perceptions of hunger and satiety and to modify behavior. Hypnosis is considered a mainstream treatment for addictions and overeating. Regardless, there are conflicting data about its effectiveness—some studies find that it adds little, if any, benefit beyond that of a placebo, whereas others conclude that hypnosis may have some initial benefit for people seeking weight loss, but that it has little sustained effect.

In "Pilot Study: Mindful Eating and Living (MEAL): Weight, Eating Behavior, and Psychological Outcomes Associated with a Mindfulness-Based Intervention for People with Obesity" (*Complementary Therapies in Medicine*, vol. 18, no. 6, December 2010), Jeanne Dalon et al. report the results of a pilot study of a six-week group program that provides mindfulness training—meditation, mindful eating, and group discussion, with emphasis on awareness of body sensations, emotions, and triggers to overeat—to people who are obese. The researchers find that subjects receiving this intervention showed statistically significant increases in measures of mindfulness and thoughtful restraint around eating, and statistically significant decreases in weight, impulsive and binge eating, depression, and perceived stress. Dalon et al. conclude that this pilot study suggests that an "eating focused mindfulness-based intervention can result in significant changes in weight, eating behavior, and psychological distress in obese individuals." In "Does Mindfulness Matter? Everyday Mindfulness, Mindful Eating and Self-Reported Serving Size of Energy Dense Foods among a Sample of South Australian Adults" (*Appetite*, vol. 67, August 2013), Monica Beshara, Amanda D. Hutchinson, and Carlene Wilson report that mindful eating is connected to serving size moderation, supporting the premise that mindfulness does change eating behaviors.

According to Asker E. Jeukendrup and Rebecca Randell of the University of Birmingham, in "Fat Burners: Nutrition Supplements That Increase Fat Metabolism" (*Obesity Reviews*, vol. 12, no. 10, October 2011), a number of nutritional supplements such as caffeine, carnitine, chromium, conjugated linoleic acid, forskolin, fucoxanthin, green tea, and kelp are promoted as "fat burners" and are being used to promote weight loss. Jeukendrup and Randell observe that some of these supplements have demonstrated some benefit but have not yet been rigorously tested. Caffeine and green tea have demonstrated fat metabolism–enhancing properties; however, evidence is lacking for the others. As a result, health care professionals cannot definitively recommend their use.

In "Eight Weeks of Supplementation with a Multiingredient Weight Loss Product Enhances Body Composition, Reduces Hip and Waist Girth, and Increases Energy Levels in Overweight Men and Women" (*Journal of the International Society of Sports Nutrition*, vol. 10, no. 1, April 2013), Hector L. Lopez et al. evaluate the effectiveness of a multi-ingredient supplement containing vitamins, raspberry ketone, caffeine, capsaicin, garlic, ginger, and Citrus aurantium. One group of subjects followed a calorie-restricted diet, had exercise training, and took the supplement. A second group followed the same diet and exercise plan but did not take the supplement. Lopez et al. find that after eight weeks, subjects taking the supplement lost significantly more weight and body fat and their waist and hip circumference decreased more than subjects who did not take the supplement.

MIGHT WEIGHT LOSS BE HARMFUL?

Successful weight-loss treatments generally result in improved health: reduced blood pressure, reduced triglycerides, reduced total cholesterol and LDL cholesterol, and increased HDL cholesterol. Weight loss of as little as 5% to 10% of initial weight produces measurable health benefits and may prevent illnesses among people at risk. These findings suggest that treatment should not exclusively focus on the medical consequences of obesity, but that obesity itself should be treated. National Institutes of Health guidelines recommend weight loss for people with a BMI greater than 30 and for people with a BMI greater than 25 with two or more obesity-related risk factors. The guidelines also recommend that for people with a BMI of between 25 and 30 without other risk factors, the focus should be on prevention of further weight gain, rather than on weight loss.

There is evidence, however, that weight cycling—repeated cycles of weight gain and loss, a not uncommon occurrence among people trying to lose weight—is associated with metabolic and cardiovascular health problems. In "Weight Cycling Increases T Cell Accumulation in Adipose Tissue and Impairs Systemic Glucose Tolerance" (*Diabetes*, vol. 62, no. 9, September 2013), Emily K. Anderson et al. indicate that weight cycling may contribute to metabolic problems by impairing glucose tolerance and insulin sensitivity. This in turn increases risk for diabetes and cardiovascular disease.

Kevin Y. Taing, Chris I. Ardern, and Jennifer L. Kuk question whether weight cycling increases the risk of death. In "Effect of the Timing of Weight Cycling during Adulthood on Mortality Risk in Overweight and Obese Postmenopausal Women" (*Obesity*, July 14, 2011), the researchers analyze data of 47,473 overweight and obese women aged 50 to 79 years. The women were classified as stable (WgtV) or as a weight-gainer or -loser (WgtC) based on weight changes during early adulthood (18 to 35 years), middle age (35 to 50 years), and later (50 years to current age) adulthood. Those with weight changes of less than 5% during all three periods were classified as being stable weight. Weight-gainers were those with at least one period of weight gain (greater than 5%) without a period of weight loss (greater than or equal to 5%), and weight-losers were those with at least one period of weight loss without a period of weight gain. Those who experienced both a period of weight gain and loss were termed WgtC. Those classified as WgtC and WgtV throughout adulthood did not have higher mortality risk than weight-stable women when the age period of weight change was not considered. However, when the age periods were analyzed, increased mortality risk was observed for every 11 pounds (5 kg) of weight gain during early or middle age or for every 11 pounds of weight loss since middle age or late adulthood. Taing, Ardern, and Kuk suggest that simply looking at WgtC and WgtV by weight changes across adulthood may not accurately assess mortality risk—the age at which the weight changes occur may influence whether the weight change poses increased risk.

Is It Really Dangerous to Be Overweight?

The health risks and consequences of obesity are well understood, but the risk of death associated with overweight remains unclear. In "Association of All-Cause Mortality with Overweight and Obesity Using Standard Body Mass Index Categories" (*JAMA*, vol. 309, no. 1, January 2, 2013), Katherine M. Flegal et al. estimate the relationship between BMI and risk of death associated with normal weight, overweight, and obesity. The researchers find that compared with normal weight, overweight (BMI 25 to 29.9) was associated with a significantly decreased risk of death. People who were somewhat obese (BMI 30 to 34.9) had roughly the same mortality level as people of normal weight. People with a BMI of 35 or higher had a higher risk of death than people of normal weight.

David Faeh et al. analyzed data from 9,853 Swiss men and women aged 25 to 74 years to determine the relationship between BMI and mortality and published their findings in "Obesity but Not Overweight Is Associated with Increased Mortality Risk" (*European Journal of Epidemiology*, vol. 26, no. 8, August 2011). The researchers indicate that obesity, but not overweight, was associated with an increased mortality risk, which was largely attributable to an increased risk of death from cardiovascular disease and cancer. Faeh et al. conclude that public health interventions should "focus on preventing normal- and overweight persons from becoming obese."

CHAPTER 7
THE ECONOMICS OF OVERWEIGHT AND OBESITY

The economic impact of obesity is considerable. In "Economic Costs of Overweight and Obesity" (*Best Practice & Research: Clinical Endocrinology & Metabolism*, vol. 27, no. 2, April 2013), Thomas Lehnert et al. report that up to 20% of total annual U.S. health care expenditures, around $190 billion, are spent on obesity-related health care. The researchers assert that the direct health care costs for overweight individuals are about 10% greater than costs for normal weight individuals. Obese individuals have even higher direct health care costs compared with normal weight individuals. Those with class I obesity (those with a body mass index [BMI; body weight in kilograms divided by height in meters squared] of 30 to 34.9) had annual costs around 23% higher, class II obesity (BMI of 35 to 39.9) was associated with 45% higher annual costs, and class II obesity (BMI 40 or higher) led to 81% higher annual costs. Persons with class III obesity, despite accounting for a relatively small proportion of the total population of people who are overweight, incur a substantial amount of the total direct health care costs associated with overweight and obesity. Examples of direct health care costs are physician office visits, hospital and nursing home charges, prescription drug costs, and special hospital beds to accommodate obese patients. The indirect costs of overweight and obesity are measured in terms of decreased earnings: lost wages and lower productivity resulting from the inability to work because of illness or disability, as well as the value of future earnings lost by premature mortality (death). Estimates of indirect costs vary, but several studies suggest that the monetary loss resulting from lost productivity is several times larger than direct health care costs.

According to Y. Claire Wang et al., in "Health and Economic Burden of the Projected Obesity Trends in the USA and the UK" (*Lancet*, vol. 378, no. 9793, August 27, 2011), the economic losses attributable to health care costs and lost productivity are projected to increase. By 2020 three out of four Americans will be overweight or obese and by 2030 there will be an additional 65 million obese adults in the United States. Obesity-related health care costs are attributable not only to increased risk for type 2 diabetes, cardiovascular diseases, and several forms of cancer but also to costly and disabling conditions such as osteoarthritis, asthma, infertility, and sleep apnea. Along with health care costs and lost productivity, there are indirect costs as a result of decreased years of disability-free life, increased mortality before retirement, early retirement, and disability benefits.

There are other economic consequences and personal costs of obesity: obese workers may earn less than their healthy-weight counterparts because of job discrimination. Also, many insurance companies, particularly in the life insurance sector, charge higher premiums with increasing degrees of overweight. When obesity compromises physical functioning and limits activities of daily living, affected individuals may require assistance from home health aides, durable medical equipment such as walkers or wheelchairs, or other costly adaptations to accommodate disability.

THE HIGH COST OF OVERWEIGHT AND OBESITY

Because overweight and obesity have been linked to an increased risk for many chronic conditions, it may be argued that some percentage of the costs attributed to arthritis, cancer, diabetes, heart disease, and stroke are also attributable to obesity. It is important to remember that estimates of the medical care costs, direct and indirect as well as total cost of overweight and obesity in the United States, vary depending on how the conditions are defined, whether overweight and obesity are considered together or separately, and which costs and obesity-related conditions are included in the estimates and projections.

According to Eric A. Finkelstein et al., in "Annual Medical Spending Attributable to Obesity: Payer- and Service-Specific Estimates" (*Health Affairs*, vol. 28, no. 5, September–October 2009), annual medical care expenditures attributable to overweight and obesity doubled between 1998 and 2006. During this period obesity (BMI of 30 or higher) increased by 39%, prompting an 89% increase in health care costs attributable to obesity. Finkelstein et al. estimate that the direct cost of overweight and obesity in 2006 was 9.1% of the total U.S. health care expenditures, up from 6.5% in 1998. Of this 9.1%, roughly 3.7% was attributable to overweight and 5.3% to obesity. An obese person incurred about 42% more costs than a healthy-weight person, which translates into $1,429 more (per obese person) per year for medical care. The majority of these dollars were spent treating obesity-related diseases and disorders.

According to Finkelstein et al., the estimated cost increase associated with being overweight was 14.5% ($247) and ranged from 11.4% ($53) for out-of-pocket spending to 15.1% ($271) for Medicaid (a federal and state health care program for people below the poverty level). The average increase in annual medical spending associated with obesity was 37.4% ($732) and ranged from 26.1% ($125) for out-of-pocket spending to 36.8% ($1,486) for Medicare (a medical insurance program for older adults and people with disabilities) and 39.1% ($864) for Medicaid. Obesity was responsible for nearly $40 billion of increased medical spending through 2006, including $7 billion in Medicare prescription drug costs.

Finkelstein et al. observe that the lifetime costs of overweight and obesity borne by the government are likely to be greater than the lifetime costs imposed by smokers. Furthermore, the results of this study reveal that obese people who live to age 65 have much larger annual Medicare expenditures than their normal-weight peers.

In *Obesity and Its Relation to Mortality and Morbidity Costs* (December 2010, http://www.soa.org/assets/DownloadAsset.aspx?id=30063), Donald F. Behan et al. estimate that the economic cost of overweight and obesity in the United States and Canada was $300 billion in 2009, with just $30 billion attributed to Canada. Roughly $220 billion is attributed to obesity, the remaining $80 to overweight. Behan et al. attribute $127 billion to health care costs, $49 billion to loss of productivity resulting from early death, $43 billion to disability of active workers, and $72 billion to loss of productivity of totally disabled workers.

In "Obesity and Severe Obesity Forecasts through 2030" (*American Journal of Preventive Medicine*, vol. 42, no. 6, June 2012), Eric A. Finkelstein et al. predict that between 2010 and 2030 the prevalence of obesity in the United States will increase 33% and clinically severe obesity will increase 130%. The researchers observe that if these increases do not occur, and obesity prevalence remains at about the 2010 levels, then the savings in health care expenditures over the two decades would be $549 billion.

Wang et al. concur with Finkelstein et al. and offer projections for 2030 that are based on current trends of BMI in the U.S. population. The researchers forecast an excess of 8 million cases of diabetes, 6 million to 8 million cases of heart disease and stroke, and more than 1.5 million cases of cancer. This forecast translates into an increase in annual medical costs of treating obesity-related disorders from $28 billion per year in 2020 to $66 billion per year in 2030.

The Impact of Obesity Costs on a State Economy

The high costs of obesity have prompted states to fund obesity prevention and control efforts. For example, in "State- and Payer-Specific Estimates of Annual Medical Expenditures Attributable to Obesity" (*Obesity*, vol. 20, no. 1, January 2012), Justin G. Trogdon et al. report that from 22% of the state-level costs of obesity in Virginia to 55% of the costs in Rhode Island are financed by Medicare and Medicaid. The researchers calculate that without obesity-related expenses, the states' annual medical expenditures would be reduced by 6.7% to 10.7%.

Assessing the Costs of Treating Childhood and Adolescent Obesity

In "Payment for Obesity Services: Examples and Recommendations for Stage 3 Comprehensive Multidisciplinary Intervention Programs for Children and Adolescents" (*Pediatrics*, vol. 128, suppl. 2, September 1, 2011), Wendy Slusser et al. explain that "health insurers and hospitals often have to evaluate coverage of obesity care services on a case-by-case basis, which creates a barrier between patients and providers." The researchers interviewed several hospital-based programs and find that most programs fell short of operating expenses. For example, the Duke Children's Health Lifestyles Program is funded by grants and clinic-visit payments and revenue is about 10% less than operating expenses each year. Approximately 40% of reimbursement is from Medicaid, 30% from private insurance such as BlueCross, BlueShield, and Aetna, 20% from managed care plans, and 10% from the Duke employee health plan.

Slusser et al. observe that recent research demonstrates that obesity interventions, especially those with intensive treatment regimens, are effective. The results of these studies support the premise that effective treatment approaches obesity as a chronic condition that requires ongoing care. The U.S. Preventive Services Task Force reviewed childhood and adolescent obesity interventions and found that medium- to high-intensity comprehensive behavioral interventions were most effective in the treatment of obesity. Slusser et al. indicate that "no statewide or national efforts are testing models of payment packages for children treated by a multidisciplinary team.... However, these efforts are desperately needed, given the near-doubling of hospital admissions and an associated increase in costs from $125.9 million in 1999 (adjusted for inflation) to $237.6 million in 2005 among US children aged 2 to 19 years with a diagnosis of obesity." They assert that intensive obesity interventions should be reimbursed, consistent with the White House Task Force on Childhood Obesity report *Solving the Problem of Childhood Obesity within a Generation: White House Task Force on Childhood Obesity Report to the President* (May 2010, http://www.letsmove.gov/white-house-task-force-childhood-obesity-report-president), which states that "federally funded and private insurance plans should cover services necessary to prevent, assess, and provide care to overweight and obese children."

In "Treatment of Childhood and Adolescent Obesity: An Integrative Review of Recent Recommendations from Five Expert Groups" (*Journal of Consulting and Clinical Psychology*, vol. 81, no. 2, 2013), Daniel S. Kirschenbaum and Kristen Gierut explain that that cost-effective treatments are urgently needed, stating, "even if all of the professional counselors in the United States devoted themselves only to treating obesity in children and adults (over 100 million potential clients), they could not keep up with the demand. Even if the numbers could work, consider the cost for such services on such a massive scale. Those numbers do not work either." The researchers consider self-help groups such as Weight Watchers and outpatient cognitive behavioral therapy, especially when delivered by telephone or via the Internet, as effective for adolescents and relatively low-cost. More costly treatment such as therapeutic summer camps have produced promising results but are not covered by insurance. Kirschenbaum and Gierut acknowledge that bariatric surgery is effective treatment for limited numbers of extremely overweight young people when all other approaches fail.

Medicare and Medicaid Coverage for Obesity Treatment

Medicare is a program run by the U.S. federal government that provides subsidized health care to Americans aged 65 years and older who paid into the system when they were younger (and certain other individuals). It is the single largest health insurance provider in the country. Medicaid provides subsidized health insurance to people who could not otherwise afford health care. The second-largest health insurance provider in the country, it is operated jointly by the federal government and state governments, with many details of the program varying from state to state.

Although Medicare and Medicaid spend billions of dollars on obesity-related illnesses, these government programs offer only limited coverage for treatment of obesity itself. In "Decision Memo for Intensive Behavioral Therapy for Obesity" (November 29, 2011, http://www.cms.gov/), the Centers for Medicare and Medicaid Services (CMS) announced that Medicare would begin covering intensive behavioral therapy for obesity, consisting of obesity screening and dietary assessment, behavioral counseling, and behavioral therapy to promote sustained weight loss through diet and exercise. As of 2014 Medicare covered one face-to-face visit every week for the first month followed by one face-to-face visit every other week for months two through six. If the beneficiary met the weight-loss requirement, a loss of at least 6.6 pounds (3 kg) over the course of the first six months of intensive therapy, then one face-to-face visit every month for months seven through twelve was also covered.

Bariatric (weight-loss) surgery is covered by Medicare for patients with a BMI of 35 or more who have comorbidities (additional disorders, such as diabetes or heart disease) and who have failed to lose weight in a medical weight-loss program. Medicare Part D is the primary means through which prescription drugs are covered under Medicare. When someone enrolls in Medicare Part D, they choose from different drug coverage plans available in their area. Weight-loss drugs are not included in the list of drugs that Medicare requires all plans to cover, but some plans do include them as an added benefit.

In view of the high prevalence of obesity among the populations covered by Medicaid, and the significant Medicaid expenditures for obesity-related illnesses, many health care industry observers believe it is shortsighted that some states specifically exclude coverage of anti-obesity products in their Medicaid programs. According to Christine C. Ferguson of the STOP Obesity Alliance at the George Washington University, in "State Survey of Coverage of Obesity Interventions Finds Coverage of Treatment Options Limited for Overweight and Obese Populations across the United States" (May 2011, http://www.stopobesityalliance.org/wp-content/assets/2011/05/Spring-2011-Obesity-and-the-States-Bulletin-FINAL.pdf), coverage varied widely as of 2011. For example, California covered weight-loss drugs and the full spectrum of bariatric surgical procedures, while Arizona excluded weight-loss drugs and bariatric surgical procedures from coverage. Overall, Ferguson reports that 27 states did not cover weight-loss drugs under Medicaid and 7 did not cover bariatric surgery. Some health care analysts and advocacy groups, including the Obesity Society (formerly the American Obesity Association), contend that it is difficult to reconcile limited coverage of obesity in light of Medicaid coverage for inpatient and outpatient alcohol detoxification and rehabilitation, chemical dependency treatment and drug rehabilitation, and services for sexual impotence.

In "Medicaid Coverage for Weight Loss Counseling May Make 'Cents'" (*Journal of Internal Medicine*, vol. 28, no. 1, January 2013), Sara N. Bleich and Bradley J. Herring assert that coverage of screening and behavioral weight-loss programs in the Medicaid program may be crucial for cost containment. Screening for obesity without also covering the cost of weight-loss counseling may not reduce obesity rates because a weekly fee for a program such as Weight Watchers may be unaffordable for people at or near poverty. Bleich and Herring opine, "Coverage of commercial weight-loss programs like Weight Watchers by the Medicaid program may not solve the problem of obesity, but—given the magnitude of the epidemic—even modest reductions in weight can lead to significant health benefits and reduced costs."

Private Insurance

In "Obamacare Requires Most Insurers to Tackle Obesity" (usatoday.com, July 4, 2013) Nanci Hellmich reports that the Patient Protection and Affordable Care Act (ACA) requires private health insurance providers to help obese patients try to lose weight but that "exactly how they do it is up to the individual plans." The ACA stipulates that screening and counseling must be covered with no patient cost-sharing, no deductibles or co-payments; health plans, however, vary in terms of covered services. Some plans offer counseling by telephone, others offer visits with a health coach, a dietician, or group counseling sessions, and some refer patients to programs such as Weight Watchers. Many health plans are reported to be adopting the same coverage provided by Medicare.

George Loewenstein, David A. Asch, and Kevin G. Volpp report in "Behavioral Economics Holds Potential to Deliver Better Results for Patients, Insurers, and Employers" (*Health Affairs*, vol. 32, no. 7, July 2013) that many employers, insurers, and health care providers use incentives to encourage patients to take better care of themselves. Loewenstein, Asch, and Volpp opine that many such programs may not be effective because in their existing forms they require people to have high levels of expertise, motivation and self-control to modify their behaviors. Instead, they propose that incentive programs offer people small and frequent payments for positive health and lifestyle behaviors, under the premise that highly visible rewards such as these will be more effective, and cheaper, than typical incentives such as a reduction in a health care premium.

The Pharmacy Benefit Management Institute (PBMI), an independent organization that is not affiliated with any employee benefits program or pharmaceutical manufacturer, periodically surveys employers to determine the extent, cost, and coverage of their pharmacy benefits. It publishes the survey data and trends in *Prescription Drug Benefit Cost and Plan Design Report*. The PBMI explains in *2012–2013 Prescription Drug Benefit Cost and Plan Design Report* (2013, http://www.pbmi.com/BenefitDesign.asp) that in 2013 nearly half of employers (47%) excluded weight-loss drugs from their coverage. Just 12% of employers surveyed offered complete, unlimited coverage of weight-loss drugs.

OVERWEIGHT WORKERS MAY PAY MORE FOR HEALTH INSURANCE COVERAGE. As John Tozzi reports in "Will Workplace Wellness Screenings under Obamacare Improve Health?" (Businessweek.com, May 16, 2013), as of 2014 the ACA authorizes employer-provided health plans to charge high premiums to people who are obese (as well as people with certain other conditions or behaviors, such as smoking). The higher premiums are intended to encourage people to take action to become healthier. This approach is closely tied to the rise of workplace wellness plans. The specifics of wellness plans vary from one company to another, but in general they involve rewarding employees for participating in health screenings and activities intended to improve their health, or penalizing them for not doing so.

As Tozzi notes, the use of premium incentives to encourage weight loss is controversial. It is unclear if they genuinely motivate people to take action, or if they just shift costs onto less-healthy employees. What is clear is that the trend toward wellness programs is strong, with 61% of companies reporting that they rewarded employees for participating in such programs in 2012, up from 36% in 2009.

In "CVS Pharmacy Wants Workers' Health Information, or They'll Pay a Fine" (ABCNews.go.com, March 20, 2013), Steve Osunsami describes measures that go further than charging overweight and obese workers more for health insurance and health care services. Osunsami reports that beginning in May 2014, CVS Pharmacy requires employees enrolled in its health plan to submit their weight, body fat, and blood glucose levels each month or pay a $50 fine each month. Richard Besser, ABC News' chief health and medical editor, explains that programs such as this one are intended to improve employee health and reduce employer costs, however critics view it as penalizing workers and say the policy is coercive and discriminatory.

FUNDING OBESITY RESEARCH

Table 7.1 shows National Institutes of Health (NIH) funding for research into a variety of diseases and research areas for fiscal years (FYs) 2009 to 2012, as well as estimates for FYs 2013 and 2014. Baseline

TABLE 7.1

Estimates of funding for various research, conditions, and disease categories, fiscal years 2009–14

Research/disease areas (Dollars in millions and rounded)	Fiscal year 2009 actual (Non-ARRA)	Fiscal year 2009 actual (ARRA)[j]	Fiscal year 2010 actual (Non-ARRA)	Fiscal year 2010 actual (ARRA)[j]	Fiscal year 2011 actual	Fiscal year 2012 actual	Fiscal year 2013 estimated	Fiscal year 2014 estimated
Acute respiratory distress syndrome	$103	$17	$110	$22	$96	$98	$98	$98
Adolescent sexual activity	+	+	$80	$7	$69	$76	$76	$77
Agent Orange & Dioxin	$13	$2	$11	$1	$8	$8	$8	$8
Aging	$3,015	$554	$2,517	$443	$2,572	$2,593	$2,591	$2,596
Alcoholism	$441	$75	$454	$65	$452	$455	$458	$460
Allergic rhinitis (hay fever)	$4	$1	$3	$1	$7	$7	$7	$7
ALS	$43	$13	$47	$12	$44	$44	$44	$44
Alzheimer's disease	$457	$77	$450	$79	$448	$503	$484	$562
American Indians/Alaska Natives	$169	$19	$151	$16	$136	$170	$153	$153
Anorexia	$8	$2	$9	$2	$11	$14	$14	$14
Anthrax	$102	$13	$118	$12	$87	$84	$84	$84
Antimicrobial resistance	$251	$52	$356	$66	$369	$377	$379	$379
Aphasia	$22	$3	$21	$1	$21	$24	$25	$25
Arctic	$28	$6	$34	$3	$28	$23	$23	$23
Arthritis	$246	$65	$249	$59	$231	$258	$260	$260
Assistive technology	$249	$43	$250	$48	$250	$237	$239	$240
Asthma	$284	$51	$244	$33	$221	$229	$230	$231
Ataxia telangiectasia	$13	$2	$12	$1	$13	$11	$11	$11
Atherosclerosis	$495	$112	$544	$104	$475	$477	$480	$480
Attention deficit disorder (ADD)	$71	$13	$66	$15	$55	$60	$60	$60
Autism	$132	$64	$160	$58	$169	$192	$193	$192
Autoimmune disease	$879	$138	$856	$125	$869	$867	$871	$872
Basic behavioral and social science	$1,410	$206	$1,163	$198	$1,173	$1,215	$1,213	$1,216
Batten disease	$5	$2	$5	$1	$4	$4	$4	$4
Behavioral and social science	$3,471	$582	$3,526	$603	$3,573	$3,682	$3,685	$3,708
Biodefense[a]	$1,755	$213	$1,794	$221	$1,803	$1,791	$1,802	$1,804
Bioengineering	$3,155	$569	$3,166	$760	$3,303	$3,498	$3,482	$3,516
Biotechnology	$5,619	$1,051	$5,682	$1,203	$5,823	$6,089	$6,127	$6,154
Brain cancer	$234	$42	$274	$36	$280	$281	$283	$284
Brain disorders	$3,538	$685	$3,847	$619	$3,864	$3,968	$3,992	$3,993
Breast cancer	$722	$111	$763	$61	$715	$800	$805	$808
Burden of illness	$43	$11	$48	$8	$40	$84	$85	$85
Cancer	$5,629	$1,120	$5,823	$803	$5,448	$5,621	$5,649	$5,671
Cardiovascular	$2,008	$396	$2,144	$398	$2,049	$2,040	$2,051	$2,052
Cerebral palsy	$21	$4	$19	$3	$23	$42	$42	$42
Cervical cancer	$84	$15	$93	$8	$119	$112	$113	$113
Charcot-Marie-Tooth Disease	$14	$2	$15	$1	$13	$13	$13	$13
Child abuse and neglect research	$32	$5	$32	$5	$30	$32	$33	$32
Childhood leukemia	$47	$12	$55	$12	$59	$77	$77	$78
Chronic fatigue syndrome (ME/CFS)	$5	$0	$6	$0	$6	$5	$5	$5
Chronic liver disease and cirrhosis	$274	$37	$284	$45	$303	$288	$289	$290
Chronic obstructive pulmonary disease	$96	$18	$118	$15	$108	$101	$102	$102
Climate change	$4	$2	$4	$2	$6	$8	$8	$8
Climate-related exposures and conditions[k]	$179	$35	$188	$23	$155	$157	$158	$158
Clinical research	$10,336	$1,854	$10,720	$1,540	$10,503	$10,951	$11,018	$11,068
Clinical trials	$2,966	$485	$3,286	$356	$3,093	$3,208	$3,194	$3,201
Colo-rectal cancer	$281	$48	$291	$26	$313	$302	$303	$305
Comparative effectiveness research	$194	$246	$558	$320	$517	$597	$581	$583
Complementary and alternative medicine	$513	$70	$521	$55	$442	$493	$496	$497
Conditions affecting unborn children	$95	$8	$98	$21	$157	$165	$166	$167
Contraception/reproduction	$427	$65	$419	$56	$415	$448	$451	$452
Cooley's anemia	$21	$3	$20	$3	$20	$20	$20	$20
Cost effectiveness research	$52	$16	$80	$14	$71	$78	$78	$78
Crohn's disease	$55	$14	$66	$12	$67	$76	$76	$76
Cystic fibrosis	$86	$13	$86	$13	$79	$86	$86	$87
Dental/oral and craniofacial disease	$490	$75	$497	$67	$501	$516	$519	$518
Depression	$402	$48	$420	$50	$426	$429	$432	$428
Diabetes[b]	$1,030	$121	$1,046	$153	$1,076	$1,061	$1,066	$1,067
Diagnostic radiology	$976	$206	$1,073	$280	$1,071	$1,090	$1,096	$1,096
Diethylstilbestrol (DES)	$4	$1	$4	$1	$3	$3	$3	$3
Digestive diseases	$1,538	$243	$1,657	$228	$1,698	$1,719	$1,729	$1,734
Digestive diseases—(gallbladder)	$7	$1	$5	$0	$4	$11	$11	$11
Digestive diseases—(peptic ulcer)	$17	$3	$30	$3	$18	$20	$20	$20
Down syndrome	$18	$4	$22	$6	$20	$20	$20	$21
Drug abuse (NIDA only)[c]	$1,040	$135	$1,067	$125	$1,051	$1,052	$1,060	$1,072
Duchenne/Becker muscular dystrophy	$27	$6	$33	$5	$32	$34	$35	$35
Dystonia	$16	$2	$14	$1	$13	$14	$14	$14

funding for obesity increased from $745 million in FY 2009 to a projected $843 million in FY 2014. However, funding for obesity research was boosted in 2009 and 2010 by temporary funds provided through the American Recovery and Reinvestment Act. When this is taken into account, funding was $862 million in FY 2009 and $971

TABLE 7.1

Estimates of funding for various research, conditions, and disease categories, fiscal years 2009–14 [CONTINUED]

Research/disease areas (Dollars in millions and rounded)	Fiscal year 2009 actual (Non-ARRA)	Fiscal year 2009 actual (ARRA)[j]	Fiscal year 2010 actual (Non-ARRA)	Fiscal year 2010 actual (ARRA)[j]	Fiscal year 2011 actual	Fiscal year 2012 actual	Fiscal year 2013 estimated	Fiscal year 2014 estimated
Eating disorders[d]	$26	$5	$28	$4	$27	$34	$34	$34
Emerging infectious diseases	$2,080	$307	$2,118	$350	$2,190	$2,153	$2,161	$2,162
Emphysema	$28	$11	$23	$9	$22	$20	$20	$20
Endometriosis	$15	$2	$15	$1	$14	$9	$9	$9
Epilepsy	$128	$21	$134	$27	$152	$156	$157	$158
Estrogen	$235	$34	$231	$23	$227	$221	$222	$223
Eye disease and disorders of vision	$862	$129	$817	$110	$831	$841	$846	$840
Facioscapulohumeral muscular dystrophy	$3	$2	$5	$1	$6	$5	$5	$5
Fetal alcohol syndrome	$34	$7	$33	$5	$36	$32	$32	$32
Fibroid tumors (uterine)	$18	$2	$12	$2	$12	$14	$14	$14
Fibromyalgia	$11	$2	$9	$0	$11	$13	$13	$13
Food allergies	+	+	+	+	$33	$31	$31	$31
Food safety	$262	$37	$290	$35	$287	$257	$259	$259
Fragile X syndrome	$27	$5	$25	$4	$29	$27	$28	$28
Frontotemporal dementia (FTD)	$22	$2	$18	$1	$23	$26	$27	$27
Gene therapy	$221	$28	$248	$32	$248	$256	$257	$258
Gene therapy clinical trials	$11	$0	$14	$0	$14	$15	$16	$16
Genetic testing	$316	$76	$298	$121	$270	$255	$256	$257
Genetics	$7,278	$1,676	$7,473	$1,440	$7,223	$7,632	$7,678	$7,703
Global warming climate change	$3	$1	$2	$2	$5	$6	$6	$6
Headaches	+	+	$18	$1	$21	$24	$25	$25
Health disparities[e]	$2,806	$434	$2,728	$351	$2,718	$2,740	$2,757	$2,764
Health services	$1,102	$316	$1,143	$334	$1,172	$1,317	$1,264	$1,295
Heart disease	$1,202	$227	$1,329	$235	$1,236	$1,278	$1,286	$1,286
Heart disease–coronary heart disease	$426	$98	$457	$80	$437	$468	$470	$471
Hematology	$908	$151	$961	$141	$1,006	$1,091	$1,098	$1,100
Hepatitis	$178	$23	$204	$25	$208	$210	$212	$212
Hepatitis–A	$4	$0	$4	$0	$4	$2	$2	$2
Hepatitis–B	$51	$6	$66	$4	$58	$51	$51	$51
Hepatitis–C	$97	$12	$100	$12	$114	$112	$113	$113
HIV/AIDS[f]	$3,019	$319	$3,085	$322	$3,059	$3,074	$3,095	$3,122
Hodgkin's disease	$26	$1	$24	$1	$20	$21	$21	$21
Homelessness	$16	$3	$15	$3	$9	$10	$10	$10
Homicide and legal interventions	$2	$1	$1	$0	$1	$1	$1	$1
HPV and/or cervical cancer vaccines	$25	$2	$25	$2	$24	$26	$26	$26
Human fetal tissue[g]	$41	$22	$55	$24	$66	$71	$71	$71
Human genome	$1,775	$566	$1,904	$598	$1,907	$2,271	$2,284	$2,313
Huntington's disease	$57	$12	$65	$7	$56	$65	$66	$66
Hydrocephalus	+	+	+	+	+	$7	$7	$7
Hyperbaric oxygen	$3	$0	$2	$0	$2	$2	$2	$2
Hypertension	$266	$41	$251	$50	$240	$215	$216	$216
Immunization	$1,773	$191	$1,798	$231	$1,756	$1,733	$1,743	$1,746
Infant mortality/(LBW)	$246	$32	$273	$53	$286	$287	$288	$290
Infectious diseases	$3,627	$526	$3,890	$568	$3,883	$3,867	$3,885	$3,885
Infertility	$75	$17	$76	$16	$74	$74	$74	$74
Inflammatory bowel disease	$91	$22	$106	$19	$113	$121	$122	$122
Influenza	$316	$46	$308	$88	$272	$251	$252	$252
Injury–childhood injuries	$33	$3	$36	$3	$33	$37	$37	$37
Injury–trauma–(head and spine)	$161	$33	$179	$31	$166	$171	$173	$176
Injury–traumatic brain injury	$71	$15	$85	$9	$81	$79	$80	$83
Injury–unintentional childhood injury	$19	$1	$22	$1	$20	$22	$22	$22
Injury (total) accidents/adverse effects	$340	$58	$372	$46	$356	$366	$369	$372
Interstitial cystitis	$11	$1	$12	$1	$13	$10	$10	$10
Kidney disease	$570	$85	$552	$98	$557	$556	$559	$560
Lead poisoning	$11	$3	$11	$1	$10	$8	$8	$8
Liver cancer	$94	$12	$102	$10	$74	$73	$74	$74
Liver disease	$572	$79	$627	$85	$623	$632	$636	$638
Lung	$1,265	$234	$1,269	$207	$1,278	$1,286	$1,294	$1,296
Lung cancer	$178	$36	$201	$22	$221	$233	$234	$235
Lupus	$115	$19	$112	$15	$106	$108	$109	$109
Lyme disease	$25	$5	$24	$5	$28	$25	$25	$25
Lymphoma	$184	$22	$195	$14	$199	$213	$214	$215
Macular degeneration	$85	$8	$104	$9	$105	$101	$101	$100
Malaria	$110	$11	$134	$14	$145	$152	$153	$153
Malaria vaccine	$34	$3	$41	$4	$39	$40	$40	$40
Mental health	$2,129	$382	$2,246	$334	$2,275	$2,287	$2,301	$2,284
Mental retardation (intellectual and developmental disabilities (IDD))	$281	$94	$311	$87	$333	$355	$357	$356

TABLE 7.1

Estimates of funding for various research, conditions, and disease categories, fiscal years 2009–14 [CONTINUED]

Research/disease areas (Dollars in millions and rounded)	Fiscal year 2009 actual (Non-ARRA)	Fiscal year 2009 actual (ARRA)ʲ	Fiscal year 2010 actual (Non-ARRA)	Fiscal year 2010 actual (ARRA)ʲ	Fiscal year 2011 actual	Fiscal year 2012 actual	Fiscal year 2013 estimated	Fiscal year 2014 estimated
Methamphetamine	$69	$13	$73	$14	$70	$69	$69	$70
Migraines	+	+	$15	+	$16	$18	$18	$18
Mind and body	$494	$90	$549	$81	$533	$533	$536	$535
Minority healthᵉ	$2,592	$378	$2,526	$312	$2,504	$2,487	$2,503	$2,510
Mucopolysaccharidoses (MPS)	$7	$0	$8	$0	$10	$10	$10	$10
Multiple sclerosis	$137	$25	$133	$18	$122	$115	$116	$116
Muscular dystrophy	$66	$17	$74	$12	$75	$75	$75	$75
Myasthenia gravis	$9	$3	$8	$3	$9	$7	$7	$7
Myotonic dystrophy	$9	$4	$10	$2	$9	$10	$10	$10
Nanotechnologyʰ	$343	$73	$435	$76	$409	$456	$459	$461
Networking and information technology R&Dʰ	$1,174	$168	$647	$248	$551	$532	$527	$527
Neuroblastoma	+	+	+	+	$25	$34	$34	$35
Neurodegenerative	$1,553	$262	$1,571	$243	$1,622	$1,671	$1,681	$1,682
Neurofibromatosis	$17	$2	$24	$1	$23	$18	$18	$18
Neuropathy	$119	$13	$121	$10	$146	$145	$146	$146
Neurosciences	$5,320	$848	$5,515	$794	$5,548	$5,618	$5,652	$5,655
Nutrition	$1,400	$205	$1,435	$208	$1,411	$1,692	$1,702	$1,707
Obesity	$745	$117	$824	$147	$830	$836	$841	$843
Organ transplantation	$139	$32	$150	$37	$164	$150	$151	$151
Orphan drug	$441	$118	$512	$89	$749	$809	$813	$816
Osteogenesis imperfecta	$5	$1	$8	$4	$9	$9	$9	$9
Osteoporosis	$198	$21	$181	$23	$179	$181	$182	$182
Otitis media	$15	$7	$19	$2	$15	$17	$17	$18
Ovarian cancer	$102	$13	$122	$10	$138	$147	$148	$149
Paget's disease	$1	$1	$1	$0	$1	$1	$1	$1
Pain conditions–chronic	$333	$53	$360	$44	$386	$396	$399	$400
Pain research	$0	$0	$0	$0	+	$479	$482	$483
Pancreatic cancer	+	+	+	+	$112	$127	$128	$129
Parkinson's disease	$162	$24	$154	$18	$151	$154	$155	$156
Patient safety	+	+	$859	$263	$839	$845	$840	$841
Pediatric	$2,996	$505	$3,286	$479	$3,277	$3,612	$3,623	$3,630
Pediatric AIDSᶠ	$227	$20	$216	$15	$228	$219	$216	$218
Pediatric research initiative	$214	$256	$308	$148	$362	$379	$381	$382
Pelvic inflammatory disease	$3	$1	$4	$1	$4	$3	$3	$3
Perinatal–birth–preterm (LBW)	$177	$23	$183	$47	$214	$217	$219	$220
Perinatal–neonatal respiratory distress syndrome	$31	$5	$31	$3	$37	$38	$38	$38
Perinatal period–conditions originating in perinatal period	$470	$65	$542	$84	$498	$538	$541	$543
Pick's disease	$2	$0	$2	$0	$3	$2	$2	$2
Pneumonia	$108	$15	$93	$17	$117	$115	$116	$116
Pneumonia & influenza	$392	$58	$396	$102	$382	$358	$360	$361
Polycystic kidney disease	$38	$7	$35	$6	$42	$42	$42	$42
Prescription drug abuse	+	+	$29	$7	$28	$33	$33	$33
Prevention	$5,332	$844	$5,983	$849	$5,929	$5,924	$5,952	$5,967
Prostate cancer	$310	$47	$331	$31	$284	$257	$258	$259
Psoriasis	$13	$3	$13	$3	$10	$10	$10	$10
Rare diseases	+	+	+	+	$3,527	$3,623	$3,645	$3,652
Regenerative medicine	$799	$144	$820	$142	$824	$877	$882	$883
Rehabilitation	$404	$75	$458	$93	$459	$449	$452	$454
Rett syndrome	$9	$4	$13	$2	$12	$13	$13	$13
Reye's syndrome	$0	$0	$0	$0	+	$0	—	—
Rural health	$186	$42	$207	$33	$211	$231	$210	$210
Schizophrenia	$265	$85	$276	$63	$264	$268	$270	$266
Scleroderma	$21	$2	$19	$2	$25	$24	$24	$24
Screening and brief intervention for substance abuse	+	+	$26	$4	$30	$31	$31	$31
Septicemia	$92	$19	$90	$17	$91	$96	$96	$96
Sexually transmitted diseases/herpes	$250	$43	$250	$38	$259	$275	$277	$277
Sickle cell disease	$63	$14	$73	$12	$65	$65	$66	$66
Sleep research	$217	$33	$226	$22	$232	$238	$240	$239
Small pox	$94	$4	$92	$5	$41	$40	$40	$39
Smoking and health	$329	$78	$336	$55	$360	$353	$355	$357
Spina bifida	$14	$3	$12	$6	$11	$12	$12	$12
Spinal cord injury	$80	$14	$87	$16	$78	$79	$79	$79
Spinal muscular atrophy	$11	$3	$16	$3	$19	$15	$15	$15

TABLE 7.1

Estimates of funding for various research, conditions, and disease categories, fiscal years 2009–14 [CONTINUED]

Research/disease areas (Dollars in millions and rounded)	Fiscal year 2009 actual (Non-ARRA)	Fiscal year 2009 actual (ARRA)[j]	Fiscal year 2010 actual (Non-ARRA)	Fiscal year 2010 actual (ARRA)[j]	Fiscal year 2011 actual	Fiscal year 2012 actual	Fiscal year 2013 estimated	Fiscal year 2014 estimated
Stem cell research	$1,044	$187	$1,099	$187	$1,179	$1,374	$1,382	$1,385
Stem cell research–embryonic–human	$120	$23	$126	$40	$123	$146	$147	$147
Stem cell research–embryonic–non-human	$148	$29	$175	$20	$165	$164	$165	$165
Stem cell research–nonembryonic–human	$339	$58	$341	$74	$395	$504	$507	$508
Stem cell research–nonembryonic–non-human	$550	$88	$570	$74	$620	$653	$657	$658
Stem cell research–umbilical cord blood/placenta	$49	$10	$42	$8	$41	$47	$48	$48
Stem cell research–umbilical cord blood/placenta–human	$42	$9	$40	$7	$36	$43	$43	$43
Stem cell research–umbilical cord blood/placenta–non-human	$10	$1	$5	$1	$10	$8	$8	$8
Stroke	$329	$54	$337	$54	$317	$310	$312	$313
Substance abuse[i]	$1,653	$245	$1,674	$216	$1,623	$1,634	$1,644	$1,658
Substance abuse prevention	+	+	$43	$10	$44	$41	$41	$41
Sudden infant death syndrome	$22	$6	$25	$2	$23	$24	$24	$24
Suicide	$36	$15	$36	$4	$49	$44	$45	$44
Suicide prevention	+	+	$17	$2	$25	$22	$22	$22
Teenage pregnancy	$23	$5	$22	$5	$19	$18	$18	$18
Temporomandibular muscle/joint disorder (TMJD)	$15	$1	$16	$1	$18	$21	$22	$21
Tobacco	$331	$78	$339	$55	$362	$355	$357	$359
Topical microbicides	$92	$7	$84	$5	$104	$99	$99	$99
Tourette syndrome	$7	$3	$7	$0	$5	$6	$6	$6
Transmissible spongiform encephalopathy (TSE)	$43	$4	$48	$3	$46	$39	$39	$39
Transplantation	$571	$94	$574	$109	$592	$552	$555	$555
Tuberculosis	$189	$27	$189	$35	$209	$218	$219	$219
Tuberculosis vaccine	$15	$3	$13	$3	$17	$21	$21	$21
Tuberous sclerosis	$20	$3	$20	$2	$20	$23	$23	$23
Underage drinking	+	+	$75	$5	$77	$80	$81	$81
Underage drinking prevention & treatment (NIAAA only)	+	+	$56	$2	$57	$62	$62	$62
Urologic diseases	$578	$81	$563	$56	$542	$496	$499	$501
Uterine cancer	$25	$4	$26	$4	$40	$42	$42	$42
Vaccine related	$1,593	$185	$1,737	$222	$1,717	$1,691	$1,701	$1,703
Vaccine related (AIDS)[f]	$561	$35	$535	$27	$550	$557	$561	$575
Vector-borne diseases	$401	$66	$426	$68	$466	$441	$443	$443
Violence against women	$39	$2	$36	$2	$34	$36	$36	$36
Violence research	$182	$21	$174	$19	$156	$154	$155	$155
Vulvodynia	$1	$1	$2	$1	$2	$4	$4	$4
West Nile virus	$59	$7	$46	$6	$65	$29	$29	$29
Women's health[e]	$3,725	$506	$3,691	$449	$3,891	$3,833	$3,857	$3,870
Youth violence	$111	$12	$102	$10	$87	$77	$78	$78
Youth violence prevention	+	+	$32	$2	$26	$27	$27	$27

*The minimum reporting threshold for a specific disease/condition is $500,000. Reporting of $0 does not indicate that no research is being conducted.

+Indicates a new category. Funding support data not available prior to the initial year reported.

[a]Reporting for this category does not follow the standard RCDC process. The total amount reported is consistent with reporting requirements for this category to the U.S. Office of Management & Budget (OMB). The project listing does not include non-project or other support costs associated with the annual total for this category.

[b]Includes research funded from the Type 1 diabetes appropriation of $150 million. These are project listings only.

[c]Reporting for this category does not follow the standard RCDC process. Spending is reported consistent with U.S. Office of National Drug Control Policy (ONDCP) requirements (Only NIDA). The FY 2012 actual and FY 2013 estimate reported in RePORT can differ from levels identified in the FY 2014 Drug Control budget submission for those fiscal years where comparable adjustments have been applied.

[d]Reported total for this category encompasses research for anorexia, bulimia nervosa, binge eating disorders, and eating disorders not otherwise specified.

[e]Reporting for this category does not follow the standard RCDC process. This category assigns project funding according to populations tracked by gender or ethnicity. The databases used to track gender/ethnicity are complex and not currently compatible with the RCDC system.

[f]Reporting for this category does not follow the standard RCDC process. These are project listings only and non-project or other support costs associated with the annual total for the category are not included.

[g]Reporting for this category does not follow the standard RCDC process. This category uses a non-standard approach involving subject matter expert reviews of manually collected project listings.

[h]The data provided reflects funding amounts reported by the NIH RCDC process for this category. Actual and estimate levels presented on this site supersede estimates detailed in OMB MAX DE application tables that may have been based on preliminary funding support information.

[i]Reporting for this category does not follow the standard RCDC process. This category includes all spending reported under the Drug Abuse category as well as projects categorized under the broader area of Substance Abuse. These are project listings only.

[j]Separate columns are used to distinguish FY 2009 and FY 2010 actual support funded from American Recovery & Reinvestment Act (ARRA) accounts from projects funded by regular annual NIH appropriations.

[k]Prior to FY 2011, this category's title was "Health Effects of Climate Change". The title was revised to more accurately reflect the content of the research conducted and facilitate reporting spending data in response to requests tracking climate change adaptation.

Notes: ARRA = American Recovery and Reinvestment Act. MB = Myalgic encephalomyelitis. HIV = Human immunodeficiency virus. AIDS = Acquired immune deficiency syndrome. LBW = Low birth weight. R&D = Research and development. NIAAA = National Institute on Alcohol Abuse and Alcoholism. RCDC = Research, Condition, and Disease Categorization.

SOURCE: "Estimates of Funding for Various Research, Condition, and Disease Categories (RCDC)," in *NIH Categorical Spending*, U.S. Department of Health and Human Services, National Institutes of Health, April 10, 2013, http://report.nih.gov/categorical_spending.aspx (accessed November 1, 2013)

million in FY 2010, meaning that spending on obesity peaked in those years and then fell somewhat.

The Obesity Society, along with myriad medical professional organizations and advocacy groups, contends that public funding for obesity research is inadequate in view of the size and scope of this public health problem. Besides insufficient NIH funding for obesity research, the Obesity Society cites inequities in research grants that are awarded by the NIH.

WEIGHING THE PRICE THAT EMPLOYERS PAY

Obese employees incur substantially higher health care costs than normal-weight employees. Obesity significantly increases health expenditures and absenteeism. James P. Moriarty et al. estimate in "The Effects of Incremental Costs of Smoking and Obesity on Health Care Costs among Adults: A 7-Year Longitudinal Study" (*Journal of Occupational & Environmental Medicine*, vol. 54, no. 3, March 2012) that health care costs are $1,400 more for obese employees compared with their healthy-weight colleagues. Moriarty et al. find that obese workers cost $600 more than smokers.

In "Obesity & the Workplace: Direct, Indirect Costs & the Role of Wellness Education" (November 2012, http://www.asse.org/practicespecialties/healthandwellness/docs/HW_Newsletter_Vol2_No1.pdf), Thomas A. Sherwood reviews multiple studies estimating the costs of obese workers. Sherwood reports that of the $900 billion U.S. employers spend on health care annually, $75 billion is attributable to obesity. Absenteeism attributable to overweight and obesity results in a cost of $4.3 billion per year. Obese workers file more medical claims, 11.65 claims per 100 full-time equivalents (FTEs) as opposed to healthy weight employees with 5.80 claims, and their medical claims costs are higher.

Dan Witters and Sangeeta Agrawal of the Gallup Organization report in *Unhealthy U.S. Workers' Absenteeism Costs $153 Billion* (October 17, 2011, http://www.gallup.com/poll/150026/Unhealthy-Workers-Absenteeism-Costs-153-Billion.aspx) that overweight and obese workers with chronic health conditions made up 48% of full-time U.S. workers in 2011. These workers missed 450 million more days of work annually than their normal-weight peers who did not have chronic health conditions (13.9% of full-time U.S. workers). Witters and Agrawal estimate that the annual cost of lost productivity attributable to absenteeism among people who are overweight or obese and who have one or more chronic conditions was more than $113 billion in 2011. Americans who were overweight or obese but had no chronic conditions were only marginally more likely to miss work than those who were of normal weight and who had no chronic conditions.

THE HIGH COST OF LOSING WEIGHT

According to the market research firm IBISWorld Inc., from 2008 to 2013 the total revenues of the weight-loss service industry declined about 3.7% per year. In 2013 gains in per capita disposable income prompted an uptick and industry revenue was projected to increase 3.1% reaching $2.4 billion. The firm's report, "Weight Loss Services in the U.S. Industry" (July 2013, http://www.ibisworld.com/industry/default.aspx?indid=1719&partnerid=prweb), describes the industry as highly competitive with more than 29,000 companies vying for consumers.

The report explains that industry leader Weight Watchers International Inc. increased its market share significantly over the five-year period by acquiring franchises and expanding its product and service lines. By contrast the second-largest company, Nutrisystem, lost ground during the economic recession because fewer consumers purchased its meal replacement products than did the counseling and support services offered by Weight Watchers and similar companies. As a result, Nutrisystem divested or discontinued some of its operations during the same period. The third major player in the industry over the period was Jenny Craig, Inc. Its corporate owner, Nestlé SA, sold Jenny Craig to North Castle Partners, a private-equity firm, on November 7, 2013. Monica Watrous reports in "Nestle Unloads Jenny Craig" (FoodBusinessNews.net, November 7, 2013) that Jenny Craig, which had been part of Nestlé since 2006, was performing poorly. She quotes Nestlé's chief financial officer as having said in August 2013 that "the Jenny Craig business—this year as well as last year—was very much below our expectations and what they have been able to do in the last few years."

The market research firm Marketdata Enterprises Inc. reports in *U.S. Weight Loss and Diet Control Market Outlook* (13th edition, March 2013) that there were about 108 million dieters in the United States in 2012, most of whom (82%) were trying to lose weight by themselves, without the benefit of a program or special products or services.

Marketdata reports that the U.S. weight-loss industry produced revenues of $61.6 billion in 2012, up 3.8% from $58.4 billion in 2010. The firm projected a 2.6% increase in 2013. This included: commercial weight-loss centers; medically supervised weight-loss programs; prescription diet drugs; diet books; audio and video programs; web-based diet and nutrition services; low-calorie and low-carbohydrate food products; meal replacements; and over-the-counter (nonprescription) appetite suppressants. Marketdata's research indicates that the commercial weight-loss center market had $3.42 billion in revenues in 2012. Sales of diet pills and meal replacement bars and shakes increased 2% to $2.78 billion in 2012 and were projected to increase 6% per year through 2016.

Weight Watchers was the leader in the online dieting arena in 2012 according to Marketdata, with more than 1.7 million paid subscribers and revenues of $504 million. Marketdata further reports that because most paid sites had not been profitable, many were shifting to an advertising-based revenue model that enables users free access to the sites.

Marketdata claims that the most affluent dieters were purchasing home-delivered diet foods, which accounted for $858 million of the weight-loss market in 2012. Nutrisystem owned about 46% of this market in 2012 but had experienced five consecutive years of declining sales. Diet food delivery services suffered during the economic recession with the percentage of consumers purchasing this service declining from 5.8% to 4.5% in 2012.

Medical and Behavioral Treatments

The greatest proportion of all outlays for weight loss go toward food products and commercial weight-loss programs. However, behavioral interventions for weight loss, such as one-on-one counseling, involve considerable expense. Prescription drug treatment is also costly—newer drugs Qsymia and Belviq cost between $100 and $250 per month.

In "Economic Evaluation of an Internet-Based Weight Management Program" (*American Journal of Managed Care*, vol. 16, no. 4, April 1, 2010), Rafia S. Rasu et al. compare the cost of a behavioral treatment program delivered via the Internet with usual care (a face-to-face nutrition-based weight management and physical fitness program, an annual fitness assessment, and a yearly preventive health checkup with a health care provider) in a sample of overweight adults serving in the U.S. Air Force. The costs associated with the Internet intervention included distribution materials and letterhead; the cost of the training sessions; the costs of educational materials, equipment, supplies, and other items (e.g., website and computer costs); and the costs for employees (project staff) while they worked on the training sessions as well as on the baseline and follow-up appointments to measure weight. The Internet intervention involved 227 participants and the total cost per participant was $49.24, which was $15.09 lower than the per participant cost of usual treatment. Rasu et al. find that although an Internet intervention has higher initial costs, it becomes more cost effective over time, and conclude that it "is a cost-effective choice for weight management."

In "Internet Programs Targeting Multiple Lifestyle Interventions in Primary and Secondary Care Are Not Superior to Usual Care Alone in Improving Cardiovascular Risk Profile: A Systematic Review" (*European Journal of Internal Medicine*, vol. 25, no. 1, 2014), Irene L. Vegting et al. review a variety of programs targeting lifestyle interventions and find that while they may be able to partially replace face-to-face contact with health care workers, on the whole they are not as effective as one-to-one interventions and suffer from high dropout rates. However, Internet-based interventions may be cost effective when they are applied on a large scale because they have the potential to reduce the number of doctor's visits.

Long-Term Savings

Some research indicates that the costs of surgical treatment of obesity are offset by a reduction in future utilization of health care services, especially prescription drug use, and a resultant reduction in health care costs. For example, in "Bariatric Surgery: Cost-Effectiveness and Budget Impact" (*Obesity Surgery*, vol. 22, no. 4, April 2012), Lorenzo Terranova et al. review the cost efficiency of bariatric surgery. They conclude that "the additional years of lives gained through bariatric surgery may be obtained at a reasonable and affordable cost. In groups of patients with very high obesity-related health costs, like patients with type 2 diabetes, the use of bariatric surgery required an initial economic investment, but may save money in a relatively short period."

However, in "Impact of Bariatric Surgery on Health Care Costs of Obese Patients" (*JAMA Surgery*, vol. 148, no. 6, June 2013), an analysis of health insurance claims data of 29,820 patients who underwent bariatric surgery between 2002 and 2008, Jonathan P. Weiner et al. conclude that bariatric surgery does not reduce total health care costs in the short or long term. The researchers find that, compared with people who did not have the surgery, the bariatric surgery patients' costs were higher in the second and third years following the surgery but were comparable in later years. The bariatric surgery patients had lower outpatient visit and prescription drug costs but higher inpatient costs.

Community-based weight-loss programs also have the potential to save money. In "Enrolling People with Prediabetes Ages 60–64 in a Proven Weight Loss Program Could Save Medicare $7 Billion or More" (*Health Affairs*, vol. 30, no. 9, September 2011), Kenneth E. Thorpe and Zhou Yang examine the potential of a community-based weight-loss program to save money for the Medicare program. The weight-loss program in question was developed by the Centers for Disease Control and Prevention, the YMCA, and the UnitedHealth Group. Featuring trained lifestyle coaches who help people make healthier food choices and increase physical activity, the program has demonstrated the ability to help people aged 60 years and older lose weight and reduce their risk of developing diabetes by as much as 71%.

Thorpe and Yang project that Medicare could save as much as $3.7 billion over 10 years by enrolling two groups of people in the weight-loss program: people aged 60 to 64 years who have prediabetes and a BMI higher than 24, and people with the same BMI who are at risk for cardiovascular disease (high blood pressure or elevated cholesterol) independent of whether they have prediabetes. The savings could reach as much as $15.1 billion over the course of the participants' lifetime. Thorpe and Yang assert, "Our results show the potential savings to Medicare if a proven community-based approach to reducing obesity and related chronic disease were to be made available, nationwide, to high-risk individuals soon to become Medicare beneficiaries. In doing so, they also present a potential business case for the federal government to partner with the private sector in order to encourage broad enrollment in effective weight loss programs."

CATERING TO AN EXPANDING MARKET

Along with increased costs, many businesses have discovered that they must literally expand their products and services to meet the needs of overweight and obese consumers. The article "13 Oversize Products for Overweight People" (Health.com, 2013) presents an array of products that are designed to meet the needs of obese Americans, including: heavy-duty weight scales, wider toilet seats that can withstand up to 1,200 pounds (544 kg), seat-belt extenders, jumbo-sized jewelry, and bicycles that can accommodate people weighing up to 550 pounds (259 kg). The article also describes electric bed lifts designed to transfer patients up to 1,000 pounds (454 kg) from bed to wheelchair, and wider wheelchairs to accommodate patients up to 700 pounds (318 kg).

The Plus-Sized Clothing Market Is Growing

In its 2013 "Plus-Size Women's Clothing Stores in the U.S." (http://www.ibisworld.com/industry/plus-size-womens-clothing-stores.html) market research report, IBISWorld states that the $8 billion plus-sized women's clothing industry consists of more than 6,100 businesses and employs more than 39,300 workers. Like other industries it suffered during the Great Recession of 2007 to 2009 when women had less disposable income, growing only 2.1% per year from 2008 to 2013.

The article "Designers Embrace Plus-Size Market" (ABCNews.go.com, June 26, 2013) indicates that high-end designers such as Michael Kors, Calvin Klein, and Vince Camuto are designing high-fashion clothes for plus-sized women and that 100 brands were represented at Full Figured Fashion Week in 2013, up from just 12 brands in 2009. In another first, in 2013 Eden Miller, a plus-sized clothing designer, showed her Cabiria line during New York Fashion Week. In "Fashion Week Just Went Plus-Size: A Major Step for the Industry Is Decked out in Prints" (HuffingtonPost.com, September 6, 2013), Lauren Duca asserts that "Cabiria is an important development for plus-size women, who are often ignored by the industry."

In 2001 Hot Topic, a California-based company that specializes in clothing for teenagers and young women, launched a chain of six stores called Torrid that offer fashion-forward plus-sized clothing for young women. A media release from the company, "Introducing the New Torrid" (August 13, 2012, http://www.businesswire.com/news/home/20120813006314/en/Introducing-Torrid), notes that in 2012 there were 176 Torrid stores and an online store that offered an array of clothing and lingerie for young women. A 2012 advertising campaign tagline, "I am torrid," is intended to serve "as an aspirational message to voluptuous women about their inherent beauty and sexuality."

CHAPTER 8

POLITICAL, LEGAL, AND SOCIAL ISSUES OF OVERWEIGHT AND OBESITY

Under the health care law, most plans must provide obesity screening and counseling for children at no out-of-pocket charge. Insurance companies also can no longer deny insurance to a child because of a pre-existing condition, like diabetes. In order to reduce childhood obesity nationwide, we must use every resource available to encourage America's youth to adopt healthy habits that can last a lifetime. HHS provides programs and resources for all Americans to maintain or improve their health.

—Kathleen Sebelius (1948–), U.S. secretary of health and human services, in a statement about National Childhood Obesity Awareness Month (September 4, 2013, http://www.hhs.gov/news/press/2013pres/09/20130904a.html)

THE GLOBAL POLITICS OF OBESITY

At the international level, the World Health Organization (WHO) has developed a strategy to combat an escalating global epidemic of overweight and obesity throughout the world. In *Global Strategy on Diet, Physical Activity, and Health* (October 2005, http://www.who.int/dietphysicalactivity/strategy/eb11344/strategy_english_web.pdf), the WHO exhorts individuals and populations to:

- Achieve energy balance and a healthy weight

- Limit energy intake from total fats and shift fat consumption away from saturated fats to unsaturated fats and toward the elimination of trans fatty acids

- Increase consumption of fruits, vegetables, legumes, whole grains, and nuts

- Limit the intake of free sugars

- Limit salt (sodium) consumption from all sources and ensure that salt is iodized

- Engage in at least 30 minutes of regular, moderate-intensity physical activity on most days

The WHO asserts that "government is crucial in achieving lasting change in public health" and believes that governments should take the lead in initiating and developing its strategy and ensuring that it is implemented. The WHO also recommends sharply limiting the marketing of food to children and using tax and pricing policies to influence food consumption. According to the WHO, these measures are necessary to reverse the rising rates of obesity-related illnesses, including heart disease, diabetes, and cancer.

These guidelines are not, however, favored by some food manufacturers. For example, the International Sugar Organization strenuously objects to the recommendation that sugar amount to no more than 10% of food and drink calories consumed per day, calling instead for a 25% cap. Table 8.1 shows that the total U.S. consumption of caloric sweeteners spiked in 1999, 2000, 2002, and 2005, but that the overall use of caloric sweeteners has not varied significantly between 1997 and 2012.

U.S. opposition to the WHO strategy has been criticized as a clear effort to appease U.S. food and sugar suppliers. Some WHO scientists and consumer advocacy groups suggest the U.S. objections—specifically those about the recommendations to limit sugar consumption and to reconsider food advertising aimed at young children—aim to protect industries that have recently been under attack rather than to improve public health. However, the food industry itself publicly pledged to support the WHO strategy. For example, the Grocery Manufacturers of America, the world's largest association of food and drink companies, which includes PepsiCo Inc. and Hershey Foods Corp., said it was committed to working with the WHO to combat obesity.

The WHO strategy became official when it was endorsed by member states at the United Nations (UN) summit in May 2004. The strategy is not binding, but it is considered a guiding document for public health efforts

TABLE 8.1

Total estimated deliveries of caloric sweeteners for domestic food and beverage use, by calendar year, 1984–2012

Calendar year	Sugar[a]		Corn sweeteners				Honey	Other edible syrups	Total caloric sweeteners[b]
	Raw value	Refined basis	HFCS	Glucose syrup	Dextrose	Total			
					1,000 shorttons, dry basis				
1966	10,235	9,565	0	952	415	1,367	98	69	11,099
1967	10,474	9,789	3	984	428	1,415	89	50	11,342
1968	10,656	9,959	15	1,031	444	1,489	90	70	11,608
1969	10,950	10,234	33	1,061	459	1,553	101	61	11,949
1970	11,163	10,433	56	1,102	471	1,629	103	51	12,216
1971	11,345	10,603	86	1,163	482	1,731	93	52	12,478
1972	11,487	10,736	121	1,257	485	1,863	105	52	12,756
1973	11,429	10,681	218	1,384	489	2,092	95	53	12,922
1974	10,945	10,229	295	1,480	486	2,262	75	43	12,609
1975	10,302	9,628	527	1,515	473	2,515	108	43	12,294
1976	10,893	10,180	782	1,514	452	2,748	100	44	13,072
1977	11,099	10,373	1,057	1,517	429	3,003	100	44	13,519
1978	10,889	10,177	1,198	1,551	410	3,159	120	45	13,501
1979	10,756	10,052	1,660	1,519	399	3,578	117	44	13,791
1980	10,189	9,522	2,158	1,472	393	4,024	94	50	13,690
1981	9,769	9,130	2,626	1,486	390	4,501	96	46	13,773
1982	9,153	8,554	3,090	1,479	392	4,961	104	46	13,665
1983	8,812	8,236	3,655	1,523	398	5,577	116	47	13,975
1984	8,428	7,877	4,399	1,552	408	6,359	108	47	14,391
1985	8,003	7,479	5,386	1,607	418	7,411	104	50	15,045
1986	7,731	7,225	5,498	1,632	430	7,561	121	50	14,957
1987	8,103	7,573	5,792	1,679	441	7,912	104	50	15,639
1988	8,136	7,604	5,998	1,747	452	8,197	100	50	15,951
1989	8,304	7,761	5,960	1,587	438	7,985	82	50	15,878
1990	8,615	8,051	6,202	1,700	455	8,358	86	50	16,546
1991	8,622	8,058	6,376	1,776	463	8,615	92	50	16,815
1992	8,826	8,249	6,652	1,943	461	9,056	95	20	17,419
1993	8,886	8,305	7,086	2,050	481	9,617	103	20	18,044
1994	9,072	8,478	7,398	2,093	502	9,993	126	26	18,623
1995	9,258	8,652	7,676	2,176	528	10,380	120	38	19,190
1996	9,381	8,767	7,788	2,216	537	10,541	131	94	19,534
1997	9,473	8,853	8,240	2,364	511	11,116	129	81	20,179
1998	9,592	8,964	8,552	2,358	502	11,411	130	81	20,586
1999	9,905	9,257	8,897	2,281	488	11,666	147	78	21,148
2000	9,899	9,252	8,845	2,230	476	11,551	157	84	21,044
2001	9,839	9,195	8,920	2,205	469	11,595	134	101	21,025
2002	9,742	9,105	9,045	2,224	473	11,741	153	97	21,096
2003	9,468	8,848	8,849	2,209	449	11,507	146	104	20,604
2004	9,661	9,029	8,779	2,292	487	11,558	130	96	20,813
2005	9,977	9,324	8,693	2,261	481	11,435	156	94	21,008
2006	9,936	9,286	8,637	2,053	463	11,153	174	98	20,712
2007	9,876	9,230	8,417	2,067	448	10,932	141	94	20,397
2008	10,605	9,911	8,015	2,036	419	10,470	151	93	20,625
2009	10,422	9,740	7,637	1,991	417	10,045	141	90	20,016
2010	10,923	10,229	7,480	1,956	450	9,886	160	104	20,358
2011	11,148	10,418	7,276	1,908	446	9,630	169	102	20,320
2012	11,153	10,423	7,263	1,969	420	9,652	170	104	20,350

NA = Not available.

HFCS = High fructose corn syrup.

[a]Based on U.S. sugar deliveries for domestic food and beverage use.

[b]Total includes sugar, refined basis.

Notes: Per capita deliveries of sweeteners by U.S. processors and refiners and direct-consumption imports to food manufacturers, retailers, and other end users represent the per capita supply of caloric sweeteners. The data exclude deliveries to manufacturers of alcoholic beverages. Actual human intake of caloric sweeteners is lower because of uneaten food, spoilage, and other losses.

SOURCE: "Table 49. U.S. Total Estimated Deliveries of Caloric Sweeteners for Domestic Food and Beverage Use, by Calendar Year," in *Sugar and Sweeteners Yearbook Tables*, U.S. Department of Agriculture, Economic Research Service, November 1, 2013, http://www.ers.usda.gov/data-products/sugar-and-sweeteners-yearbook-tables.aspx#.UnfelZFIDY0 (accessed November 4, 2013)

on the issue worldwide. The strategy provides member states with a range of policy options to address two of the major risks responsible for the growing burden of chronic diseases that are attributable to unhealthy diet and physical inactivity. It explains how healthier diets and physical activity can help prevent and control these diseases. The strategy describes the roles of WHO member states, UN agencies, civil society, educators, and the private sector in helping to reduce the occurrence of obesity. It recommends obesity-prevention measures, including effective food and agriculture policies, fiscal policies, surveillance systems, consumer education, and nutrition labeling. The strategy also emphasizes the need for countries to develop national strategies with a long-term, sustainable perspective on making healthy choices at both the individual and community levels.

At the 63rd World Health Assembly in May 2013, the WHO endorsed a set of guidelines aimed at reducing noncommunicable (noninfectious and nontransmissible) diseases, which includes obesity. In "Follow-Up to the Political Declaration of the High-Level Meeting of the General Assembly on the Prevention and Control of Non-communicable Diseases" (http://apps.who.int/gb/ebwha/pdf_files/WHA66/A66_R10-en.pdf) the WHO advises: "developing or strengthening national food and nutrition policies and action plans and implementation of related global strategies including the global strategy on diet, physical activity and health, the global strategy for infant and young child feeding, the comprehensive implementation plan on maternal, infant and young child nutrition and WHO's set of recommendations on the marketing of foods and nonalcoholic beverages to children. Member States should also consider implementing other relevant evidence-guided strategies, to promote healthy diets in the entire population while protecting dietary guidance and food policy from undue influence of commercial and other vested interests."

Among the dietary recommendations suggested in "Follow-Up to the Political Declaration of the High-Level Meeting of the General Assembly on the Prevention and Control of Non-communicable Diseases" are reducing the content of free and added sugars in food and beverages, developing policies that engage food retailers to improve the availability, affordability and acceptability of healthier food products (plant foods, including fruit and vegetables, and products with reduced content of salt/sodium, saturated fatty acids, trans-fatty acids and free sugars), and reducing the impact of marketing of unhealthful foods to children.

In "Health, Agricultural, and Economic Effects of Adoption of Healthy Diet Recommendations" (*Lancet*, vol. 376, November 13, 2010), Karen Lock et al. consider how implementing the WHO guidelines will affect population health. Lock et al. explain that for many countries, adhering to WHO guidelines "would mean a substantial decrease in the consumption of vegetable oils (by 30%), dairy products (by 28%), animal fats (by 30%), meat (e.g., pork by 13.5% or mutton and goat by 14.5%), and sugar (by 24%), and a substantial increase in the consumption of cereals (by 31%), fruits (by 25%), and vegetables (by 21%)." The researchers conclude that the benefits of a healthy diet policy will vary in response to population dietary intake as well as agricultural production, trade, and other economic factors. Lock et al. advise the public health community to address not only the implementation of health and dietary recommendations but also social, economic, and environmental factors, such as sustainability.

Is Sugar the New Tobacco?

The WHO named sugar as one of the chief culprits in the current epidemic of obesity and obesity-related diseases, diabetes, and cardiovascular heart disease. The WHO approach to food is not, however, comparable to its strategy to combat tobacco use. The food strategy aims to provide member states and other interested stakeholders with a range of recommendations and policy options to promote healthier diets and more physical activity. It is up to member states to decide how these should be further developed and implemented at the national level. Because the strategy was endorsed at the World Health Assembly, member states are responsible for determining which specific policy options are appropriate to their circumstances. The WHO provides technical support for the implementation of programs, as requested by member states.

AMERICANS CRAVE SUGAR

The United States is the world leader in sweetener consumption and is among the top sugar producers and importers. Table 8.2 shows monthly estimates of the U.S. sugar supply and use during fiscal year 2014. Dan Bobkoff explains in "Farm Bill's Sugar Subsidy More Taxing than Sweet, Critics Say" (NPR.org, March 28, 2013) that the federal government uses import restrictions, production quotas, and loan guarantees, among other measures, to ensure that U.S. sugar producers get good prices for their crops. Bobkoff notes that in 2012 sugar prices worldwide averaged $0.26 per pound, whereas in the United States they averaged $0.43. Charles Abbott states in "UPDATE 1-Low Prices Mean Highest U.S. Sugar Subsidy Cost in Decade" (Reuters.com, October 24, 2013) that in 2013 the loan guarantee program alone cost the federal government an estimated $280 million, a consequence of falling sugar prices.

Many industry observers feel sugar subsidies undermine efforts to improve Americans' diets. For example, the editorial "For a Healthier Country, Overhaul Farm Subsidies" (ScientificAmerican.com, May 1, 2012) asserts that "public money is working at cross-purposes: backing an overabundance of unhealthful calories that are flooding our supermarkets and restaurants, while also battling obesity and the myriad illnesses that go with it. It is time to align our farm policies with our health policies."

Sugar (including sucrose, dextrose, fructose, corn syrup, and maltodextrin) is a key ingredient of many processed food products. Table 8.3 lists the names of added sugars that may be found in processed foods. Alice G. Walton reports in "How Much Sugar Are Americans Eating?" (Forbes.com, August 30, 2012) that the average American consumes about three pounds of sugar per week for a total of 130 pounds of sugar per year, or about

TABLE 8.2

Monthly estimates of fiscal year 2014 sugar supply and use, May–October 2013

	May 2013	June 2013	July 2013	August 2013	September 2013
Beginning stocks 1/	2,168	2,231	2,219	2,309	2,215
Total production	**8,584**	**8,584**	**8,643**	**8,453**	**8,703**
Beet sugar	4,840	4,840	4,890	4,800	4,950
Cane sugar	3,744	3,744	3,753	3,653	3,753
Florida	1,833	1,833	1,833	1,833	1,833
Louisiana	1,561	1,561	1,600	1,500	1,600
Texas	170	170	140	140	140
Hawaii	180	180	180	180	180
Total imports	**3,438**	**3,810**	**3,116**	**3,228**	**3,400**
Tariff-rate quota imports	1,265	1,265	1,122	1,122	1,332
Other program imports	400	400	125	110	110
Non-program imports	1,773	2,145	1,869	1,996	1,958
Mexico	1,763	2,135	1,859	1,986	1,948
Total supply	**14,190**	**14,625**	**13,978**	**13,990**	**14,318**
Exports	200	200	200	200	200
Adjustments	0	0	0	0	0
Total deliveries	**11,745**	**11,745**	**11,765**	**11,765**	**11,785**
Domestic food and beverage	11,560	11,560	11,580	11,580	11,600
Other use	185	185	185	185	185
Total use	**11,945**	**11,945**	**11,965**	**11,965**	**11,985**
Ending stocks	2,245	2,680	2,013	2,025	2,333
Stocks/use ratio	18.80	22.44	16.82	16.92	19.46

SOURCE: "Table 26. Monthly Estimates of Fiscal 2014 U.S. Sugar Supply and Use," in *Sugar and Sweeteners Yearbook Tables*, U.S. Department of Agriculture, Economic Research Service, November 1, 2013, http://www.ers.usda.gov/data-products/sugar-and-sweeteners-yearbook-tables.aspx#.Unfel ZFIDY0 (accessed November 4, 2013)

TABLE 8.3

Names for added sugars that appear on food labels

A food is likely to be high in sugars if one of these names appears first or second in the ingredient list or if several names are listed.

Brown sugar	Invert sugar
Corn sweetener	Lactose
Corn syrup	Malt syrup
Dextrose	Maltose
Fructose	Molasses
Fruit juice concentrate	Raw sugar
Glucose	Sucrose
High-fructose corn syrup	Syrup
Honey	Table sugar

SOURCE: "Box 21. Names for Added Sugars That Appear on Food Labels," in *Nutrition and Your Health: Dietary Guidelines for Americans*, 5th ed., U.S. Department of Health and Human Services and U.S. Department of Agriculture, 2000, http://www.health.gov/dietaryguidelines/dga2000/document/choose.htm (accessed November 4, 2013)

756g of sugar every five days. By contrast, in 1822, the average American consumed 45g of sugar every five days. Added sugar accounts for about 500 calories per day in the American diet. According to Walton, refined sugar has no nutritional value and its consumption is linked to the development of obesity, hypertension, depression, headaches, fatigue and other health problems.

In addition, she reports that brain scans reveal that sugar is as addictive as cocaine.

In "The Relationship of Sugar to Population-Level Diabetes Prevalence: An Econometric Analysis of Repeated Cross-Sectional Data" (*PLoS One*, vol. 8, no, 2, February 2013), Sanjay Basu et al. report that there is a direct correlation between how much sugar is available in countries' food supplies and their rates of type 2 diabetes. Countries with higher amounts of sugar in their food supply had higher rates of type 2 diabetes. Specifically, every additional 150 calories of sugar available per person per day (roughly equivalent to the sugar in a can of soda) is associated with a 1.1% increase in diabetes prevalence.

Walton observes that the American Heart Association recommends limiting sugar consumption to no more than 9.5 teaspoons per day. The average U.S. adult, however, consumes 22 teaspoons per day and the average child consumes 32 teaspoons per day. About one-third of Americans' sugar comes from soft drinks (there are 10 teaspoons of sugar in a 12 oz. [355 mL] can of Coca-Cola), about 16% from candy, 13% from cakes, cookies and pies, and 9% from dairy desserts and milk.

The health food industry has been warning the public about the perils of the overconsumption of refined sugars for more than 30 years, and mainstream nutritionists and public health professionals have joined the ranks of those calling for reduced sugar consumption. Along with ending sugar subsidies, they want to sharply limit the advertising of sugary products to children, ban the sale of soft drinks in schools, and conduct widespread community public health education programs to inform Americans about the health risks of consuming excessive amounts of refined sugars.

THE U.S. WAR ON OBESITY GAINS MOMENTUM

Besides generating international debate, the issue of obesity is receiving considerable attention from lawmakers, public health officials, and politicians throughout the United States. For example, the Trust for America's Health (TFAH is a nonprofit, nonpartisan organization working to make disease prevention a national priority) calls for a national strategy to combat obesity to address the problem. TFAH and the Robert Wood Johnson Foundation publish an annual report titled *F as in Fat: How Obesity Threatens America's Future* (2014, http://fasinfat.org), which details state and national obesity rates and policies to prevent and reduce obesity. The 2013 report describes policy accomplishments over the preceding decade, including changes to nutrition standards for school foods, improved health screenings for children, changes to improve nutrition and health counseling in the WIC program, increased understanding about how the built environment affects people's ability to eat healthful foods and be physically active, and a growth in community-based programs targeting obesity. Key recommendations include:

- All food in schools must be healthy

- Children and adults should have access to more opportunities to be physically active

- Restaurants should post calorie information on menus

- Food and beverage companies should market only their healthiest products to children

- The country should invest more in preventing disease to save money spent treating it

- America's transportation plans should encourage walking and biking

- Everyone should be able to purchase healthy, affordable foods close to home

TFAH executive director Jeffrey Levi presented the organization's concerns in a congressional briefing on September 12, 2013 (http://healthyamericans.org/health-issues/wp-content/uploads/2013/09/9-12-Jeff-Presentation-FINAL-9-5-132.pdf). These include:

- Uncertainty about whether the halt in overweight and obesity increases observed in 2012–13 can be sustained

- The financial impact of baby boomers, many of whom are obese, on Medicare

- Obesity's negative implications for education, agriculture and transportation

- Inadequate public health and prevention funding

Jennifer L. Pomeranz and Kelly D. Brownell of Yale University assert in "Advancing Public Health Obesity Policy through State Attorneys General" (*American Journal of Public Health*, vol. 101, no. 3, March 2011) that the war on obesity requires "government action at multiple levels and across disciplines." The researchers call on state attorneys general to assume lead roles to champion nutrition policy and to protect consumers, especially children, from misleading marketing and advertising practices. Attorneys general can also reach across state lines to tackle issues including food marketing in schools and the use of web-tracking and analytics that target food marketing to individual Internet users, including children. They can advocate consumer education and can issue formal written opinions about issues such as the legality of taxing sugar-sweetened beverages. Pomeranz and Brownell aver that "there is much room for greater attorney general involvement in formulating and championing solutions to this public health problem. Obesity may not be on the radar of every attorney general as a topic for their attention, so state and local advocates should contact and work with their attorneys general to support public health measures at every level."

Skirmishes in the war on obesity do not center on whether there is a problem, but on how best to address it. Participants on one side characterize the food industry, advertisers, and the media as complicit, in that they entice consumers with seductive advertising and sugary, high-calorie treats. Their opponents believe consumers should exercise personal responsibility and make their own choices about food and exercise.

FDA MOVES TO BAN TRANS FAT

In November 2013 the U.S. Food and Drug Administration (FDA) put forth a plan to eliminate trans fats from the U.S. food supply. Sabrina Tavernise observes in "F.D.A. Ruling Would All but Eliminate Trans Fats" (NYTimes.com, November 7, 2013) that the agency was proposing to reclassify partially hydrogenated oils—the source of trans fats in fried and baked goods and margarine—as no longer "generally recognized as safe." This would for all intents and purposes ban them from use in food. The FDA's move came 10 years after it first required that added trans fats be listed on food labels, which caused many companies to reformulate their products to eliminate or greatly reduce them. For instance, the Grocery Manufacturers Association voluntarily reduced the use of trans fats by more than 73% between 2005 and 2013. As a consequence of these voluntary changes, Americans' consumption of trans fats declined sharply, from an average of 4.6 grams per day in 2006 to 1 gram a day in 2012. The ban on hydrogenated oils was expected to reduce this even further. Tavernise reports, however, that some nutritionists were concerned that health benefits would not be realized if Americans replaced their consumption of trans fats with saturated fats.

JUNK FOOD IS IRRESISTIBLE—IS THE FOOD INDUSTRY TO BLAME?

In "The Extraordinary Science of Addictive Junk Food" (NYTimes.com, February 24, 2013), Michael Moss asserts that the food industry has conditioned Americans to crave unhealthy, sugary, salty, fatty, processed foods. Moss describes food industry efforts aimed at getting consumers "hooked" on convenient, inexpensive foods and their efforts to use science not only to produce highly desirable and potentially addictive foods but also to dismiss health concerns about excessive consumption of salt, sugar and fat. He refers to the sophisticated scientific and market testing that produces food that looks and tastes good but is not necessarily healthy. For example, he details the development of Lunchables—prepackaged meat, cheese and crackers with a sugary drink and candy for dessert—that were marketed to busy, working mothers as convenient alternatives to preparing homemade lunches for their children. Moss recounts criticism of Lunchables, "One article said something like, 'If you take Lunchables apart, the most healthy item in it is the napkin.'" In 2011 Kraft, the company that produces Lunchables, reduced salt, sugar, and fat in their products by 10% and replaced the candy bars with fruit, but critics remained skeptical because the ingredients in Lunchables hardly constituted healthy choices.

Does Nutrition Labeling Help Consumers Make Healthier Choices?

According to Joanna Parks of the FDA's Center for Food Safety and Applied Nutrition Use, food labels do affect what people eat. In *The Effects of Food Labeling and Dietary Guidance on Nutrition in the United States* (August 2013, http://ageconsearch.umn.edu/bitstream/149667/2/AAEA%20Nut-Label-DRAFT-IV-5-23-13.pdf), she reports that people who use the Nutrition Facts Panel (NFP) on food packages to learn about their ingredients and nutrients consume 120 fewer calories per day on average than those who do not use the labels. This may help them to regulate body weight. Parks reports that some groups of people were more likely to report using the NFP than others, including: women, people with college degrees, those with food allergies, those who think it is important to consider nutrition when making food choices, individuals who engage in vigorous leisure-time physical activity, and people who follow special diets.

In "Front-of-Package Food and Beverage Labeling: New Directions for Research and Regulation" (*American Journal of Public Health*, vol. 40, no. 3, March 2011), Jennifer L. Pomeranz of Yale University explains that the federal government regulates what sort of health claims can be made on food packaging, but that the food industry nevertheless has substantial leeway about what to put on the front of its packaging. According to Pomeranz, as of 2010 there were a wide variety of such claims being made conveying "an excessive amount of information and misinformation" and "creating consumer confusion and distrust." She notes that in October 2010 the FDA, in response to consumer complaints, suggested that front-of-package labels should display calories, serving sizes, saturated fat, trans fat, and sodium. Pomeranz reports that the following month the Grocery Manufacturers Association announced plans to develop its own front-of-package labeling guidelines. Because adherence with the FDA guidelines is voluntary, however, the food industry was free to design its own schema for labeling. Pomeranz suggests that the FDA mandate adherence to its guidelines if the industry fails to adopt science-based criteria.

In October 2011, the Institute of Medicine (IOM) released a report about consumer use and understanding of front-of-package nutrition information, *Front-of-Package Nutrition Rating Systems and Symbols: Promoting Healthier Choices* (http://books.nap.edu/openbook.php?record_id=13221). The report recommends replacing current front-of-package labels, which provide nutrition information but do not

inform consumers about the healthfulness of the product, with a simpler, graphic nutrition rating system that uses symbols on the front of food packaging to display calories per serving. It also advises describing servings in familiar measurements, such as per slice or per cup, to improve consumers' understanding, as well as showing whether a product's saturated and trans fats, sodium, and added sugar content is at or below a certain level. The IOM also recommended a ranked system using points to help consumers determine whether foods contain unhealthy amounts of saturated and trans fats, sodium, and added sugars.

The IOM observes in "Walmart Announces 'Great for You' front-of-package symbol" (February 2012, http://www.iom.edu/Reports/2011/Front-of-Package-Nutrition-Rating-Systems-and-Symbols-Promoting-Healthier-Choices/Action-Taken.aspx) that, in response to the IOM recommendations, in February 2012 Walmart debuted a new front-of-package icon to deliver nutrition information to consumers.

Another study, in which "traffic light" labeling—red for unhealthy items, yellow for less healthy items, and green for healthy items—was used to identify foods in a hospital cafeteria confirms that labels do influence purchasing behavior. In "A Traffic Light Food Labeling Intervention Increases Consumer Awareness of Health and Healthy Choices at the Point-of-Purchase" (*Preventive Medicine*, vol. 57, no. 4, October 2013), Lillian Sonnenberg et al. find that the traffic light labels "prompt people to consider their health at point-of-purchase" and help them make healthier food choices.

Can and Should Laws Change Americans' Diets?

The American legal professor John F. Banzhaf III (1940–), who campaigned against tobacco, advocates using the legal system to create change in Americans' diets. He exhorts attorneys to bring lawsuits against fast-food purveyors and junk-food manufacturers to increase consumer awareness of the role the food industry plays in promoting obesity. Banzhaf was interviewed in Morgan Spurlock's (1970–) documentary film *Super Size Me* (2004), which focuses on the fast-food industry's promotion of unhealthy eating and the director's experience subsisting on a diet of fast food for 30 days.

The Center for Consumer Freedom is an advocacy group that is supported by restaurant and food companies and that represents major corporations such as RJR Nabisco. The center marshals lawyers, publicists, and lobbyists to respond to antiobesity crusaders and derides lawsuits and legislation aimed at limiting consumers' rights to choose the foods they want to consume. It also pokes fun at the self-appointed "food police" (legislators, public health officials, and others) that is intent on modifying Americans' diets, and at mandates by the Center for Science in the

Public Interest (CSPI; a nonprofit advocacy group for nutrition, food safety, health, and other issues) to offer consumers nutritional data. It is credited with helping defeat a measure that would have required chain restaurants to offer nutritional data about their products. In "Ballot Issues up for Grabs Tomorrow" (November 4, 2013, http://www.consumerfreedom.com/2013/11/ballot-issues-up-for-grabs-tomorrow/), the Center for Consumer Freedom staunchly opposes measures that would label genetically engineered food or tax soft drinks. It asserts that physical inactivity—as opposed to the overconsumption of foods high in sugar, fat, and calories—is the primary cause of childhood obesity.

The Obesity Society Action Plan

In its position statement (June 24, 2010, http://www.obesity.org/images/pdf/Obesity2010/TOS_Washington_Times_Eradicating.pdf), the Obesity Society provides an ambitious agenda for the government and private sector that enumerates specific funding priorities, programs, and services to prevent, treat, and educate Americans. It calls for:

- A "war on obesity, not the obese." The Obesity Society asserts that this war will not be waged or won by further stigmatizing obese people and calls for efforts to end discrimination and eliminate the social stigma associated with obesity.

- Educating the public to improve awareness of obesity as "a complex disease involving genes, behavior and environment" rather than as a moral weakness.

- Informing the public about obesity, its causes, and consequences, and engaging in "a national debate on obesity, similar to past campaigns in smoking and cholesterol."

- Expanding access to professional treatment of obesity so that its medical, social, and economic consequences can be averted.

- Ensuring reimbursement for medical treatment for obesity, including drugs and surgery.

- Including nutrition education, lifestyle counseling, and obesity diagnosis and management into medical school curricula and other health professionals' training.

- Revising national policies, such as farm policies promoting the production of energy-dense foods with low nutritional value, that exacerbate the problem.

- Preventing excess weight gain in children and adults, teaching healthy behaviors and lifestyles early in life, and providing healthy school lunches.

- Building environments that encourage healthier behaviors such as walking and more physical activity at work.

- Recognizing the economic impact of obesity on medical expenditures and lost wages.

- Supporting research to address the problem by doubling funding from federal agencies including the National Institutes of Health, the U.S. Department of Agriculture (USDA), and the Centers for Disease Control and Prevention (CDC).

The Healthy, Hunger-Free Kids Act

In December 2010 President Obama signed the Healthy, Hunger-Free Kids Act into law. The act authorizes funding for federal school meal and child nutrition programs and is intended to increase access to healthful food for low-income children. The bill reauthorizes child nutrition programs for five years and includes $4.5 billion in new funding for these programs over 10 years. Furthermore, it:

- Authorizes the USDA to establish nutritional standards for all foods that are sold in schools during the school day, including vending machines, lunch lines, and school stores

- Provides increased reimbursement to schools that meet updated nutritional standards for federally subsidized lunches

- Assists communities to establish local farm-to-school networks, create school gardens, and use more local foods in schools

- Improves access to drinking water in schools

- Establishes standards for school wellness policies, including goals for nutrition promotion and education and physical activity

- Promotes nutrition and wellness in child care settings through the federally subsidized Child and Adult Care Food Program

- Supports breastfeeding through the Women, Infants, and Children program

The USDA describes its proposed school nutrition standards in "Smart Snacks in School: USDA's 'All Foods Sold in Schools' Standards" (July 16, 2013, http://www.fns.usda.gov/cnd/governance/legislation/allfoods.htm). The standards aim to ensure that all foods offered to students in school are nutritious. The standards establish limits on how many calories the food available in schools can contain, as well as how much sodium, fat, and sugar. In addition, under the standards any food sold in schools must meet at least one of four requirements: be whole-grain rich; have a fruit, vegetable, dairy product, or protein food as its first ingredient; be a "combination food" containing at least 1/4 cup of fruits or vegetables; contain 10% or more of the recommended daily value of calcium, potassium, vitamin D, or dietary fiber. Figure 8.1 compares food offered in schools before and after the new standards.

FIGURE 8.1

Snack choices before and after Smart Snacks in School nutrition standards, 2013

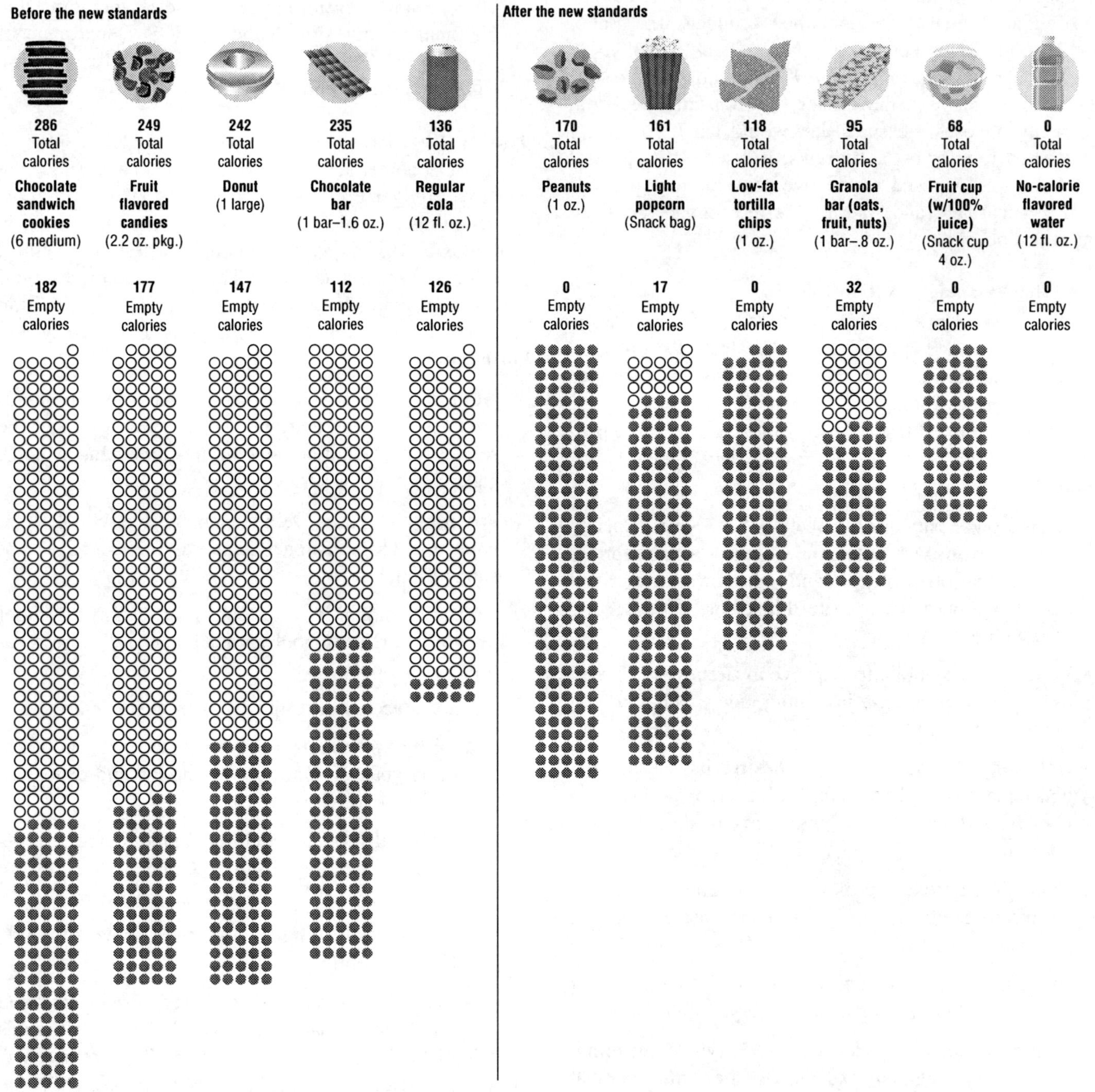

Before the new standards

286 Total calories	249 Total calories	242 Total calories	235 Total calories	136 Total calories
Chocolate sandwich cookies (6 medium)	Fruit flavored candies (2.2 oz. pkg.)	Donut (1 large)	Chocolate bar (1 bar–1.6 oz.)	Regular cola (12 fl. oz.)
182 Empty calories	177 Empty calories	147 Empty calories	112 Empty calories	126 Empty calories

After the new standards

170 Total calories	161 Total calories	118 Total calories	95 Total calories	68 Total calories	0 Total calories
Peanuts (1 oz.)	Light popcorn (Snack bag)	Low-fat tortilla chips (1 oz.)	Granola bar (oats, fruit, nuts) (1 bar–.8 oz.)	Fruit cup (w/100% juice) (Snack cup 4 oz.)	No-calorie flavored water (12 fl. oz.)
0 Empty calories	17 Empty calories	0 Empty calories	32 Empty calories	0 Empty calories	0 Empty calories

*Calories from food components such as added sugars and solid fats that provide little nutritional value. Empty calories are part of total calories.

SOURCE: "Smart Snacks in School Infographic," in *Smart Snacks in School*, U.S. Department of Agriculture, Food and Nutrition Service, November 1, 2013, http://www.fns.usda.gov/cnd/governance/legislation/allfoods_infographic.pdf (accessed November 5, 2013)

F as in Fat: How Obesity Threatens America's Future states that, in 2013, 31 states and the District of Columbia had farm-to-school programs in place that improve students' diets by bringing fresh local produce to schools. Farm-to-school programs have changed students' eating habits, not only increasing fruit and vegetable consumption but also prompting them to choose healthier foods at lunch. Many of these programs, however, applied to only a limited number of schools within the states in question.

OVERWEIGHT, OBESITY, AND THE LAW

Health care coverage and the availability of services to prevent or treat obesity vary widely. The Patient Protection and Affordable Care Act (ACA), which was signed into law in March 2010, significantly strengthens obesity-prevention efforts. The law authorizes new resources and initiatives, including screening for obesity, diet counseling for adults who are at risk for chronic diseases, and referral to intensive behavioral interventions that are intended to reduce obesity.

The ACA also provides funds through 2015 for the Childhood Obesity Demonstration Project, which was established through the Children's Health Insurance Program Reauthorization Act of 2009. The demonstration project funds programs aimed at improving children's nutrition. It is aimed at children aged 2 to 12 years who are covered by the Children's Health Insurance Program, which provides low-cost health insurance to over 7 million children of working families. The CDC observes in "Identifying Effective Strategies to Help Combat Childhood Obesity" (April 27, 2012, http://www.cdc.gov/obesity/childhood/researchproject.html) that minority children and those in low-income communities are at higher risk for obesity and its consequences.

In addition, the ACA requires chain restaurants and food establishments to disclose calorie counts and other nutritional information (fat, saturated fat, cholesterol, sodium, total carbohydrates, sugars, fiber, and total protein) for standard menu items. Vending machine operators with 20 or more machines must also disclose calorie content for many items.

Sin Taxes on Sodas and Junk Food?

Sumptuary taxes, more commonly known as sin taxes, are taxes imposed on goods at least in part because the government wants to discourage their use by forcing their prices higher. Tobacco and alcohol are subject to sin taxes in many areas. Many antiobesity activists believe that taxes on sugary soda drinks, or on junk food in general, would reduce the amount of these items that Americans consume, leading in turn to better health. Jason P. Block and Walter C. Willett assert in "Taxing Sugar-Sweetened Beverages: Not a "Holy Grail" but a Cup at Least Half" (*International Journal of Health Policy and Management*, vol. 1, no. 2, August 2013) that a tax on sugar-sweetened beverages would be likely to decrease their consumption. They also observe that when asked whether they support a soda tax that would be used to fund obesity prevention programs, about half of survey respondents favor the tax.

In "Taxing Junk Food to Counter Obesity" (*American Journal of Public Health*, vol. 103, no. 11, November 2013), Caroline Franck, Sonia M. Grandi, and Mark J. Eisenberg opine that small taxes on junk food may generate considerable revenue but are unlikely to significantly reduce the prevalence of obesity. High taxes are more likely to impact obesity rates, but are likely to be unpopular. Franck, Grandi, and Eisenberg feel that the way in which tax revenues are used to address the problem will determine whether the taxes are effective at combatting obesity.

Lawsuits Attack Food Service Industry

A number of individuals and advocacy groups have brought lawsuits against the food service industry. Some claim they deserve compensation for the damage that fattening foods have done to their health. Others focus on advertising and marketing that they feel is deceptive and misleads people into eating unhealthy products. Many attorneys and public health professionals believe such lawsuits can serve as vehicles that reverse the obesity epidemic, in part because the media attention generated by such lawsuits motivates food companies to produce healthier products and to reconsider marketing and advertising practices.

The first class-action suit was the widely publicized case of Caesar Barber, a 56-year-old New Yorker weighing 270 pounds (122 kg), who claimed that four fast-food restaurants (McDonald's, Burger King, Wendy's, and KFC) jeopardized his health by promoting high-calorie, high-fat, and salty menu items. In "Whopper of a Lawsuit: Fast-Food Chains Blamed for Obesity, Illnesses" (ABCNews.com, July 26, 2002), Geraldine Sealey reports that Barber filed the lawsuit in the New York State Supreme Court "on behalf of an unspecified number of other obese and ill New Yorkers who also feast on fast food." According to Sealey, Barber's suit alleged that the fast-food restaurants, where he ate "four or five times a week even after suffering a heart attack, did not properly disclose the ingredients of their food and the risks of eating too much." Barber's suit was dismissed, so he filed for a second time. His second suit was also dismissed, and he was barred from filing for a third time.

Pelman v. McDonald's Corporation (237 F. Supp. 2d 512, 543 [S.D.N.Y. 2003]) was a similar case, in which two teenagers sought class action status to sue McDonald's on the grounds that the company had misled them into thinking that its food was healthier than it really was, and as a consequence they had developed obesity and related disorders. The case ended in dismissal in 2010, after nearly 10 years of legal wrangling. In "Where's the Beef?—The Challenges of Obesity Lawsuits" (BloombergLaw.com, 2013), Saul Wilensky and Kerry C. O'Dell explain that the courts sided with McDonald's in *Pelman* for a number of reasons, among them the fact that to prevail the plaintiffs would need to show that McDonald's food was the specific cause of their health problems, not just one factor among many. They opine that similar lawsuits will most likely fail as well.

Legislation Protects Food Industry Interests

The food industry contends that Americans choose what they eat and should not be able to blame the food industry if their personal choices have unhealthy consequences. State and federal legislators who agree with this viewpoint have enacted or attempted to enact so-called Commonsense Consumption Acts (CCAs). In general, CCAs bar civil lawsuits seeking recovery for obesity-related health harms. Some in the media call these laws "cheeseburger bills," and in "Beyond Cheeseburgers: The Impact of Commonsense Consumption Acts on Future Obesity-Related Lawsuits" (*Food and Drug Law Journal*, vol. 68, no. 3, 2013), Cara L. Wilking and Richard A. Daynard report that CCAs were enacted in 25 states between 2004 and 2012. In 16 states the CCAs conferred broad civil immunity for claims stemming from long-term consumption of food.

In October 2005 the U.S. House of Representatives passed a bill that would prevent most obesity or weight-related claims against the food industry and make it harder for consumers to sue restaurants and food retailers for serving fattening fare. The legislation, however, did not receive a vote in the U.S. Senate, so it did not become law. The act had been reintroduced three times as of January 2014, without success.

Wilking and Daynard discuss the rationale behind CCAs in their article. As an example, they describe how Colorado's rationale for its CCA states that obesity and other health problems result from "poor choices that are habitually made" by individuals, and that it asserts that "excessive litigation restricts the wide range of choices otherwise available to individuals who consume products responsibly."

Those in favor of CCAs contend that the central issue is "common sense and personal responsibility" and generally subscribe to the opinion that obesity is an individual health issue as opposed to a larger societal and public health problem. Opponents of legislation limiting liability suggest that it is unrealistic to expect consumers to assume personal responsibility when food companies do not disclose relevant information about their products, such as the number of calories and fat content. Wilking and Daynard argue that CCAs are not truly motivated by a desire to prevent frivolous lawsuits; instead they claim that CCAs aim to "limit legally and factually sound litigation, which might eventually have harmed industry's bottom line and forced it to change its practices."

THE FOOD INDUSTRY RESPONDS TO PUBLIC OUTCRY

Mounting pressure on the food industry to change its marketing practices and offer healthier products has had some success. For example, in September 2012 McDonald's began posting calorie counts on its menus,

before the ACA deadline for doing so. It also debuted some more healthful offerings, including an egg-white McMuffin, a grilled chicken option Happy Meal, and accompaniments of fruits and vegetables. In 2013 McDonald's also introduced a calorie-counting app. In "McDonald's Menu to Post Calorie Data" (NYTimes.com, September 12, 2012), Stephanie Strom quotes Margo Wootan, director of nutrition policy at the Center for Science in the Public Interest, who praised the company's efforts by saying, "They are such a huge restaurant and there are so many people that eat their food, so this is a really positive step.... It will help their customers get more familiar with calorie counts and make decisions about what they eat based on them, and it will probably improve McDonald's menu over time."

One year later, McDonald's promised to offer options that are lower in fat, salt, or sugar content than its traditional fare, especially on its children's menu. For example, it offered premium wraps, which feature grilled (rather than fried) chicken rolled into a flour tortilla with lettuce, tomatoes and cucumbers, and added more fruit, vegetable and whole-grain offerings. In "With Tastes Growing Healthier, McDonald's Aims to Adapt Its Menu" (NYTimes.com, September 26, 2013), Stephanie Strom reports that the company will also promote fruit and vegetable consumption on the packaging for its children's meals as well as providing nutrition information.

In "Profits and Pandemics: Prevention of Harmful Effects of Tobacco, Alcohol, and Ultra-processed Food and Drink Industries" (*Lancet*, vol. 381, no. 9867, February 2013), Rob Moodie et al. assessed the effectiveness of self-regulation, public-private partnerships, and public regulation of unhealthy commodities: tobacco, alcohol, and energy-dense ultra-processed food. The researchers assert that:

- Transnational corporations are major drivers of non-communicable disease epidemics and profit from increased consumption of tobacco, alcohol, and ultra-processed food and drink (so-called unhealthy commodities).

- Alcohol and ultra-processed food and drink industries use strategies similar to those of the tobacco industry to undermine effective public health policies and programs.

- Unhealthy commodity industries should have no role in the formation of national or international policy for noncommunicable disease policy.

- Despite the common reliance on industry self-regulation and public-private partnerships to improve public health, there is no evidence to support their effectiveness or safety.

Moodie et al. point out that these three industries have all employed the same tactics—presenting biased research findings, co-opting policy makers and health professionals, and lobbying politicians and public official to oppose public regulation—to undermine public health interventions. The researchers note that to deflect claims that their products harm health, companies in these industries often point to factors outside their areas of expertise. For example, food and beverage corporations point to physical inactivity as the culprit in the obesity epidemic. Moodie et al. conclude "the only evidence-based mechanisms that effectively prevent harm caused by unhealthy commodity industries are public regulation and market intervention."

FOOD INDUSTRY INITIATIVES

In "The Role and Challenges of the Food Industry in Addressing Chronic Disease" (*Global Health*, vol. 6, May 28, 2010), Derek Yach et al. state that the food industry is doing much to reduce the burden of overweight and obesity-related diseases. The researchers cite as examples "global public commitments to address food reformulation, consumer information, responsible marketing, promotion of healthy lifestyles, and public-private partnerships." They also present PepsiCo's pledge to increase the amount of whole grains, fruits, vegetables, nuts, seeds, and low-fat dairy in its product portfolio and to increase the range of foods and beverages that offer solutions for managing calories.

PepsiCo states in *2012 Annual Report* (2012, http://www.pepsico.com/download/PEP_Annual_Report_2012.pdf) that it eliminated the use of partially hydrogenated cooking oils in its snacks and also reduced their saturated fat levels and sodium content. In addition, the company stated it was offering more baked products. In 2012 PepsiCo debuted Quaker Real Medleys—oatmeal with other whole grains, fruits and nuts in a portion-controlled serving, It also continued to sell reduced-calorie orange juice and introduced juice that contains a serving of fruit and vegetables in an eight-ounce glass.

In "Food Industry: Friend or Foe?" (*Obesity Reviews*, vol. 15, no. 1, January 2014), Derek Yach of the Vitality Institute in New York, New York, calls for collaboration between the public and private sectors to address nutrition issues and provide healthy, sustainable food. Yach observes that neither sector fully understands or appreciates the efforts of the other. For example, he cites the tremendous efforts made by companies to reformulate their products to met standards for salt, sugar, and saturated fat content. He feels that public sector efforts to inform consumers about the dangers of excessive consumption of salt, sugar and saturated fat would strengthen companies' motivation and ability to supply these healthier food products. Yach notes that inexpensive commodities in the American diet are those that have been heavily subsidized over decades. More expensive foods such as fruits and vegetables have increased in cost over time. Yach favors making healthier choices more affordable rather than imposing taxes on unhealthy foods. He suggests public-private collaboration to improve the taste of foods with reduced sodium and fat and asks that public funds such as those allocated to the NIH be used to research cost-effective, sustainable diet and lifestyle solutions rather than drug treatment of diet and weight-related disorders.

Yach notes that corporate innovation and commitment to healthier foods have been rewarded by investors who understand the long-tem importance of improving consumers' health. He points out that companies do not have to sacrifice profits to combat obesity and promote health. They can succeed in selling less volume if they can sell products with similar value. For example, a quality product with a smaller serving size can have a higher profit margin than a bargain-sized product of lesser quality. Yach concludes, "When common interests and outcomes are at stake, private-public engagement is more likely to achieve faster and more sustainable results than relying on governments to act alone."

THE HEALTHY WEIGHT COMMITMENT FOUNDATION AND CHILDHOOD OBESITY

In October 2009 a group of 41 retailers, nongovernmental organizations, and food and beverage manufacturers launched the Healthy Weight Commitment Foundation (HWCF), a national initiative intended to reduce the rate of obesity, especially among children and adolescents. In the press release "Retailers, NGOs, and Food and Beverage Industry Launch National Initiative to Help Reduce Obesity" (2009, http://www.prnewswire.com/), the HWCF explains that members of the foundation, which include the Campbell Soup Co., General Mills Inc., Kellogg Co., Nestlé USA, Ralston Foods/Post Foods, and PepsiCo, invested $20 million in the initiative. The initiative targets three key audiences—markets, the workplace, and schools—and with a nationwide public education campaign that focuses on ways to help people reach and maintain a healthy weight by balancing calories consumed with calories expended through physical activity.

By 2014 the HWCF (http://www.healthyweightcommit.org/about/overview/) had a membership of more than 250 retailers, food and beverage manufacturers, restaurants, sporting goods companies, insurance companies, trade associations, nongovernmental organizations, and professional sports organizations. The HWCF Together Counts program is encourages families to eat meals and participate in physical activities together to help prevent obesity and promote good health. The Together Counts website (http://www.togethercounts.com/) provides families with tools to track their progress and compare them with the results in their community and across the United States. The site also offers tips and advice to promote participation and a mobile application that enables participants to log and track their progress.

WEIGHT-BASED DISCRIMINATION

Nearly everyone who is overweight or obese has experienced some form of bias, from disapproving glances and unsolicited advice about how to lose weight, to the seemingly unending stream of "fat jokes" and the unflattering and even humiliating portrayal of overweight people in the media. The pervasive anti-fat bias in American culture and negative attitudes toward obese individuals have resulted in stigmatization and clear instances of discrimination.

In "The Stigma of Obesity: A Review and Update" (*Obesity*, vol. 17, no. 5, May 2009), Rebecca M. Puhl and Chelsea A. Heuer of Yale University find that the prevalence of weight discrimination increased by 66% between 1995 and 2006 and describe it as comparable to rates of racial discrimination. Systematic discrimination against obese individuals occurs in at least three areas: education, employment, and health care. Evidence also points to discrimination in adoption proceedings, jury selection, and housing.

Puhl and Heuer observe that obese people suffer discrimination in many aspects of life. For example, in the workplace they may be "the target of derogatory humor and pejorative comments from co-workers and supervisors," and in educational settings obese students often experience teasing, taunts, and derision from peers. Health care professionals and educators have been found to hold and promote negative stereotypes about people who are obese, and the media, especially television and film, continue to stigmatize overweight and obese characters. Puhl and Heuer assert that overweight people "remain one of the last acceptable targets of humor and ridicule in North American television and film." Even the news media participates by blaming obese people for contributing to "rising fuel prices, global warming, and causing weight gain in their friends."

Several studies find distinct anti-fat bias in children as young as age three and increasingly negative stereotypic attitudes as children age. Puhl and Heuer observe that an analysis of 25 popular videos and 20 popular books for young children attributed many "desirable traits such as sociability, kindness, happiness, and success" to thin female characters, whereas overweight characters were "commonly depicted as evil, unattractive, unfriendly, and cruel."

Overweight and obese job applicants and workers may be subjected to weight-based discrimination in employment. Many studies document discrimination in hiring practices, especially when the positions sought involved public contact, such as sales or direct customer service. Obese workers face inequities in wages, benefits, and promotions, and several studies confirm that the economic penalties are greater for women than for men. Overweight women earn less doing the same work as their normal-weight counterparts and have dimmer prospects for promotion. The courts have considered cases in which workers contended that their job terminations were weight-related. The outcomes of these cases indicate that termination can occur because of employer prejudice and arbitrary weight standards.

In "New Developments in the Law for Obesity Discrimination Protection" (*Obesity*, vol. 21, no. 3, March 2013), Jennifer L. Pomeranz and Rebecca M. Puhl observe that amendments to the Americans with Disabilities Act of 1990 (ADA) that went into effect in 2009 broaden the definition of disability. The courts now consider severe obesity an impairment using the ADA definition of disability. Pomeranz and Puhl believe that additional protections are warranted and suggest legislation comparable to the Age Discrimination in Employment Act, which prohibits employment discrimination based on age. They believe that "without improved legislation, weight discrimination will continue to prevent equal opportunities, reinforce disparities, and reduce quality of life for millions of individuals affected by obesity."

Weight Bias among Health Professionals

Anti-fat bias among health care professionals may discourage obese people from seeking medical care and compromise the care they receive. Although research indicates that obese patients often delay or cancel medical appointments for a variety of reasons, including fear about being weighed or undressing in front of health professionals, speculation exists that presumed or real prejudice on the part of health professionals may also deter them from seeking medical care.

In "Implicit and Explicit Anti-fat Bias among a Large Sample of Medical Doctors by BMI, Race/Ethnicity and Gender" (*PLoS ONE*, vol. 7, no. 11, November 2012), Janice A. Sabin, Maddalena Marini, and Brian A. Nosek sought to determine the prevalence of negative attitudes about weight among physicians. Bias was assessed using the Implicit Associations Test (IAT), a timed test that analyzes the automatic associations respondents make about particular attributes. For example, the IAT helped identify whether test takers held negative attitudes and stereotypical views about obese people, such as considering them to be lazy, unmotivated, sluggish, or worthless. About two-thirds of the physicians who took the test were in the normal body mass index (BMI; body weight in kilograms divided by height in meters squared) range and they demonstrated a strong implicit, or unconscious, anti-fat bias.

Sabin, Marini, and Nosek explain that implicit bias may predict discriminatory behavior even among people who have no intention of discriminating.

Rebecca M. Puhl, Joerg Luedicke, and Carlos M. Grilo find that students training in the health professions they questioned—physician associates, clinical psychologists, and physicians in psychiatric residencies—reported significant weight bias. In "Obesity Bias in Training: Attitudes, Beliefs, and Observations among Advanced Trainees in Professional Health Disciplines" (*Obesity*, October 2013) the researchers report that students say obese patients are targets of negative attitudes and insulting humor by peers (63%), health care providers (65%), and instructors (40%).

OBESE AMERICANS RECEIVE FEWER PREVENTIVE HEALTH SERVICES. Ironically, people who are obese and usually receive more medical care for chronic diseases related to obesity may also receive fewer preventive services. Does bias contribute to this disparity in preventive care? In "Preventive Care and Health Behaviors among Overweight/Obese Men in HMOs" (*American Journal of Managed Care*, vol. 18, no. 1, January 2012), Virginia P. Quinn et al. examine the association between BMI and laboratory tests for cholesterol, glucose, and diabetes control, as well as screening exams for colorectal and prostate cancer. Quinn et al. find no weight-related differences in laboratory tests but do find that despite comparable access to care, overweight and obese men were less likely to be screened for colorectal and prostate cancer. This finding is alarming in view of the fact that overweight and obese men are at greater risk for colorectal cancer and may be at greater risk for aggressive forms of prostate cancer.

Quinn et al. suggest that educating health care providers may help to reduce these disparities in care. The researchers observe, "Education also can help clinicians be sensitive to the stigmatizing experiences heavier patients deal with in the medical setting, and the importance of their attitude and choice of words when treating these patients."

Airlines Consider Their Options

In June 2002 Southwest Airlines became the center of a fiery debate when the airline decided to strengthen its enforcement of a policy established in 1980 of requesting and requiring passengers who must occupy two airplane seats because of excessive girth to purchase both tickets. The policy allows passengers to be reimbursed for the additional seat if their flight is not full. The National Association to Advance Fat Acceptance, an advocacy group, and other consumer groups called the move discriminatory. Regardless, Southwest Airlines is not the only airline with this policy; Continental, Northwest, and other commercial carriers also require large-sized passengers to pay for two seats.

In 2003 the Federal Aviation Administration (FAA) proposed requiring all passengers on small airlines to be weighed in along with their luggage. The FAA asserted that before takeoff the pilot must calculate the weight of the aircraft as well as that of its passengers, luggage, and crew to determine which seats passengers should occupy to ensure proper balance. For this reason it is vital to know exact passenger and luggage weights on small planes, where several people with a few extra pounds can tilt the plane away from its center of gravity. Although operators of smaller commuter airlines acknowledged the safety issue, they were reluctant to support the FAA recommendation because they feared that weighing people would discourage them from using commuter airlines, many of which were already strapped financially.

In May 2003 the FAA ruled that airlines must assume that passengers weigh between 190 and 195 pounds (86 and 88 kg), depending on the season. At the same time, checked bags on domestic flights were adjusted from an estimated 25 pounds (11 kg) to 30 pounds (14 kg). The 30-pound estimate for checked bags on international flights remained unchanged. The requirement followed shortly after the crash of a commuter plane that killed all 21 people aboard. Investigators suspect the propeller plane was slightly above its maximum weight on takeoff, with most of the weight toward the tail. The weight distribution problem was compounded by a maintenance error that made it difficult to lower the nose with the control column. After the 19-seat plane rose above the ground, its nose pointed dangerously skyward; the pilots were unable to level it off, and the plane spun to the ground.

In "How Long until All Airlines Charge More for Fat People?" (BusinessInsider.com, April 5, 2013), Alex Davies reports that Samoa Airlines is the first airline to charge passengers based on how much they and their luggage weigh. The policy helps offset the cost of fuel for heavier passengers and ensures that the airline's small planes, which hold just 12 passengers each, do not exceed their maximum take-off weights. Davies notes that while this policy may work well for a small operation with few flights and passengers, it would be unwieldy for larger carriers to implement. He also asserts that it would be unpopular and might generate protests arguing that the policy is discriminatory.

In "Pay-as-You-Weigh Pricing of an Air Ticket: Economics and Major Issues for Discussions and Investigations" (*Journal of Revenue & Pricing Management*, vol. 12, no. 2, March 2013), Bharat P. Bhatta of Sogn og Fjordane University College in Sogndal, Norway, observes that policies that charge heavier passengers more but do not offer discounts to lighter passengers only benefit the airlines while harming passengers and society at large. Instead, Bhatta favors a model with average, high, and low weight fares, based on whether a passenger is of average weight, above a specific weight, or below a specific weight.

Laws against Weight Discrimination

The San Francisco Human Rights Commission reports in "Compliance Guidelines to Prohibit Weight and Height Discrimination" (http://www.sf-hrc.org/Modules/ShowDocument.aspx?documentid=159) that on July 26, 2001, it unanimously approved historic guidelines for implementing a height-weight antidiscrimination law, and the city became the first jurisdiction in the United States to offer guidelines on how to prevent discrimination based on weight or height.

The strength of the ordinance was tested in 2003, when Jennifer Portnick, a 240-pound (109-kg) aerobics instructor, was refused a job at Jazzercise Inc., an international dance-fitness organization based in Carlsbad, California, and brought her case before the San Francisco Human Rights Commission. She eventually reached an agreement with the company to drop a requirement about the appearance of instructors. It was the first case settled under the San Francisco ordinance, which has become known as the "Fat and Short Law."

Patricia Leigh Brown reports in "240 Pounds, Persistent, and Jazzercise's Equal" (NYTimes.com, May 8, 2002) that Portnick's attorney, Sondra Solovay, the author of *Tipping the Scales of Justice: Fighting Weight-Based Discrimination* (2000), said Portnick was "geographically lucky" to have filed her case in one of just four jurisdictions in the country that outlawed weight-based discrimination at the time.

In "Legal Largesse or Big, Fat Failure: Do Weight-Discrimination Laws Improve Employment Outcomes for the Obese?" (January 14, 2011 http://papers.ssrn.com/sol3/papers.cfm?abstract_id=2396667), Jennifer Bennett Shinall of the Vanderbilt University Law School notes that as of early 2014 there were 10 jurisdictions in the United States that had laws to protect people from workplace anti-obesity discrimination. They were the cities of San Francisco; Urbana, Illinois; Madison, Wisconsin; Binghamton, New York; Santa Cruz, California; and Washington, D.C.; the state of Michigan; and the counties of Harford, Howard, and Prince George in Maryland. Shinall's analysis of these jurisdictions' laws finds that Madison and Urbana make it easier for discrimination victims to seek relief than do other locations. In those two cities complaints are mediated by commissions, which means complainants do not need lawyers and the process is quick, easy, and inexpensive. Shinall suggests these cities may serve as models for others wishing to combat weight discrimination.

The Origins of Stigma and Bias

Rebecca M. Puhl and Kelly D. Brownell of Yale University observe in the landmark study "Psychosocial Origins of Obesity Stigma: Toward Changing a Powerful and Pervasive Bias" (*Obesity Reviews*, vol. 4, no. 4, November 2003) that many people intensely dread the possibility of becoming obese. In one survey 24% of women and 17% of men said they would sacrifice three or more years of their life to be thin. There are reports of women who choose not to become pregnant because they fear gaining weight and becoming fat. Others smoke cigarettes in an effort to remain thin or reject the advice that they quit smoking because they fear they will gain weight should they quit. This powerful fear of fat, coupled with widespread perceptions that overweight people lack competence, self-control, ambition, intelligence, and attractiveness, create a culture in which it is socially acceptable to hold negative stereotypes about obese individuals and to discriminate against them.

One explanation of the origin of weight stigma is that traditionally Americans believe in self-determination and individualism—people get what they deserve and are responsible for their circumstances. In this context, when overweight is viewed as a consequence of controllable behaviors, it is possible to understand that if an individual believes overweight people are to blame for their weight, then they should be stigmatized. Other research findings—that many Americans view life as predictable, with effort and ability inevitably producing the desired outcomes, and that attractive people are deemed good and believed to embody many positive qualities—support this theory. Interestingly, researchers find that in other countries the best predictors of anti-fat attitudes were cultural values that held both negative views about overweight and the belief that people are responsible for their life outcome.

Several other theories about the origins of weight stigma have been proposed. Conflict theory suggests that prejudice arises from conflicts of interest between groups and struggles to acquire or retain resources or power. Social identity theory posits that groups develop their social identities by comparing themselves to other groups and designating other groups as inferior. Integrated threat theory proposes that stigmatized groups are perceived as a threat. Proponents of this theory suggest that overweight and obese people threaten deeply held cultural values of self-discipline, self-control, moderation, and thinness. Another theory, evolved dispositions theory, proposes that members of a group will be stigmatized if they threaten or undermine group functioning. This evolutionary adaptation may predispose people to shun obese individuals because they are at increased health risk and may not be able to make sufficient contributions to the group's welfare because of weight-related illness or disability.

Reducing Weight Bias and Stigma

In the landmark study "Demonstrations of Implicit Anti-fat Bias: The Impact of Providing Causal Information and Evoking Empathy" (*Health Psychology*, vol. 22, no. 1, January 2003), Bethany A. Teachman et al. wondered if anti-fat bias would be reduced when people were told that an individual's obesity resulted largely from genetic factors rather than from overeating and lack of exercise. The researchers assigned study participants to one of three groups. The first group received no information about the cause of obesity; the second group was given an article asserting that the principal cause of obesity was genetic; and the third group was given an article that attributed most obesity to overeating and lack of physical activity. As the researchers anticipated, the group told that obesity was controllable—resulting from overeating and inactivity—revealed the greatest amount of bias. However, to their surprise, Teachman et al. find that the group informed that obesity was primarily genetic in origin did not have significantly lower levels of bias than either the control group that had received no prior information or the group informed that obesity was caused by overeating and inactivity.

Teachman et al. also wanted to find out whether eliciting empathy for obese people would significantly reduce negative attitudes. The researchers hypothesized that by sharing written stories about weight-based discrimination with study participants they would feel empathy with the subjects in the stories, which they would then generalize to the entire population of obese people. Although some study participants in the group that read the stories displayed lower bias, the majority did not have lower bias than the control group that had not read the stories of discrimination. The researchers speculate that the stories describing negative evaluations of an obese person might actually have served to reinforce rather than diminish bias.

Puhl and Brownell note that the increasing prevalence of obesity has not acted to reduce weight bias. They also refute the notion that stigma is necessary to motivate overweight and obese people to lose weight. They reiterate that dieting is not associated with long-term weight loss, regardless of the individual's motivation. Furthermore, they indicate that stigma can lead to discrimination and exert a harmful influence on health and quality of life. Puhl and Brownell assert that unless stigma is reduced, obese people will continue to contend with prejudice and discrimination.

Although few studies have evaluated the effectiveness of strategies to reduce weight stigma, a variety of initiatives have produced varying degrees of attitudinal change. These approaches include:

- Educating participants about external uncontrollable causes such as the biological and genetic factors that contribute to obesity.

- Teaching and encouraging young children to practice size acceptance.

- Improving attitudes by combining efforts to elicit empathy with education about the uncontrollable causes of obesity.

- Encouraging direct personal contact with overweight and obese individuals to dispel negative stereotypes.

- Changing individuals' beliefs by exposing them to opposing attitudes and values held by a group that they consider important. This approach, which is called social consensus theory, relies on the observation that after learning that a group does not share the individuals' beliefs, they are more likely to modify their beliefs to be similar to those expressed by the group they respect or wish to join.

Puhl and Brownell describe the results of their experiments using social consensus theory to modify attitudes toward obese people. They conducted experiments with university students in which participants reported their attitudes toward obese people before and after the researchers offered them varying consensus opinions of other students. In one experiment, participants who were told that other students held more favorable attitudes about obese people reported significantly fewer negative attitudes and more positive attitudes about obese people than they had before they learned about the opinions of other students. Furthermore, they also changed their ideas about the causes of obesity, favoring the uncontrollable causes after they were told the other students believed obesity was attributable to these causes.

A second experiment confirmed that the power to alter the participants' beliefs depended on whether the source of the opposing beliefs was an in-group or out-group. Not surprisingly, participants' attitudes toward obese people were more likely to change when the information they were given came from a source they valued—an in-group. In a third experiment the researchers compared attitudinal change produced by social consensus with other methods to reduce stigma, including one in which participants were given written material about the controllable or uncontrollable causes of obesity. Puhl and Brownell find that social consensus theory was as effective as or more effective than any of the other methods they applied. They state that social consensus theory also offers an explanation about why obese individuals themselves express negative stereotypes—they want to belong to the valued social group and choose to accept negative stereotypes to align themselves with current culture. Furthermore, by accepting prevailing cultural values and beliefs, they not only resemble the in-group more closely but also distance themselves from the out-group, where identity and membership are defined by being overweight or obese.

Although Puhl and Brownell consider social consensus a promising approach to reducing weight bias and stigma, they caution that there are many unanswered questions about its widespread utility and effectiveness. They conclude that "an ideal and comprehensive theory of obesity stigma would identify the origins of weight bias, explain why stigma is elicited by obese body types, account for the association between certain negative traits and obesity, and suggest methods for reducing bias. Existing theories do not yet meet all these criteria."

Weight Bias in the Media

Puhl and Heuer describe how the media take a dim view of people who are obese, often casting them as "targets of humor and ridicule." The researchers point out that in recent years news reports have attributed a host of ills to people who are obese, ranging from playing a role in rising fuel prices and global warming to causing weight gain among their friends. Children's entertainment also consistently presents thin characters in a positive light and overweight characters negatively. Because most American adults are overweight or obese, it would be helpful to see overweight and obese people in lead roles and cast in a flattering light, as opposed to being in television reality shows, "where the entire cast is trying desperately to become thin."

In "Female Stars Step Off the Scale" (NYTimes.com, October 11, 2012), Alessandra Stanley asserts that television is no longer averse to overweight and obesity and that the presence of overweight characters reflects "a changing American norm." Although reality shows such as *The Biggest Loser* chronicle weight-loss efforts, other shows—such as *The Mindy Project*, *Mike & Molly*, *Girls*, *Curvy Girls*, and *Awkward*—feature characters who are overweight and unapologetic. These characters are not overly concerned with or obsessing about losing weight. Supporters of these shows believe they are realistic and inspiring, because their characters are not defined by their weight.

Stanley observes that the changing norm has also extended to films. In *Bachelorette* (2012), Rebel Wilson (1986–) plays an overweight bride who marries a handsome groom. Melissa McCarthy (1970–), star of *Mike & Molly*, received an Academy Award for her performance in *Bridesmaids* (2011), and also starred in *Identity Thief* (2013) and *The Heat* (2013).

Advocacy Groups Promote Size and Weight Acceptance

Our vision [is] a society in which people of every size are accepted with dignity and equality in all aspects of life. Our mission [is] to eliminate discrimination based on body size and provide fat people with the tools for self-empowerment though public education, advocacy, and support.

—National Association to Advance Fat Acceptance (2013)

There is a robust social movement that advocates size and weight acceptance with the overarching goal of assisting people to have a positive body image at any weight and to achieve health at any size. Nearly all the organizations that champion size acceptance characterize society's preoccupation with dieting and weight loss as unhealthy and unproductive, citing statistics about diet failures, the dangers of weight cycling (the repeated loss and regain of body weight), and low self-esteem. The size acceptance movement proposes that it is possible to be fit and fat simultaneously, and that health and beauty are attainable at all weights. It also works to reduce "fat phobia," anti-fat bias, and weight-based discrimination.

The International Size Acceptance Association (ISAA) promotes size acceptance and aims to end size discrimination throughout the world by means of advocacy and visible, lawful actions. The ISAA asserts that people of all sizes can become more fit and is committed to helping people of all sizes strive for higher levels of fitness and improvement in their overall quality of life. Similarly, the ISAA observes that everyone can benefit from healthier food choices and is committed to helping inform the public about healthy nutrition.

The Council on Size and Weight Discrimination, a nonprofit advocacy organization working to end "sizism," bigotry, and discrimination against people who are heavier than average, focuses its advocacy efforts on affecting changes in medical treatment, job discrimination, and media images. The council's basic principles were derived from the "Tenets of the Nondiet Approach" (Karin Kratina, Dayle Hayes, and Nancy King, *Moving away from Diets: Healing Eating Problems and Exercise Resistance*, 2003) and focus on:

- Total health enhancement and well-being, rather than on weight loss or achieving a specific "ideal weight"

- Self-acceptance and respect for the diversity of bodies that come in a wide variety of shapes and sizes, rather than on the pursuit of an idealized weight at all costs

- The pleasure of eating well, based on internal cues of hunger and satiety (the feeling of fullness or satisfaction after eating), rather than on external food plans or diets

- The joy of movement, encouraging all physical activities, rather than on prescribing a specific routine of regimented exercise

The council exhorts people to free themselves from weight obsession and the effects of negative body image, to learn about issues such as weight discrimination and eating disorders, and to become an educated consumer and seek out health care providers who are competent and unbiased. It also advocates interrupting sizism—pointing out instances of weight discrimination of negative stereotypes and expressing the opinion that "fat jokes" and derogatory stereotypes are both wrong and hurtful.

The National Association to Advance Fat Acceptance (NAAFA; 2013, http://www.naafaonline.com/dev2/about/index.html) is a nonprofit, volunteer civil rights organization dedicated to eliminating discrimination based on body size and providing people with the "tools for self-empowerment through advocacy, public education, and support." Founded in 1969, the NAAFA has assumed a proactive role in protesting social prejudice, bias, and discrimination and in working with the Federal Trade Commission to stop diet fraud. The organization also seeks to improve legal protection for people who are overweight and obese by educating lawmakers and serving as a national legal clearinghouse for attorneys challenging size discrimination.

In an ongoing effort to counter discrimination, the organization has issued statements that are aimed at preventing overweight and obese children from suffering from bullying in school. In October 2011 the NAAFA (http://issuu.com/naafa/docs/) released guidelines for health care providers who treat people who are overweight and obese. The guidelines detail respectful treatment of overweight and obese patients and advise health care providers to:

- Weigh patients in a private setting

- Ensure that patients have access to waiting room seating, examination room facilities, and durable medical equipment that comfortably accommodates them

- Not assume that all the patient's health problems are caused by excess weight

- Not assume that patients want weight-loss counseling or information

In a letter dated February 12, 2013, (http://www.naafaonline.com/newsletterstuff/oldnewsletterstuff/February%202013%20NAAFA%20Newsletter.html), the NAAFA wrote to the U.S. secretary of the treasury, Timothy Geithner (1961–); the U.S. acting secretary of labor, Seth Harris (1962–); and the U.S. secretary of health and human services, Kathleen Sebelius, to express its objections to provisions of the ACA that it felt would encourage employers to discriminate against employees based on weight. Specifically, it objected to the idea of employers offering employees enrolled in their wellness plans different levels of rewards based on factors such as weight and BMI.

CHAPTER 9

DIET AND WEIGHT-LOSS LORE, MYTHS, AND CONTROVERSIES

One of the challenges facing public health professionals as they seek to combat obesity among Americans is helping consumers to distinguish myths, lore, legends, and outright fraud from accurate, usable information about nutrition, diet, exercise, and weight loss. Some of these inaccuracies are so long-standing and deeply rooted in American culture that even the most educated consumers unquestioningly accept them as facts. Others began with a kernel of truth but have been so wildly distorted or misinterpreted that they are confusing, misleading, or entirely erroneous. The rapid influx and dissemination of information about the origins of overweight and obesity and the conflicting accounts of how best to treat these problems compound the challenge. With media reports and advertisements trumpeting different diets nearly every week, it is no wonder that Americans are confused about diet and weight loss.

The fiction that people who are overweight or obese are lazy and weak-willed is among the most harmful myths because it serves to promote stigma, bias, and discrimination. Another common misconception is that it is equally easy or difficult for all people to lose weight. There are biological and behavioral factors that affect an individual's body weight, and people vary in terms of genetic propensity to become overweight, basal metabolic rate (BMR), and the number of fat cells. BMR, often referred to simply as the metabolic rate, is the number of calories an individual expends at rest to maintain normal body functions. BMR changes with age, weight, height, diet, and exercise habits (and varies based on gender) and has been found to vary by as much as 1,000 calories per day. Differences in metabolic rate explain, in part, why not all people who adhere to the same diet achieve the same results in terms of pounds lost or rate of weight loss.

Another factor that produces variation in weight loss is the number of fat cells in the dieter's body. Although fat cells do not determine body weight, they are affected by weight gain and act to limit weight loss because their number cannot be decreased. For example, a normal-weight person has about 40 billion fat cells, whereas an individual who weighs 250 pounds (113 kg) with a body mass index (BMI; body weight in kilograms divided by height in meters squared) of 40 may have as many as 100 billion fat cells. Weight loss causes fat cells to shrink in size but does not decrease their number. As a result, individuals with twice as many fat cells as normal-weight people may be able to shrink their fat cells to a normal size, but even when they have attained a healthy weight they will still have twice as many fat cells.

DIET AND WEIGHT-LOSS MYTHS

It is impossible to recount all the fantastic and improbable claims that have been made over the years. This section considers some of the most persistent myths about diet, exercise, and weight loss.

Small Changes in Caloric Intake or Expenditure Produce Large, Long-Term Weight Loss

MYTH. Small changes in energy intake (consuming fewer calories) or expenditure (burning more calories) will, over time, produce large, long-term weight loss.

FACT. According to Krista Casazza et al., in "Myths, Presumptions, and Facts about Obesity" (*New England Journal of Medicine*, vol. 368, no. 5, January 2013), national health guidelines assert that small, sustained changes in daily behavior such as walking for 20 minutes or eating 10 fewer potato chips will continue to promote the same weight loss over long periods. Casazza et al. point out that this myth arose as a result of the premise that a 3,500-calorie deficit always results in a one-pound weight loss. Recent research demonstrates that many factors influence changes in body composition in response to reduced caloric intake or increased expenditure. For example, the "3,500 fewer calories equals a one-pound weight loss" premise predicts that if people walk one mile per day, burning 100 calories, then over five years they will lose 50 pounds. The truth is, assuming that the participants did not consume more calories to compensate for those expended, their total weight loss would be just 10 pounds, largely because as they lose weight, their calorie requirements also decrease.

Rate of Weight Loss

MYTH. People who lose large amounts of weight quickly do not fare as well as those who have slow, gradual weight loss.

FACT. Casazza et al. observe that this myth likely originated in response to the use of very-low-calorie diets (fewer than 800 calories per day) in the 1960s. The researchers note that in weight-loss studies, large, rapid weight loss is associated with lower weight in the long term. When the results of rapid weight loss that came from very-low-calories diets was compared with weight loss resulting from low-calorie diets, short-term weight loss was greater among those on very-low-calorie diets—16.1% of body weight lost compared with 9.7% on low-calorie diets. At the follow-up at the end of one year, there was no significant difference in total weight loss between the two groups of dieters. Casazza et al. acknowledge that although it is not yet known why some dieters have larger initial weight loss than others, advising dieters that slow weight loss is preferable has the potential to hamper the success of their weight-loss efforts.

Physical Education in School Is Key to Preventing Childhood Obesity

MYTH. Traditional physical education (PE) classes play a vital role in preventing or reducing childhood obesity.

FACT. According to Casazza et al., conventional PE classes have not demonstrated the ability to prevent or reduce childhood obesity. Even schools in which students attended PE classes more frequently and schools that promoted PE were not found to influence the prevalence of obesity nor did they reduce BMI of students. Although it is likely that there is a frequency, intensity, and duration of PE that would help to prevent or reduce obesity, the necessary formula has not yet been determined, and even if it were known, might not be feasible in conventional schools.

Sexual Activity Burns Hundreds of Calories

MYTH. Sexual activity burns between 100 and 300 calories for each participant.

FACT. Casazza et al. report that the average episode of sexual activity has a duration of about six minutes and a young man might burn about 21 calories during sexual intercourse. The researchers point out that just by sitting and watching television, the young man would have spent about one-third of those calories, which would mean the benefit of energy expenditure attributable to sexual activity is about 14 calories.

Eating at Night

MYTH. Eating after 8:00 p.m. causes weight gain.

FACT. Weight gain or loss does not depend on the time of day food is consumed—excess calories are stored as fat whether they are consumed midmorning or just before bedtime. In general, weight is governed by the amount of food consumed (measured in total calorie count) and the amount of physical activity expended during the day.

Some nutritionists and dieticians view breakfast as the most important meal of the day and advise dieters to eat breakfast regularly, based on the assumption that skipping breakfast will lead to overeating later in the day. Casazza et al. question this advice, noting that two rigorous studies found no difference in weight between people who ate breakfast and those who did not.

Anne de la Hunty, Sigrid Gibson, and Margaret Ashwell reviewed 14 studies about the relationship of breakfast habits to body weight in children and adolescents and reported the results in "Does Regular Breakfast Cereal Consumption Help Children and Adolescents Stay Slimmer? A Systematic Review and Meta-Analysis" (*Obesity Facts*, vol. 6, no. 1, 2013). The researchers found that although energy intake was higher among regular breakfast cereal eaters, they had lower BMIs compared with those who ate breakfast cereal infrequently. Nevertheless, the researchers find that the results did not establish a causal relationship, and cited a need for further research to determine whether other factors were in play.

Natural Weight-Loss Products

MYTH. Organic, natural, or herbal weight-loss products are safer than synthetic (produced in the laboratory) over-the-counter (nonprescription) or prescription drugs.

FACT. Simply because products are organic or naturally occurring does not necessarily mean they are effective, risk-free, or safe. For example, in "An Evidence-Based Review of Fat Modifying Supplemental Weight Loss Products" (*Journal of Obesity*, October 2011), Amy M. Egras et al. explain that a 2008 survey found that more than one-third of adults who tried to lose weight had used a dietary supplement to assist their weight loss. Although dietary supplements are widely used, there are very little data on the safety and efficacy of these products. Dietary supplements are considered food and not drugs, so the U.S.

Food and Drug Administration (FDA) does not regulate them as it does prescription medications. When a dietary supplement is found to be unsafe after being sold, the FDA can then determine whether to remove it from the market. The first time the FDA withdrew a dietary supplement for weight loss from the market was in 2004, when serious health risks were associated with the use of ephedra.

Egras et al. analyze studies that tested dietary supplements for weight loss and find evidence that some supplements such as conjugated linoleic acid (an unsaturated fatty acid in the milk and meat of cows, sheep, and goats), pyruvate (a substance that naturally occurs in apples, beer, and red wine that helps to produce energy), and *Irvingia gabonensis* (a supplement derived from the African mango) have demonstrated some potential benefit for weight loss. The researchers conclude that more research is necessary "to draw any definitive conclusions on the use of dietary supplements for weight-loss."

In "How Safe Is the Use of Herbal Weight-Loss Products Sold over the Internet?" (*Human and Experimental Toxicology*, vol. 32, no. 1, January 2013), Bora Ozdemir et al. obtained nine herbal weight-loss products sold over the Internet and analyzed their ingredients. Although all of the products were advertised as purely herbal, three contained sibutramine, a weight-loss drug that was withdrawn from the market in 2010 because it was associated with increased risk for heart attack and stroke. Also, three of the products examined contained caffeine and three contained caffeine and temazepam, a drug used to treat anxiety and insomnia. The researchers also found toxic and trace elements in some of the herbal products.

Low-Fat and Low-Carbohydrate Foods

MYTH. Low-fat, nonfat, and low carbohydrate mean few or no calories.

FACT. Low-fat or nonfat food is usually lower in calories than the same sized portion (as measured by weight) of the full-fat food; a food product, however, can contain zero grams of fat and still have a high calorie content. Many fat-free foods replace the fat with sugar or other sweeteners and contain just as many or more calories as full-fat versions. Although most fruits and vegetables are naturally low in fat and calories, processed low-fat or nonfat foods may be high in calories because extra sugar (or other sweeteners), flour, or starch thickeners have been added to enhance the low-fat foods' taste or texture.

Similarly, low-carbohydrate foods are often higher in calories than their "regular" counterparts because their fat content is higher. Many foods that are naturally low in carbohydrates such as meat, butter, and cheese are also calorie-dense. Many nutritionists suggest limiting the consumption of low-carbohydrate versions of foods, such as low-carbohydrate frozen desserts, because they not only contain as many or more calories per serving than regular frozen desserts but are also often sweetened with artificial sweeteners that lack any nutrients.

Eliminating Starchy Foods

MYTH. Pasta, potatoes, and bread are fattening foods and should be eliminated or sharply limited when trying to lose weight.

FACT. Potatoes, rice, pasta, bread, beans, and some starchy vegetables such as squash, yams, sweet potatoes, turnips, beets, and carrots are not innately fattening. (They are often fattening because of the "extras" that are served with them, such as butter, sour cream, margarine, or cheese.) These foods are rich in complex carbohydrates, which are important sources of energy. Furthermore, foods that are high in complex carbohydrates are often low in fat and calories because carbohydrates contain only four calories per gram, compared with the nine calories per gram contained by fats. In "A Randomized Trial of a Low-Carbohydrate Diet vs Orlistat Plus a Low-Fat Diet for Weight Loss" (*Archives of Internal Medicine*, vol. 170, no. 2, January 25, 2010), William S. Yancy Jr. et al. report the results of a study in which dieters on a low-carbohydrate diet lost the same amount of weight as dieters on a low-fat, high-carbohydrate diet. The 146 overweight or obese subjects were randomly assigned to one of the two diets and the diet drug orlistat, and after 48 weeks both diets helped subjects lose about 10% of their initial, pre-diet weight. The diets were comparable in terms of adherence, and both groups decreased their calorie consumption by about 29% from the baseline.

A plant-based, low-fat diet that includes extra-virgin olive oil and nuts has benefits beyond weight loss or management. In "Primary Prevention of Cardiovascular Disease with a Mediterranean Diet" (*New England Journal of Medicine*, vol. 368, no. 14, April 2013), Ramoón Estruch et al. report that among persons at high risk for cardiovascular disease, a Mediterranean diet supplemented with extra-virgin olive oil or nuts reduced the incidence of major adverse cardiovascular events, such as heart attack and stroke.

Genetic Destiny

MYTH. People from families in which many members are overweight or obese are destined to become overweight.

FACT. It is true that studies of families find similarities in body weight and that immediate relatives of obese people are at an increased risk for overweight and obesity, compared with people with normal-weight family members. Although it is generally accepted that genetic susceptibility or predisposition to overweight or obesity is a factor, researchers believe environmental and behavioral factors make equally strong, if not stronger, contributions to the development of obesity. As a result, people from overweight or obese families may have to make a concerted effort to maintain healthy body weight and prevent weight gain, but they are not destined to become overweight or obese simply by virtue of the genes they inherited.

Exercise Alone

MYTH. Exercise is a better way to lose weight than dieting.

FACT. Although there are many health benefits from exercise, weight loss is not generally considered a direct benefit. Research consistently demonstrates that for weight loss, diet trumps exercise because it is simpler to reduce caloric intake significantly through diet than to increase caloric expenditure significantly through exercise. For example, if a 155-pound (70-kg) person wants to reduce his or her consumption by 400 calories per day, it might be achieved by simply eliminating dessert and reducing portion sizes. In contrast, expending 400 calories per day requires considerable effort. To burn 400 calories a 155-pound person has to spend an hour bicycling 10 miles per hour (16 km/hr), ice skating at 9 miles per hour (14.5 km/hr), or water skiing or walking uphill at about 3.5 miles per hour (5.6 km/hr). Many studies, however, demonstrate that exercise is an important way to prevent overweight and maintain weight loss.

D. Enette Larson-Meyer et al. combined calorie restriction with exercise and reported their findings in "Caloric Restriction with or without Exercise: The Fitness versus Fatness Debate" (*Medicine and Science in Sports and Exercise*, vol. 42, no. 1, January 2010). The researchers randomly assigned 36 otherwise healthy overweight adults to a 25% caloric restricted diet alone or to a 25% energy deficit regime produced equally by calorie restriction and exercise—12.5% by decreasing food intake and 12.5% by increasing energy expended through regular aerobic exercise.

Subjects in both groups lost about the same amount of weight and visceral fat; the calorie restriction and exercise group, however, had improved insulin sensitivity, low-density lipoprotein and cholesterol levels, and diastolic blood pressure. Larson-Meyer et al. conclude that "results of the current study suggest that beyond changes in fatness, combining caloric restriction with exercise is important for increasing aerobic fitness and optimizing improvements in risk factors for diabetes and cardiovascular disease."

Eating Disorders

MYTH. Eating disorders occur exclusively among middle- and upper-class white females.

FACT. Like many myths about diet, weight, and nutrition, this one is based on fact: an estimated 90% of people with anorexia nervosa or bulimia nervosa are female. The National Eating Disorders Association (NEDA; 2013, http://www.nationaleatingdisorders.org/silent-epidemic) estimates that 30 million Americans suffer from eating disorders and one-third of them are men.

In "Why Men Should Be Included in Research on Binge Eating: Results from a Comparison of Psychosocial Impairment in Men and Women" (*International Journal of Eating Disorders*, vol. 45, no. 2, March 2012), Ruth H. Striegel et al. report that although binge eating disorder has been associated with women, a significant number of men suffer from this disorder. The researchers estimate that among the 4 million Americans with an eating disorder, between 5% and 10% of men and about 11% of women are binge eaters. Because more men than previously thought are affected, Striegel et al. call for efforts "to raise awareness of the clinical significance of binge eating in men so that this group can receive appropriate screening and treatment services."

NEDA notes that reports of eating disorders among racial and ethnic minorities and older adults are on the rise. In "Classification and Correlates of Eating Disorders among Blacks: Findings from the National Survey of American Life" (*Journal of Health Care for the Poor and Underserved*, vol. 24, no. 1, February 2013), Jacquelyn Y. Taylor et al. note that although the rates of anorexia and bulimia are lower than among whites, there are high rates of binge eating among African American adults and adolescents.

Older adults are affected too. Survey results presented by Danielle Gagne et al., in "Eating Disorder Symptoms and Weight and Shape Concerns in a Large Web-Based Convenience Sample of Women Ages 50 and Above: Results of the Gender and Body Image Study (GABI)" (*International Journal of Eating Disorders*, vol. 45, no. 7, November 2012), indicate that of women over the age of 50 years, 13% have symptoms of eating disorders, 62% feel that their weight or shape has a negative effect on their life, and well over two-thirds (70%) are attempting to lose weight.

Freshmen in College Gain Weight

MYTH. College freshmen gain an average of 15 pounds (6.8 kg) during their first year of school.

FACT. Historically, college students were warned about the "freshman 15," the 15 pounds that students supposedly gain during their first year of college, presumably because freed from the constraints of healthful eating at home, they subsist on a diet of unhealthy food. Jay L. Zagorsky and Patricia K. Smith, however, dispel the myth of freshman weight gain in "The Freshman 15: A Critical Time for Obesity Intervention or Media Myth?" (*Social Science Quarterly*, vol. 92, no. 5, December 2011). The researchers analyze data from 7,418 college freshmen and find that first-year students, both male and female, gained an average of 2.5 to 3.5 pounds (1.1 to 1.6 kg) during their first year in college. Zagorsky and Smith also find that this weight gain is only one-half pound more than that gained by people of the same age who are not attending college.

WHY DIETS FAIL

Historically, diets have been considered to have "failed" when lost weight is regained. Many nutritionists and obesity researchers believe diets fail because most are not sustainable. The more restrictive the diet, the less likely an individual will be to remain faithful to it because, in general, people cannot endure extended periods of hunger and deprivation. Diets may also fail because they neglect to teach dieters new eating habits to assist them in maintaining their weight loss. Most overweight people gained their excess weight by consuming more calories per day than they needed. Dieting creates a temporary deficit of calories or specific macronutrients such as carbohydrates or fat. Because the weight-loss diet is viewed as a temporary measure with a beginning and an end, at its conclusion most dieters return to their previous eating habits and often regain the lost weight or gain even more weight. Many nutritionists and dieticians who work with people who are overweight or obese assert that diets do not fail; instead, dieters fail to learn how to eat properly to prevent weight regain.

Consumers are not the only ones who believe that diets are doomed to fail. Many health professionals and researchers cite the statistic that 95% of diets fail. This oft-cited statistic has been attributed to Albert James Stunkard (1922–), the director emeritus of the Obesity Society (formerly the American Obesity Association). Stunkard put forth the 95% failure rate based on research he performed in 1959, which involved advising 100 overweight patients to diet, with no follow-up or support to increase their adherence to the diet. In "Whether Obesity Should Be Treated?" (*Health Psychology*, vol. 12, no. 5, September 1993), Kelly D. Brownell of Yale University observes that this statistic has been widely applied even though it is quite dated, was not confirmed by subsequent studies, and involved only subjects in university-based research programs.

The article "New Diet Winners: We Rate the Diet Books and Plans" (*Consumer Reports*, vol. 72, no. 6, June 2007) observes that only more recently have successful dieters been studied to learn from their successes and incorporate them into more effective, and ideally sustainable, weight-loss plans. It cites as an example the new emphasis on achieving satiety without consuming too many calories by consuming low-density foods. This article and other recent research may help dispel the myth that dieters are doomed to fail. For example, in "Psychobehavioural Factors Are More Strongly Associated with Successful Weight Management Than Predetermined Satiety Effect or Other Characteristics of Diet" (*Journal of Obesity*, June 2012), Leila Karhunen et al. find that neither foods with higher satiety value nor the type of diet contribute to better weight management. Instead, Karhunen et al. find that better self-control of eating behavior, such as a decrease in binge eating, is associated with success in weight management.

Improving Long-Term Weight Loss

Research demonstrates that dieters find it challenging to maintain weight loss; nevertheless, research refutes the 95% failure rate. In "Effects of Dietary Composition on Energy Expenditure during Weight-Loss Maintenance" (*JAMA*, vol. 307, no. 24, June 2012), Cara B. Ebbeling et al. observe that just one in six overweight and obese adults report ever having maintained a 10% weight loss for one year. Although one explanation for this lack of success may be that the motivation to adhere to a restricted diet erodes over time, another is that weight loss provokes biological adaptations—a decline in energy expenditure and an increase in hunger—that encourage weight regain.

Ebbeling et al. compared the effects of three weight-loss maintenance diets—a low-fat diet, a low glycemic index (a measure of a food's ability to raise blood glucose) diet, and a very-low-carbohydrate diet—on energy expenditure, hormones, and other health indicators. The researchers find that energy expenditure during weight-loss maintenance differed significantly for the three diets. The low-fat diet produced changes in energy expenditure and leptin (a hormone that signals satiety) that favor weight regain. By contrast, the very-low-carbohydrate diet had the most beneficial effects on energy expenditure but also exerted potentially harmful effects on other health indicators such as inflammation. The low glycemic index diet had comparable but smaller benefits than the very-low-carbohydrate diet, while appearing to not increase inflammation, which suggests that it may be a better approach for weight-loss maintenance.

Because there is considerable variation in individuals' responses to dietary interventions and some interventions may benefit individuals or population subgroups more than others, nutrigenetics (using genetic information to custom-tailor a weight-loss diet) may be used to custom-tailor weight-loss diets and weight-maintenance efforts, which in turn may improve their success. In "The Future Direction of Personalised Nutrition: My Diet, My Phenotype, My Genes" (*Proceedings of the Nutrition Society*, vol. 72, no. 2, May 2013), Michael J. Gibney and Marianne C. Walsh indicate that personalized nutrition using genetic data enables individuals to choose the optimal diet for weight loss based on complex interactions between diet, genes, and the environment.

Approaches to enhance motivation focus on two areas: improved social supports and tangible financial incentives. Strategies to improve social supports emphasize including spouses or significant others in the weight-loss process to teach them to provide social support for their partner's weight-loss efforts. Such strategies demonstrate modest success as do contracts in which groups agree to aim for individual or group weight loss.

Alfredo R. Paloyo et al., in "The Causal Link between Financial Incentives and Weight Loss: An Evidence-Based Survey of the Literature" (*Journal of Economic Surveys*, January 2013), review available research to determine whether financial incentives are effective inducements to lose weight. The researchers considered nine studies. Some of the studies used positive monetary incentives, some used negative monetary incentives, and some combined positive and negative incentives for weight loss. Only five of the studies reported that financial incentives improved weight loss and none determined that weight lost this way was maintained.

Financial incentives may encourage people to lose weight, but such incentives do not appear to prevent weight regain. In "Financial Incentives for Extended Weight Loss: A Randomized, Controlled Trial" (*Journal of General Internal Medicine*, vol. 26, no. 6, June 2011), Leslie K. John et al. analyze data from a 32-week-long weight-loss program—24 weeks of weight loss followed by eight weeks of weight maintenance. Sixty-six program participants were given the goal of losing 1 pound (0.5 kg) per week and received a financial incentive for achieving this weight loss. To assess longer-term maintenance following the 32-week intervention, participants returned for a weigh-in approximately 36 weeks after they completed the 32-week program. The researchers find that the incentive did promote weight loss and maintenance through the 32-week program; after the program ended, however, there was significant weight regain. John et al. conclude that "future research is needed to devise techniques that promote sustained weight loss over longer periods."

Teaching patients skills that are useful for weight maintenance as opposed to weight loss emphasizes that there are two distinctly different sets of strategies: one set focuses on weight loss and the other set focuses on maintaining a stable energy balance around a lower weight. The most commonly used model for teaching maintenance-specific skills is relapse prevention, which involves teaching people to identify situations in which lapses in behavioral adherence are likely to occur, to plan strategies in advance to prevent lapses, and to get back on track should they occur. Relapse prevention is based on the idea that breaking the so-called rules in terms of remaining faithful to diet and exercise programs may often lead to negative psychological reactions that in turn prompt reversion to pre-weight-loss behaviors.

Brent Van Dorsten and Emily M. Lindley of the University of Colorado, Denver, review in "Cognitive and Behavioral Approaches in the Treatment of Obesity" (*Medical Clinics of North America*, vol. 95, no. 5, September 2011) research about long-term weight maintenance using relapse prevention strategies after weight loss. The researchers report that long-term contact with treatment providers is an important factor in successful weight maintenance. Long-term follow-up contacts may be face-to-face, via telephone, Internet, or e-mail. Although the optimal frequency of contacts to support weight maintenance is not yet known, the frequency of weighing is another factor identified by successful weight-loss maintainers. The use of personal trainers and monetary incentives for weight loss as well as group work-site competitions also demonstrate the capacity to promote long-term engagement with, and adherence to, weight-loss programs.

WEIGHT-LOSS SCHEMES DEFRAUD CONSUMERS

The marketing of so-called fat-burning pills, potions, and products to Americans seeking effortless weight loss has a long history. Peter N. Stearns, in *Fat History: Bodies and Beauty in the Modern West* (1997), and Laura Fraser, in *Losing It: False Hopes and Fat Profits in the Diet Industry* (1998), offer detailed histories of magical cures and weight-loss fads. At the beginning of the 20th century products such as obesity belts and chairs that delivered electrical stimulation, as well as corsets, tonics, and mineral waters, claimed to cause weight loss.

Diet pills appeared in 1910 with the introduction of weight-loss tablets that contained arsenic (a poisonous metallic element), strychnine (a plant toxin formerly used as a stimulant), caffeine, and pokeberries (formerly used as a laxative). During the 1920s cigarette makers promoted their product as a diet aid, urging Americans to smoke rather than eat. During the 1930s diet pills containing dinitrophenol, a chemical used to manufacture explosives, dyes, and insecticides, enjoyed brief popularity after it was observed that factory workers making munitions lost weight. Their popularity was short lived as cases of temporary blindness and death became attributed to their use.

The second half of the 20th century saw the proliferation of questionable, and often entirely worthless, weight-loss devices and gimmicks, including inflatable suits to "sweat off pounds," diet drinks and cookies, and slimming creams, patches, shoe inserts, and wraps to reduce fat thighs and abdomens. Even though the claims made for many of these products sounded too good to be true, unsuspecting Americans spent billions of dollars in the hope of achieving quick, easy, and permanent weight loss.

The promotion of dubious and potentially dangerous weight-loss products continued during the second decade of the 21st century. In 2013 alone, the FDA issued consumer alerts about 17 products marketed for weight loss that contained drugs or other potentially harmful ingredients. The agency has also issued warning letters, seized products, and criminally prosecuted people responsible for illegal diet products. For example, in "Tainted Weight Loss Products" (2014, http://www.fda.gov/Drugs/ResourcesForYou/Consumers/BuyingUsingMedicineSafely/Medication HealthFraud/ucm234592.htm), the FDA explains that many dietary supplements marketed as weight-loss aids are actually powerful drugs that may carry significant risks to unsuspecting consumers. The FDA notes that "consumers may unknowingly take products laced with varying quantities of approved prescription drug ingredients, controlled substances, and untested and unstudied pharmaceutically active ingredients."

Use of Over-the-Counter Weight-Loss Products

In "The Effect of Deceptive Advertising on Consumption of the Advertised Good and Its Substitutes: The Case of Over-the-Counter Weight Loss Products" (February 2013, http://ftp.iza.org/dp7247.pdf), John Cawley, Rosemary Avery, and Matthew Eisenberg report that over-the-counter (OTC) weight-loss products have been used by 20% of adult women, 10% of adult men, 14% of adolescent females, and 7% of adult males. About one-third of people who have ever made a serious weight-loss attempt have used an OTC weight-loss product. The researchers observe that about half of Americans mistakenly believe that OTC weight-loss products are evaluated for safety and efficacy before they are marketed.

Cawley, Avery, and Eisenberg analyzed information on Americans' consumption, magazine reading, and television viewing and measured individual exposure to ads for OTC weight-loss products. They also calculated the percentage of the ads that contained at least one deceptive statement and analyzed the impact of exposure to advertising, including deceptive ads, on the likelihood that an OTC weight-loss product was used in the 12 months prior to the study. The researchers find that deceptive television advertising of OTC weight-loss products reduces the probability that better-educated

women will purchase these products; deceptive print advertising, however, increases the likelihood that men will buy them. Deceptive advertising that is unbelievable may unintentionally suggest to consumers that the product is questionable, discouraging consumption.

A promising finding from this research is that deception may make consumers suspicious of the advertised product, prompting them to substitute an established approach such as diet, exercise, or professional counseling, for the advertised product. Deceptive ads for questionable products that make weight loss seem easy may unintentionally make weight loss in general seem simpler. Cawley, Avery, and Eisenberg conclude, "Advertising, and even deceptive advertising, of questionable products apparently has the potential of a beneficial unintended consequence of inspiring people to undertake healthy and responsible approaches to weight loss."

Weighing the Claims

In May 2000 the Partnership for Healthy Weight Management, a coalition of scientific, academic, health care, government, commercial, and public interest representatives, initiated consumer and media education programs that aimed not only to increase public awareness of the obesity epidemic in the United States but also to promote responsible marketing of weight-loss products and programs. The partnership published a consumer guide *Finding a Weight Loss Plan That Works for You* (December 2009) designed to help overweight and obese consumers find weight-loss solutions to meet their needs. The guide contains a checklist that enables consumers to compare weight-loss plans based on a variety of criteria. (See Table 9.1.) It also advises consumers about how to select weight-loss programs and services based on specific information from potential providers.

The Federal Trade Commission (FTC) described eight broad categories of advertising claims, in *Deception in Weight-Loss Advertising Workshop: Seizing Opportunities and Building Partnerships to Stop Weight-Loss Fraud* (December 2003, http://www.ftc.gov/os/2003/12/031209weightlossrpt.pdf). The following section considers these advertising claims and assessments of them. It also draws on an analysis of the FTC report by Stephen Barrett in "Impossible Weight-Loss Claims: Summary of an FTC Report" (December 16, 2003, http://www.quackwatch.org/01QuackeryRelatedTopics/PhonyAds/weightlossfraud.html), and "Being Fooled by Empty Diet Promises" (2013, http://www.accessdata.fda.gov/scripts/video/drugs.cfm?yid=wcdO6dDnUKE), a video prepared by the FDA.

No Diet or Exercise Required

CLAIM. The advertised product causes substantial weight loss without exercise or diet.

TABLE 9.1

Checklist for evaluating weight-loss products and services

Use this checklist to gather and compare information from all weight loss programs you're considering.

Make several copies of the blank form so you can fill out one for each program. A provider's willingness to give you this information is an important factor in choosing a program. If you need help to evaluate the information you gather, talk with your primary health care provider or a registered dietitian.

Program name _____
Address _____
Phone number _____

In this program, my daily caloric intake will be: _____

My daily caloric intake is determined by: _____
I   will   will not be evaluated initially by program staff.

The evaluation will be made by (check all that apply):
Physician   Nurse   Registered dietitian   Other company-trained employee

My progress is supervised by (check all that apply):
Physician   Nurse   Licensed psychologist
Registered dietitian   Company-trained employee

I will   will not be evaluated by a physician during the course of my treatment.

During the first month, my progress will be monitored:
Weekly   Biweekly   Monthly   Other _____

After the first month, my progress will be monitored:
Weekly   Biweekly   Monthly   Other _____

My weight loss plan includes (check all that apply):
Nutrition information about healthy eating   At least 1,200 calories/day for women or 1,400 calories/day for men
Suggested menus and recipes   Keeping food diaries or other monitoring activities
Portion control   Liquid meal replacements
Prepackaged meals   Dietary supplements (vitamins, minerals, botanicals, herbals)
Prescription weight loss drugs   Help with weight maintenance and lifestyle changes
Surgery

My plan includes regular physical activity that is (check both if both apply):
Supervised (at the program site)   _____ times per week, _____ minutes per session.
Unsupervised (on my own time)   _____ times per week, _____ minutes per session.

The physical activity includes (check all that apply):
Walking   Swimming   Stationary cycling
Strength training   Aerobic dancing   Other _____

The weight loss plan includes (check all that apply):
Family counseling   Group support   Lifestyle modification advice
Weight maintenance advice   Weight maintenance counseling
The staff explained the risks associated with this weight loss progam. They are:

_____
_____

The staff explained the costs of this program. (Check all that apply and fill in the blanks.)
I will be charged a one-time entry fee of $ ___.
I will be charged $ ___ per visit.
Food replacements will cost about $ ___ per month.
Prescription weight loss drugs will cost about $ ___ per month.
Vitamins and other dietary supplements will cost about $ ___ per month.
Diagnostic tests are required and will cost about $ ___ .
Other costs include _____ at $ ___.

Total cost for this program $____

The program gave me information about:
The health risks of being overweight.   The difficulty many people have maintaining weight loss.
The health benefits of weight loss.   How to improve my chances at maintaining my weight.

Other information to ask for:
Participants in this program have lost an average of ___ lbs. over ___ months/years.
Participants in this program have kept off ___ % of their weight loss for ___ years.

This information is based on the following (check one):
All participants.
Participants who completed the program.
Other _____

Notes: _____
_____

SOURCE: "Checklist for Evaluating Weight Loss Products and Services," in *Finding a Weight Loss Program That Works for You*, Federal Trade Commission, The Partnership for Healthy Weight Management, December 28, 2009, http://www.mhhe.com/socscience/hpp/fahey7e/wellness_worksheets/wellness_worksheet_083.html (accessed March 19, 2014)

TABLE 9.2

Examples of claims that promise weight loss without diet or exercise

"Awesome attack on bulging fatty deposits... has virtually eliminated the need to diet." (Konjac root pill)

"They said it was impossible, but tests prove [that] my astounding diet-free discovery melts away... 5, 6, even 7 pounds of fat a day." (ingredients not disclosed)

"The most powerful diet pill ever discovered! No diet or workout required. The secret weight-loss pill behind Fitness models, Show Biz and Entertainment professionals! No prescription required to order." (ingredients not disclosed)

"Lose up to 30 lbs . . . No impossible exercise! No missed meals! No boring foods or small portions!" (plant extract fucus vesiculosus)

"Lose up to 8 to 10 pounds per week... [n]o dieting, no strenuous exercise." (elixir purportedly containing 16 plant extracts)

"My 52 lbs of unwanted fat relaxed away without dieting or grueling exercise." (hypnosis seminar)

"No exercise... [a]nd eat as much as you want—the more you eat, the more you lose, we'll show you how." (meal replacement)

SOURCE: Richard L. Cleland et al., "Table 5. Lose Weight without Diet or Exercise Claims," in *Weight-Loss Advertising: An Analysis of Current Trends*, Federal Trade Commission, September 2002, http://www.ftc.gov/sites/default/files/documents/reports/weight-loss-advertisingan-analysis-current-trends/weightloss_0.pdf (accessed November 11, 2013)

EXAMPLES. "U.S. patent reveals weight loss of as much as 28 pounds in 4 weeks . . . . Eat all your favorite foods and still lose weight. The pill does all the work," and "Lose up to 2 pounds daily without diet or exercise." Table 9.2 contains other examples of comparable claims.

ASSESSMENT. Products purporting to cause weight loss without diet or exercise would either need to cause malabsorption (impair the absorption) of calories or to increase metabolism. Because the number of calories that can be malabsorbed is limited to 1,200 to 1,300 calories per week, or about 0.3 of a pound (0.1 kg) per week, malabsorption alone is unlikely to lead to substantial weight loss. Similarly, there is no thermogenic (heat-producing) agent, such as ephedrine combined with caffeine, able to boost metabolism enough to produce weight loss without diet or exercise. In fact, the mechanism by which ephedrine products appear to assist weight loss is by suppressing appetite rather than by speeding metabolism. Furthermore, although green tea extract was found to increase metabolism, it was by a scant 4%.

No Restrictions on Eating

CLAIM. Users can lose weight while still enjoying unlimited amounts of high-calorie foods.

EXAMPLE. "Eat All the Foods You Love and Still Lose Weight (Pill Does All the Work)."

ASSESSMENT. This claim was viewed as a variation of the assertion that dieters can lose weight without reducing caloric intake or increasing exercise, because this claim states that users not only can lose weight without reducing caloric intake but also may increase caloric intake and still lose weight. The assembled experts concurred that if this claim were true, it would defy the laws of physics.

Permanent Weight Loss

CLAIM. The advertised product causes permanent weight loss.

EXAMPLES. "Take it off and keep it off. You won't gain the weight back afterwards because your weight will have reached an equilibrium," and "People who use this product say that even when they stop using the product, their weight does not jump up again."

ASSESSMENT. Even if a product caused weight loss through a reduction of calories, appetite suppression, or malabsorption, weight would be regained once use of the product stopped and calorie consumption returned to previous levels. Researchers and health professionals have repeatedly observed that dieters tend to regain weight lost over time once the diet, intervention, or other treatment ends. According to the Food and Nutrition Board of the National Academy of Sciences, "Many programs and services exist to help individuals achieve weight control. But without continuing vigilance and a strategy for weight maintenance, many dieters who complete weight-loss programs and lose approximately 10% of their body weight regain two-thirds of it back within 1 year and almost all of it back within 5 years." Furthermore, there are no published scientific studies supporting the claim that a nonprescription drug, dietary supplement, cream, wrap, device, or patch can cause permanent weight loss.

Fat Blockers

CLAIM. The advertised product causes substantial weight loss through the blockage or absorption of fat or calories.

EXAMPLES. "[The named ingredient] can ingest up to 900 times its own weight in fat, that's why it's a fantastic fat blocker," and "The Super Fat Fighting Formula inhibits fats, sugars and starches from being absorbed in the intestines and turning into excess weight, so that you can lose pounds and inches easily."

ASSESSMENT. Science does not support the possibility that these products cause sufficient malabsorption of fat or calories to result in substantial weight loss. The FTC has challenged deceptive fat-blocker claims for some of the most popular diet products on the market. The evidence supports the position that consumers cannot lose substantial weight through the blockage of absorption of fat. It is not scientifically feasible for a nonprescription drug, dietary supplement, cream, wrap, device, or patch

Examples of claims that promise fast results

"This combination of plant extracts constitutes a weight-loss plan that facilitates what is probably the fastest weight loss ever observed from an entirely natural treatment." (elixir purportedly containing 16 plant extracts)

"Just fast and easy, effective weight loss!" (fucus vesiculosus)

"Lose 10 lbs. in 8 Days!" (apple cider vinegar)

"Rapid weight loss in 28 days!" (ephedra)

"Knock off your unwanted weight and fat deposits at warp speeds! You can lose 18 pounds in one week!" (ingredients not disclosed)

"Clinically proven to cause rapid loss of excess body fat." (phosphosterine)

"Two clinically proven fat burning formulations that are guaranteed to get you there fast or it costs you absolutely nothing." (ingredients not disclosed)

SOURCE: Richard L. Cleland et al., "Table 4. Representative Claims That Promise Fast Results," in *Weight Loss Advertising: An Analysis of Current Trends*, Federal Trade Commission, September 2002, http://www.ftc.gov/ sites/default/files/documents/reports/weight-loss-advertisingan-analysis-current-trends/weightloss_0.pdf (accessed November 11, 2013)

to cause substantial weight loss through the blockage of absorption of fat or calories.

Quick Weight Loss

CLAIM. The user of the advertised product can safely lose more than 3 pounds (1.4 kg) per week for periods exceeding four weeks. Table 9.3 shows claims that promise unbelievably rapid results.

EXAMPLE. "Lose three pounds per week, naturally and without side effects."

ASSESSMENT. Significant health risks are associated with medically unsupervised, rapid weight loss over extended periods. Basically, "the more restrictive the diet, the greater are the risks of adverse effects associated with weight loss." One documented risk is the increased incidence of gallstones. The claim that consumers using products such as these without medical oversight can safely lose more than 3 pounds per week for a period of more than four weeks is not feasible.

Weight-Loss Creams and Patches

CLAIM. The advertised product that is worn on the body or rubbed into the skin causes substantial weight loss.

EXAMPLES. "Lose two to four pounds daily with the Diet Patch," and "Thigh Cream drops pounds and inches from your thighs."

ASSESSMENT. Diet patches and creams that are worn or applied to the skin have not been proven to be safe or effective. Furthermore, their alleged mechanisms of action are not scientifically credible.

Guaranteed Success

CLAIM. The advertised product causes substantial weight loss for all users.

EXAMPLE. "Lose excess body fat. No willpower required. Works for everyone no matter how many times you've tried and failed before."

ASSESSMENT. This claim assumes that overweight and obesity arise from a single cause or are amenable to a single solution. Because the causes of overweight and obesity are thought to be genetic factors and environmental conditions, and contributing factors such as diet, metabolic rate, level of physical activity, and adherence to weight-loss treatment vary, it is unlikely that one product will be effective for all users. Even FDA-approved prescription drugs for weight loss have a high level of nonresponders, and surgical treatment for obesity is not successful 100% of the time. The claim that a nonprescription drug, dietary supplement, cream, wrap, device, or patch will cause substantial weight loss for all users is not scientifically feasible.

Targeted Weight-Loss Products

CLAIM. Users of the advertised product can lose weight from only those parts of the body where they wish to lose weight.

EXAMPLE. "And it has taken off quite some inches from my butt (5 inches) and thighs (4 inches), my hips now measure 35 inches. I still wear the same bra size though. The fat has disappeared from exactly the right places."

ASSESSMENT. Small published studies of aminophylline cream indicate that its use may cause the redistribution of fat from the thighs to other fat stores; it has not, however, been shown to cause fat loss. Even if some products were capable of causing more weight loss from certain areas of the body, no part would be spared completely—fat is lost from all fat stores throughout the body.

Campaign Targets Phony Weight-Loss Claims

Another FTC education initiative aims to assist the media to voluntarily screen weight-loss product ads containing claims that are "too good to be true." The media were targeted for intensive education not only because broad-based public education has proven largely inadequate to protect consumers from persuasive messages trumpeting easy weight loss but also to acknowledge the media's powerful ability to reduce weight-loss fraud by sharply limiting the dissemination of obviously false weight-loss advertising. In December 2003 the FTC launched its Red Flag campaign to assist the media to reduce deceptive weight-loss advertising and promote positive, reliable advertising messages about weight loss.

The FTC (http://www.ftc.gov/news-events/press-releases/2003/12/ftc-releases-guidance-media-false-weight-loss-claims) defines Red Flag claims as those that promise to:

- Cause weight loss of two pounds or more a week for a month or more without dieting or exercise
- Cause substantial weight loss no matter what or how much the consumer eats
- Cause permanent weight loss (even when the consumer stops using product)
- Block the absorption of fat or calories to enable consumers to lose substantial weight
- Safely enable consumers to lose more than three pounds per week for more than four weeks
- Cause substantial weight loss for all users
- Cause substantial weight loss by wearing it on the body or rubbing it into the skin

The FTC also launched a website (http://www.consumer.ftc.gov/articles/0061-weighing-claims-diet-ads#thetruth) to help consumers identify false weight-loss claims.

The FTC continues to file actions to stop false and unsupported weight-loss claims. For example, the FTC reports in a media release, "FTC Charges HCG Marketer with Deceptive Advertising" (October 30, 2013, http://www.ftc.gov/news-events/press-releases/2013/10/ftc-charges-hcg-marketer-deceptive-advertising) that it filed suit against Kevin Wright and his companies, HCG Platinum and Right Way Nutrition, LLC, which market human chorionic gonadotropin (HCG) for weight loss. Claiming that consumers will lose substantial amounts of weight using HCG and adhering to a very-low-calorie diet (500–800 calories per day), the companies charge from $60 to $149 for a 30-day supply of their formulas. The product is marketed through retail stores such as Rite Aid and Walgreens and through Internet advertising and social media such as Facebook.

The FTC notes that the companies claim that two of their three formulas are homeopathic—the active ingredients are diluted to undetectable levels. The products' packaging and advertising, according to the FTC, make unsubstantiated claims that "the products cause consumers to lose a pound a day, are safe to use, and are clinically proven to burn fat, reduce weight, and lower cholesterol." The FTC suit asserts that the companies sold more than $13 million of their products since 2010 and asks the companies to surrender money received in response to deceptive advertising.

FTC actions not only stop purveyors of weight-loss products from making unsubstantiated claims but also seek compensation for consumers. For example, in a July 11, 2013, media release, "FTC Mails Refund Checks to Consumers Who Bought Skechers' Shape-Ups and Other 'Toning' Shoes" (http://www.ftc.gov/news-events/press-releases/2013/07/ftc-mails-refund-checks-consumers-who-bought-skechers-shape-ups), the FTC reports that under the terms of the FTC settlement in accordance with a class-action lawsuit, more than 509,000 checks were mailed to consumers who bought toning shoes from Skechers USA, Inc. The FTC charged the company with deceptive advertising that claimed its shoes would "help people lose weight, and strengthen and tone their buttocks, legs and abdominal muscles."

DO VERY-LOW-CALORIE DIETS INCREASE LONGEVITY?

Although many Americans are overweight, some people are experimenting with very-low-calorie diets in the hope that by remaining extremely thin they will stave off disease and live longer. Advocates of extreme caloric restriction (CR) contend that sharply reducing caloric intake creates biochemical changes that slow the aging process, which theoretically should increase life expectancy.

Most people would find it impossible to adhere to semi-starvation diets, but there is scientific evidence—such as Luigi Fontana and Samuel Klein's "Aging, Adiposity, and Calorie Restriction" (JAMA, vol. 297, no. 9, March 7, 2007) and Arthur V. Everitt and David G. Le Couteur's "Life Extension by Calorie Restriction in Humans" (Annals of the New York Academy of Sciences, vol. 1114, October 2007)—that subsistence diets increase the life span of fruit flies, worms, spiders, guppies, mice, and hamsters by between 10% and 40%. In theory, semi-starvation prolongs life by reducing metabolism (how quickly glucose is used for energy) in an evolutionary adaptation to conserve calories during periods of famine. Dieters are familiar with this process—they know from experience that as they eat less, their metabolic rate drops, which makes losing weight increasingly more difficult. CR adherents experience comparable drops in metabolic rate—one study found that their body temperature dropped by a full degree. Proponents of CR assert that although metabolism is vital for life, it is also destructive because it produces unstable molecules known as free radicals that can damage cells through a process called oxidation.

CR adherents report immediate health benefits including increased mental acuity, reduced need for sleep, sharply reduced cholesterol and fasting blood sugar levels, weight loss, and reduced blood pressure. The regimen is clearly not easy, and even its staunchest advocates, such as members of the Caloric Restriction Society, concede that many people who practice CR experience constant hunger, obsessions with food, mood disorders such as irritability and depression, and lowered libido (sex drive). CR can also cause people to feel cold, and even with adequate vitamin and mineral supplementation it can cause some people to suffer from osteoporosis (decreased bone mass) and hair loss. Jon Gertner reports in "The Calorie-Restriction Experiment" (NYTimes.com, October 7, 2009) that the majority of subjects in the Calerie study achieved their weight-loss goals and were maintaining their weight loss by sticking to their diet. He notes, however, that CR is a challenging undertaking and one that most Americans would forgo. Gertner opines that "living a life of less in a culture of more—is extremely difficult to achieve and even more difficult to maintain. Americans' seemingly inexorable slide toward obesity tends to indicate as much: for the majority of us, the desire to eat can easily overwhelm personal willpower and (so far) any messages from public-health campaigns."

In "Why Dietary Restriction Substantially Increases Longevity in Animal Models but Won't in Humans" (*Ageing Research Reviews*, vol. 4, no. 3, August 2005), John P. Phelan and Michael R. Rose challenge the notion that CR will increase longevity. The researchers conclude that severely restricting calories over decades may add a few years to a human life span but will not enable humans to live to 125 years or more. Phelan and Rose developed a mathematical model based on the known effects of calorie intake and life span that shows that people who consume the most calories have a shorter life span. It also shows that if people severely restrict their calories over their lifetime, their life span increases by between 3% and 7%, which is far less than the 20-plus years some hoped could be achieved by drastic CR. The researchers suggest that "longevity is not a trait that exists in isolation; it evolves as part of a complex life history, with a wide range of underpinning physiological mechanisms involving, among other things, chronic disease processes." They advise Americans to "try to maintain a healthy body weight, but don't deprive yourself of all pleasure. Moderation appears to be a more sensible solution."

Everitt and Le Couteur confirm that although short-term CR does improve specific markers that are associated with longevity, such as deep body temperature and plasma insulin levels, CR is unlikely to offer markedly increased longevity. The researchers cite as evidence the Okinawans, the longest-lived people on the earth, who consume 40% fewer calories than the average American and live just four years longer. Everitt and Le Couteur surmise that "the effects of CR on human life extension are probably much smaller than those achieved by medical and public health interventions, which have extended life by about 30 years in developed countries in the 20th century, by greatly reducing deaths from infections, accidents, and cardiovascular disease."

Although model organism and animal studies demonstrate positive responses to CR, it is not yet known whether CR will extend the human life span. Daniel L. Smith Jr., Tim R. Nagy, and David B. Allison of the University of Alabama, Birmingham, observe in "Calorie Restriction: What Recent Results Suggest for the Future of Ageing Research" (*European Journal of Clinical Investigation*, vol. 40, no. 5, May 2010) that preliminary data from a seven-year study confirm many of the metabolic and physiologic responses that have been observed in animals. These responses include reductions in body weight, subcutaneous fat, visceral fat, lean muscle mass, insulin, energy expenditure, and core body temperature and improved lipid profiles. Smith, Nagy, and Allison opine that independent of whether CR confers longevity benefits, it is likely to play a role in disease prevention and healthy aging.

In "Ageing: Mixed Results for Dieting Monkeys" (*Nature*, vol. 489, no. 7415, September 2012), Steven N. Austad of the University of Texas Health Science Center at San Antonio' Barshop Institute for Longevity and Aging Studies reports the results of calorie restriction in rhesus monkeys. Although the 57 calorie-restricted monkeys were healthier in terms of cholesterol and triglyceride levels (indicators of reduced risk for cardiovascular disease) and muscle loss and suffered lower rates of diseases, they did not live longer than the 64 monkeys in the control group that were not calorie restricted.

CHAPTER 10
PREVENTING OVERWEIGHT AND OBESITY

Many obesity researchers and health professionals believe the most effective way to win the war on obesity is to intensify efforts to prevent overweight and obesity among children, adolescents, and adults. They assert that over time prevention is far more cost effective than the expenditures that are associated with weight-loss efforts and medical treatment of obesity-related diseases. They also observe that prevention is a preferable strategy because there is no universally effective long-term treatment that consistently produces and maintains weight loss.

The landmark report *Surgeon General's Call to Action to Prevent and Decrease Overweight and Obesity, 2001* (2001, http://www.cdc.gov/nccdphp/dnpa/pdf/Call toAction.pdf) calls for the design and implementation of interventions to prevent and decrease overweight and obesity, both individually and collectively. It asserts that effective actions must occur at many levels and acknowledges that—although individual behavioral change is at the core of all strategies to reduce overweight and obesity—to be optimally effective, efforts must not be limited to individual behavioral change.

The report recommends actions to modify group influences by initiating prevention programs that target families, communities, employers and workers, the health care delivery system, and the media, as well as changes in public policy. Furthermore, the report calls for concerted efforts and predicts that actions to prevent and reduce overweight and obesity will fail unless changes are made at every level of U.S. society. Characterizing these problems as societal rather than as individual, the report observes that individual behavioral change is possible only in "a supportive environment with accessible and affordable healthy food choices and opportunities for regular physical activity." The report also warns that actions aimed exclusively at individual behavioral change that do not consider social, cultural, economic,

and environmental influences will be counterproductive, serving only to reinforce negative stereotypes, bias, and stigmatization of people who are overweight or obese.

Many public health professionals believe environmental and policy interventions are the most promising strategies for generating and maintaining healthy nutrition and physical activity behaviors in Americans. Environmental interventions are those actions that modify availability of, access to, pricing of, or education about foods at the places where they are purchased. Policy interventions legislate, regulate, or, through formal or informal rules, serve to guide individual and collective behavior. Examples of environmental and policy initiatives that have met with success include:

- Increasing the availability of fruits and vegetables at school and workplace cafeterias and adding fresh fruit to refrigerated vending machines

- Replacing soft drinks in school vending machines with fruit juices and water

- Instituting daily physical education requirements for students

- Providing point-of-purchase nutrition information at restaurants and grocery stores to encourage healthy food choices

- Allowing workers adequate break time and a location where nursing mothers can express milk so their babies can continue to accrue the health benefits of breastfeeding even after their mothers return to work

In the annual status report *National Prevention, Health Promotion, and Public Health Council* (July 1, 2013, http://www.surgeongeneral.gov/initiatives/prevention/2013-npc-status-report.pdf), the U.S. surgeon general Regina Benjamin (1956–) lists prevention initiatives to help Americans lead healthier lives through better nutrition and regular physical activity. Benjamin describes several actions to promote healthy eating and physical activity, including:

- Working together, the U.S. Department of Defense (DOD) and the U.S. Department of Agriculture (USDA) have increased access to fresh fruits and vegetables for millions of students. The DOD Fresh Fruit and Vegetable program enables schools to buy U.S.-grown fresh produce.

- The U.S. Department of Veterans Affairs (VA) is providing menus that include freshly prepared foods, fresh fruits and vegetables, whole grains, and lower-sodium, gluten-free, and low-fat baked items. The VA changed the vending machine choices in its facilities to include more healthful options and is offering farmers' markets on VA medical center campuses.

- The VA operates 44 Healthy Teaching Kitchens to teach veterans and their families how to select and prepare healthy foods.

- The President's Council on Fitness, Sports, and Nutrition (PCFSN) promotes the Healthy People 2020, the 10-year national objective for improving the health of all Americans. The PCFSN Physical Activity Outreach initiative included radio, television, and print public service announcements to educate parents and caregivers about the importance of regular physical activity for kids and its positive impact on academic performance.

- The U.S. Department of Health and Human Services (HHS) launched the Presidential Youth Fitness Program, a free program that teaches students the skills they need to be physically active; 23,000 schools have adopted the program.

- The U.S. Department of Transportation (DOT) promotes safety education for state agencies to educate older adults about pedestrian safety and to promote safe, active living among this population. The DOT offers free online training about safe walking and bicycling through the Livable Communities webinar series.

PREVENTION EFFORTS TARGET FAMILIES, COMMUNITIES, WORK SITES, AND SCHOOLS

Public health education, communication, and other programs aimed at families and communities are identified as the cornerstone of prevention efforts. In *National Prevention, Health Promotion and Public Health Council*, Benjamin describes various national prevention programs. For example, the Corporation for National and Community Service promotes healthy communities via programs that involve youth in physical activity and teach them the importance of nutrition. The HHS Community Transformation Grant program helps create safe

recreational space to enable children to have increased opportunities for physical activity and improves access to more healthful food and beverages in school vending machines.

In the community, schools offer ideal settings and multiple opportunities for preventing overweight and obesity by educating children about, and engaging them in, healthy eating and physical activity. To reinforce their messages concerning the importance of school physical activity and nutrition programs, schools can ensure that breakfast and lunch programs meet nutrition standards and provide food options that are low in fat, calories, and added sugars. Other ways to improve student health and nutrition include offering healthy snacks in vending machines and school stores and providing all students with quality daily physical education to cultivate the knowledge, attitudes, skills, behaviors, and confidence needed to be physically active for life.

One way to consider how Americans relate to food and physical activity and how to improve diet and activity levels is to use a social-ecological model that looks at the population demographics, environments, organizations, values, and culture that influence nutrition and physical-activity decisions. Public health officials use this model to show how all elements of society combine to shape an individual's food and physical activity choices, which in turn influence calorie balance and risk for overweight and obesity. Figure 10.1 displays the myriad influences on an individual's food and physical activity decisions.

Community Strategies to Prevent Obesity

In *Strategies to Prevent Obesity and Other Chronic Diseases: The CDC Guide to Strategies to Increase the Consumption of Fruits and Vegetables* (2011, http://www.cdc.gov/obesity/downloads/FandV_2011_WEB_TAG508.pdf), the Centers for Disease Control and Prevention (CDC) identifies the following 10 environmental- and policy-level strategies that communities and local governments can use to plan and monitor changes to help prevent obesity:

1. Promote food policy councils as a way to improve the food environment at state and local levels

2. Improve access to retail stores that sell high-quality fruits and vegetables or increase the availability of high-quality fruits and vegetables at retail stores in underserved communities

3. Start or expand farm-to-institution programs in schools, hospitals, workplaces, and other institutions

4. Start or expand farmers' markets in all settings

5. Start or expand community supported agriculture programs in all settings

FIGURE 10.1

Factors shaping nutrition and physical activity decisions

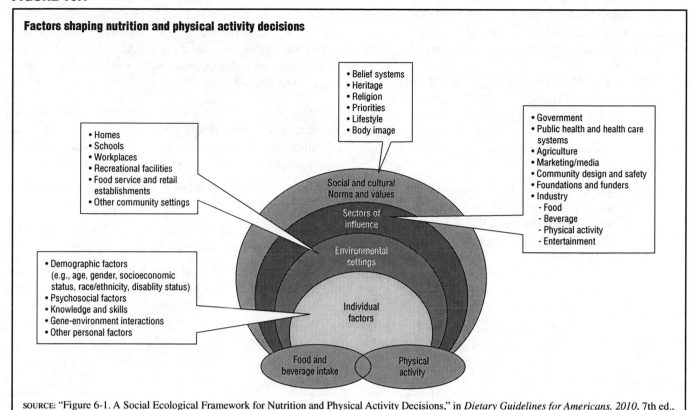

- Belief systems
- Heritage
- Religion
- Priorities
- Lifestyle
- Body image

- Homes
- Schools
- Workplaces
- Recreational facilities
- Food service and retail establishments
- Other community settings

- Government
- Public health and health care systems
- Agriculture
- Marketing/media
- Community design and safety
- Foundations and funders
- Industry
  - Food
  - Beverage
  - Physical activity
  - Entertainment

- Demographic factors (e.g., age, gender, socioeconomic status, race/ethnicity, disablity status)
- Psychosocial factors
- Knowledge and skills
- Gene-environment interactions
- Other personal factors

Social and cultural Norms and values

Sectors of influence

Environmental settings

Individual factors

Food and beverage intake

Physical activity

SOURCE: "Figure 6-1. A Social Ecological Framework for Nutrition and Physical Activity Decisions," in *Dietary Guidelines for Americans, 2010*, 7th ed., U.S. Department of Health and Human Services and U.S. Department of Agriculture, December 2010, http://www.cnpp.usda.gov/Publications/ DietaryGuidelines/2010/PolicyDoc/PolicyDoc.pdf (accessed November 13, 2013)

6. Ensure access to fruits and vegetables in workplace cafeterias and other food service venues

7. Ensure access to fruits and vegetables at workplace meetings and events

8. Support and promote community and home gardens

9. Establish policies to incorporate fruit and vegetable activities into schools as a way to increase consumption

10. Include fruits and vegetables in emergency food programs

Similarly, in *Strategies to Prevent Obesity and Other Chronic Diseases: The CDC Guide to Strategies to Increase Physical Activity in the Community* (2011, http:// www.cdc.gov/obesity/downloads/PA_2011_WEB.pdf), the CDC presents 10 strategies aimed at increasing physical activity:

1. Community-wide campaigns—large-scale multimedia campaigns in concert with support and self-help groups, physical activity counseling, and risk factor screening and education at work sites, schools, and community health fairs

2. Point-of-decision prompts to encourage use of stairs—signs posted beside elevators and escalators to encourage people to use nearby stairs instead

3. Individually adapted health behavior change programs—custom-tailored strategies that respond to an individual's interests and preferences

4. Enhanced school-based physical education—engaging students in moderate to vigorous physical activity

5. Social support interventions in community settings— building, strengthening, and maintaining social networks that support physical activity behavior change

6. Creation of or enhanced access to places for physical activity combined with informational outreach activities—creating or improving access to exercise facilities and walking trails, providing programs that educate people about physical exercise, and offering screenings and referrals to other types of services

7. Street-scale urban design and land-use policies— activities include improving street lighting and increasing ease and safety of street crossings

8. Community-scale urban design and land-use policies—actions include improving the continuity and connectivity of streets, sidewalks, and bicycle lanes

9. Active transport to school—interventions designed to encourage and support youth walking, bicycling, or skating to school

10. Transportation and travel policies and practices—encouraging walking, bicycling, and public transportation use, increasing the safety of walking and bicycling, reducing car use, and improving air quality

Federally Funded National Nutrition Education

Together, the USDA and the HHS update *Nutrition and Your Health: Dietary Guidelines for Americans* every five years. First published in 1980, the guidelines serve as the basis for federal food and nutrition education programs.

In December 2010 the seventh version of the dietary guidelines, *Dietary Guidelines for Americans, 2010* (http://health.gov/dietaryguidelines/dga2010/DietaryGuidelines2010.pdf), was released. According to the USDA and the HHS, in the press release "USDA and HHS Announce New Dietary Guidelines to Help Americans Make Healthier Food Choices and Confront Obesity Epidemic" (January 31, 2011, http://www.cnpp.usda.gov/Publications/DietaryGuidelines/2010/PolicyDoc/PressRelease.pdf), the updated dietary guidelines emphasize reducing calorie consumption and increasing physical activity in an effort to prevent and reverse the nation's obesity epidemic. They urge Americans to consume more vegetables, fruits, whole grains, fat-free and low-fat dairy products, and seafood and to consume less sodium, saturated and trans fats, added sugars, and refined grains.

The 2010 dietary guidelines present 23 key recommendations for the general population and six additional recommendations for specific populations, such as pregnant women. The guidelines advise Americans to reduce:

- Consumption of sodium to less than 2,300 milligrams per day and cholesterol to less than 300 milligrams per day

- Saturated fats by replacing them with monounsaturated and polyunsaturated fats

- Consumption of trans fatty acids by sharply limiting the intake of partially hydrogenated oils and other solid fats (see Figure 10.2, which shows commonly used solid fats and oils and their composition in terms of saturated fat, monounsaturated fat, and polyunsaturated fat)

FIGURE 10.2

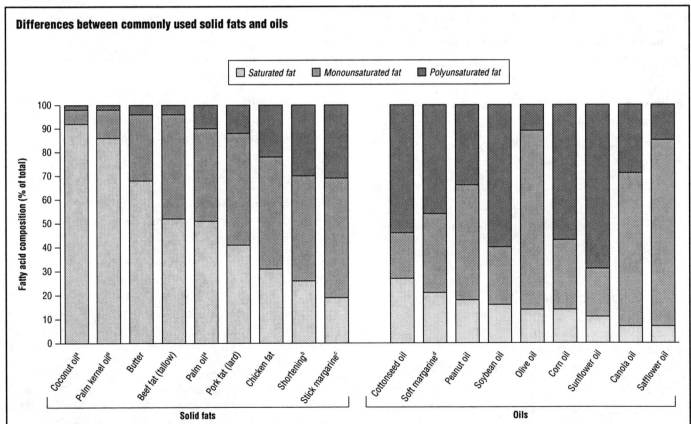

Differences between commonly used solid fats and oils

[a]Coconut oil, palm kernel oil, and palm oil are called oils because they come from plants. However, they are semi-solid at room temperature due to their high content of short-chain saturated fatty acids. They are considered solid fats for nutritional purposes.
[b]Partially hydrogenated vegetable oil shortening, which contains transfats.
[c]Most stick margarines contain partially hydrogenated vegetable oil, a source of transfats.
[d]The primary ingredient in soft margarine with no transfats is liquid vegetable oil.

SOURCE: "Figure 3-3. Fatty Acid Profiles of Common Fats and Oils," in *Dietary Guidelines for Americans, 2010*, 7th ed., U.S. Department of Health and Human Services and U.S. Department of Agriculture, December 2010, http://health.gov/dietaryguidelines/dga2010/dietaryguidelines2010.pdf (accessed November 14, 2013)

FIGURE 10.3

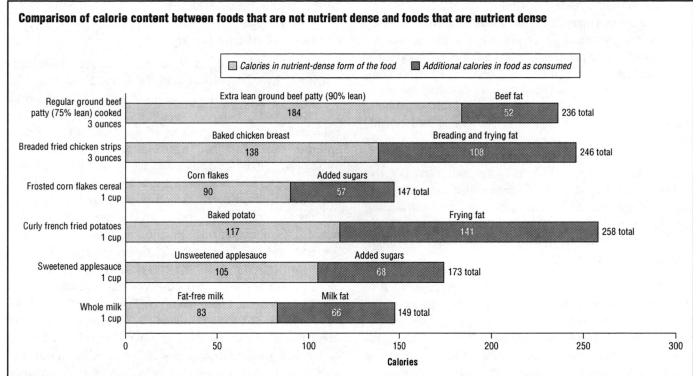

Comparison of calorie content between foods that are not nutrient dense and foods that are nutrient dense

☐ Calories in nutrient-dense form of the food   ▨ Additional calories in food as consumed

Food		
Regular ground beef patty (75% lean) cooked 3 ounces	Extra lean ground beef patty (90% lean) 184 — Beef fat 52	236 total
Breaded fried chicken strips 3 ounces	Baked chicken breast 138 — Breading and frying fat 108	246 total
Frosted corn flakes cereal 1 cup	Corn flakes 90 — Added sugars 57	147 total
Curly french fried potatoes 1 cup	Baked potato 117 — Frying fat 141	258 total
Sweetened applesauce 1 cup	Unsweetened applesauce 105 — Added sugars 68	173 total
Whole milk 1 cup	Fat-free milk 83 — Milk fat 66	149 total

Calories (scale: 0, 50, 100, 150, 200, 250, 300)

SOURCE: "Figure 5-2. Examples of the Calories in Food Choices That Are Not in Nutrient Dense Forms and the Calories in Nutrient Dense Forms of These Foods," in *Dietary Guidelines for Americans, 2010*, 7th ed., U.S. Department of Health and Human Services and U.S. Department of Agriculture, December 2010, http://health.gov/dietaryguidelines/dga2010/dietaryguidelines2010.pdf (accessed November 14, 2013)

- Intake of refined grains and refined grain products with solid fats, added sugars, and sodium

- Alcohol consumption—one drink per day for women and two for men

The guidelines advise Americans to increase the consumption of:

- Nutrient-dense foods (e.g., fruits, lean meats and poultry, and eggs prepared without added solid fats, sugars, starches, and sodium) that provide the full range of essential nutrients and fiber, without excessive calories (see Figure 10.3, which compares the calorie content in some commonly consumed nutrient-dense foods with foods that are not nutrient dense)

- Vegetables (especially dark green, red, and orange vegetables), beans, peas, and fruits

- Whole grains and fat-free or low-fat dairy or fortified soy beverages

- Fish and other seafood

- A variety of foods high in protein, including eggs, beans, peas, soy products, and unsalted nuts and seeds

- Foods that are rich in potassium, dietary fiber, calcium, and vitamin D, including vegetables, fruits, whole grains, and dairy

The guidelines advise "appropriate calorie balance during each stage of life—childhood, adolescence, adulthood, pregnancy and breastfeeding, and older age." Women who may become pregnant are advised to choose foods that are rich in iron and folate and to take 400 micrograms of folic acid per day. Women who are pregnant are advised to take an iron supplement and those who are pregnant or breastfeeding are cautioned to limit their consumption of white tuna to just 6 ounces per week and to avoid eating tilefish, shark, swordfish, and mackerel, because these fish contain high mercury content. Adults aged 50 years and older are encouraged to choose foods that are fortified with vitamin B12, such as fortified cereals, or to take dietary supplements to ensure adequate B12 intake.

MyPlate Is Also for Children

In June 2011 MyPlate replaced MyPyramid for Kids, which, like the food pyramid for adults, provided guidance for children's diets. (See Figure 5.2 in Chapter 5.) The website ChooseMyPlate.gov replaces much of the information that was formerly available on MyPyramid.gov and, to engage children, includes a coloring sheet for children. It also has an interactive feature to help with meal planning. MyPlate is part of a larger communications initiative based on the 2010 dietary guidelines to help consumers of all ages make better food choices.

The dietary guidelines observe that healthy diets and adequate physical activity are vitally important for children in view of the fact that risk factors for adult chronic diseases are increasingly found in younger ages. The guidelines assert that "eating patterns established in childhood often track into later life, making early intervention on adopting healthy nutrition and physical activity behaviors a priority." The guidelines advise that young children consume between 1,000 and 2,000 calories per day and older children and adolescents between 1,400 and 3,200 calories per day. Table 10.1 shows the estimated calories needed of children, adolescents, and adults by sex and physical activity level. The proportion of recommended macronutrients (carbohydrate, fat, and protein) changes with advancing age. For example, children aged one to three years require less protein and more fat in their diet than do older children. (See Table 5.1 in Chapter 5.)

Children aged six years and older are encouraged to play hard and be more physically active to meet the government's recommended 60 minutes of exercise per day. Although the guidelines do not offer specific recommendations about the duration of physical activity for children aged two to five years, they advise that young children should play actively several times each day. Because children and teens are often active in short bursts of time rather than for sustained periods, these short bursts accumulate to meet physical activity requirements.

Praise and Criticism for MyPlate

Like MyPyramid, MyPlate has garnered praise and criticism. In "Why It's Good That the Food Pyramid Became a Plate" (Atlantic.com, June 3, 2011), Marion Nestle of New York University praises the new icon, explaining that it is easy enough for a child to use. Nestle approves of the fact that vegetables are the largest sector on the plate, that vegetables and fruits together consume half the plate, and that dairy foods are off to the side so they may be considered discretionary. Nestle also likes the fact that unless one chooses a very large plate, there's no need to count servings or measure portion sizes. She has just one criticism of MyPlate: its categorization of protein as a food group. Nestle explains that "protein is a nutrient, not a food," and observes that "protein is not exactly lacking in American diets. The average American consumes twice the protein needed." Nestle is concerned that Americans may equate protein exclusively with meat rather than with a larger group of foods including beans, nuts, poultry, fish, grains, and dairy (which have separate sectors on the plate) that are also sources of protein in American diets.

TABLE 10.1

Estimated calorie needs by age, sex, and physical activity

Estimated amounts of calories needed to maintain calorie balance for various gender and age groups at three different levels of physical activity. The estimates are rounded to the nearest 200 calories. An individual's calorie needs may be higher or lower than these average estimates.

Gender	Age (years)	Physical activity level[a]		
		Sedentary	Moderately active	Active
Child (female and male)	2–3	1,000–1,200[b]	1,000–1,400[b]	1,000–1,400[b]
Female[c]	4–8	1,200–1,400	1,400–1,600	1,400–1,800
	9–13	1,400–1,600	1,600–2,000	1,800–2,200
	14–18	1,800	2,000	2,400
	19–30	1,800–2,000	2,000–2,200	2,400
	31–50	1,800	2,000	2,200
	51+	1,600	1,800	2,000–2,200
Male	4–8	1,200–1,400	1,400–1,600	1,600–2,000
	9–13	1,600–2,000	1,800–2,200	2,000–2,600
	14–18	2,000–2,400	2,400–2,800	2,800–3,200
	19–30	2,400–2,600	2,600–2,800	3,000
	31–50	2,200–2,400	2,400–2,600	2,800–3,000
	51+	2,000–2,200	2,200–2,400	2,400–2,800

Notes: Based on Estimated Energy Requirements (EER) equations, using reference heights (average) and reference weights (healthy) for each age/gender group. For children and adolescents, reference height and weight vary. For adults, the reference man is 5 feet 10 inches tall and weighs 154 pounds. The reference woman is 5 feet 4 inches tall and weighs 126 pounds. EER equations are from the Institute of Medicine's *Dietary Reference Intakes for Energy, Carbohydrate, Fiber, Fat, Fatty Acids, Cholesterol, Protein, and Amino Acids*. Washington (DC): The National Academies Press; 2002.
[a]Sedentary means a lifestyle that includes only the light physical activity associated with typical day-to-day life. Moderately active means a lifestyle that includes physical activity equivalent to walking about 1.5 to 3 miles per day at 3 to 4 miles per hour, in addition to the light physical activity associated with typical day-to-day life. Active means a lifestyle that includes physical activity equivalent to walking more than 3 miles per day at 3 to 4 miles per hour, in addition to the light physical activity associated with typical day-to-day life.
[b]The calorie ranges shown are to accommodate needs of different ages within the group. For children and adolescents, more calories are needed at older ages. For adults, fewer calories are needed at older ages.
[c]Estimates for females do not include women who are pregnant or breastfeeding.

SOURCE: "Table 2-3. Estimated Calorie Needs per Day by Age, Gender, and Physical Activity Level," in *Dietary Guidelines for Americans, 2010*, 7th ed., U.S. Department of Health and Human Services and U.S. Department of Agriculture, December 2010, http://health.gov/dietaryguidelines/dga2010/dietaryguidelines2010.pdf (accessed November 14, 2013)

Walter Willett of the Harvard School of Public Health indicates in "Out with the Pyramid, in with the Plate" (June 2011, http://www.hsph.harvard.edu/nutritionsource/what-should-you-eat/plate-replaces-pyramid/index.html) that the MyPlate icon is an improvement over previous nutrition icons and praises its effort to coax Americans to consume a diet that is more plant based. Although Willett believes the plate is better than the pyramid, he is also concerned about the information it lacks, asking, "What type of grain? What sources of proteins? What fats are used to prepare the vegetables and the grains?"

The Physicians Committee for Responsible Medicine (PCRM) concurs in "Breaking News! USDA Replaces Food Pyramid with MyPlate" (June 2011, http://www.pcrm.org/media/online/jun2011/breaking-news-usda-replaces-food-pyramid-with) with Nestle about the protein portion of the plate, observing that beans, whole grains, and vegetables contain protein. The PCRM objects to the inclusion of dairy, which is often a source of fat and cholesterol, and opines that there are more healthful sources of dietary calcium. Furthermore, the PCRM nutritionist Kathryn Strong asserts that "the USDA's new plate icon couldn't be more at odds with federal food subsidies. The plate icon advises Americans to limit high-fat products like meat and cheese, but the federal government is subsidizing these very products with billions of tax dollars and giving almost no support to fruits and vegetables." Nearly two-thirds (63%) of federal agricultural subsidies support meat and dairy production and less than 1% of subsidies support the cultivation of fruits and vegetables.

In "What's on Your Plate? MyPlate Replaces the Food Pyramid" (Shape.com, June 2011), Jennifer Walters laments that MyPlate fails to address Americans' tendency to snack, does not suggest that fruits be eaten to increase fiber intake rather than consumed as juice, does not specify that grains should be whole grain, does not emphasize the importance of eating vegetables in a variety of colors, and does not indicate that protein may be derived from foods other than meat.

Knowledge and Use of MyPlate Guidelines

MyPlate debuted in June 2011 and in 2013 Florence O. Uruakpa et al. surveyed consumers to determine whether they were aware of the move from MyPyramid to MyPlate and to find out whether MyPlate had influenced their dietary choices. In "Awareness and Use of MyPlate Guidelines in Making Food Choices" (*Procedia Food Science*, vol. 2, 2013), the researchers report that 80% of survey respondents said they were familiar with MyPlate and 43% knew that MyPlate had replaced MyPyramid. More than two-thirds noticed that the food group "meat and beans" had been renamed "protein" on MyPlate. Although just 12% of respondents said they had visited the ChooseMyPlate.gov website, nearly half said

they would likely visit the website. Because less than half (43%) of respondents thought that MyPlate would influence their food choices, Uruakpa et al. suggest that health care professionals and guidelines may need to direct consumers to the MyPlate website to increase their familiarity and comfort with the recommended food choices.

Fruits & Veggies: More Matters

Founded in 1991, the 5 a Day for Better Health Program was jointly sponsored by the National Cancer Institute and the Produce for Better Health Foundation (PBH), a nonprofit consumer-education foundation representing the fruit and vegetable industry. In 2007 the program was renamed the National Fruit and Vegetable Program. To reflect the changes and recommendations made in the dietary guidelines that were released in 2010, the PBH revamped the program and gave it a new name: Fruits & Veggies: More Matters (http://www.fruitsand veggiesmatter.org).

The Fruits & Veggies: More Matters initiative (2013, http://www.fruitsandveggiesmorematters.org) aims to increase fruit and vegetable consumption. Its objective is to help "Americans increase fruit & vegetable consumption for better health." Studies indicate that the majority of U.S. adults and adolescents are not eating the recommended two or more servings of fruit and three or more servings of vegetables per day. For example, in "Promoting Healthy Food Consumption: A Review of State-Level Policies to Improve Access to Fruits and Vegetables" (*Wisconsin Medical Journal*, vol. 111, no. 6, December 2012), Carlyn Hood, Ana Martinez-Donate, and Amy Meinen observe that 86% of adults and 91.5% of adolescents do not consume the recommended five daily servings of fruits and vegetables.

Along with reducing the risk for heart disease, high blood pressure, stroke, many cancers, and diabetes, diets rich in fruits and vegetables can help prevent overweight and obesity. Fruits and vegetables are naturally low in calories and fat, and their high water and fiber content produce feelings of satiety (the feeling of fullness or satisfaction after eating). Combined with an active lifestyle and a low-fat diet, eating greater amounts of fruits and vegetables and fewer high-calorie foods at meals can help control weight.

The Fruits & Veggies: More Matters initiative offers information about the benefits of eating fruits and vegetables, recipes, interactive tools, and information about how to use fruits and vegetables to help consumers manage their weight. For example, Table 10.2 shows fruit and vegetable choices that total 100 calories or fewer. In "100-Calorie Comparison Chart" (2014, http://www.fruitsandveggiesmorematters.org/100-calorie-comparison), the PBH illustrates how substituting fruits or vegetables for high-calorie snacks such as muffins, corn chips, or cookies

TABLE 10.2

Servings of fruit and vegetables with 100 calories or less

- a medium-size apple (72 calories)
- a medium-size banana (105 calories)
- 1 cup steamed green beans (44 calories)
- 1 cup blueberries (83 calories)
- 1 cup grapes (100 calories)
- 1 cup carrots (45 calories), broccoli (30 calories), or bell peppers (30 calories) with 2 tbsp. hummus (46 calories)

SOURCE: Adapted from "My NASA Center," in *Employee Orientation*, National Aeronautics and Space Administration, 2013, http://employeeorientation.nasa.gov/mycenter/default.htm (accessed January 9, 2014)

enablers dieters to eat more. For example, two cups of strawberries or cantaloupe contain the same 100 calories as two 2-inch (5-cm) chocolate chip cookies or three-eighths of a doughnut.

State and Community Funding for Prevention Efforts

The CDC Division of Nutrition, Physical Activity, and Obesity aims to help states prevent obesity and other chronic diseases by focusing on poor nutrition and inadequate physical activity. The division assists states in developing and implementing nutrition and physical activity interventions, and sponsoring initiatives to help populations balance caloric intake and expenditure, increase physical activity, improve nutrition by increasing consumption of fruits and vegetables, reduce television time, and increase breastfeeding.

According to the HHS, in "American Recovery and Reinvestment Act Prevention and Wellness Initiative: Communities Putting Prevention to Work" (March 19, 2010, http://www.cdc.gov/chronicdisease/recovery/PDF/HHS_CPPW_CommunityFactSheet.pdf), 44 communities received funding for obesity prevention programs totaling $230 million in 2010. The dollar amount of the awards ranged from $16.1 million for the County of San Diego Health and Human Services Agency in California and $15.9 million each for the Cook County Department of Public Health/Public Health Institute of Metropolitan Chicago, Illinois, and the County of Los Angeles Department of Public Health in California, to $1 million for the Cherokee Nation Health Service Group in Oklahoma and $900,000 for the Pueblo of Jemez, New Mexico.

In "Communities Putting Prevention to Work" (October 25, 2013, http://www.cdc.gov/nccdphp/dch/programs/CommunitiesPuttingPreventiontoWork/action/nutrition.htm), the CDC lists examples of obesity prevention community initiatives, such as the Hamilton County, Ohio, school district, which used its funding to provide more healthful foods and beverages for 99,000 students at 180 schools.

IS NUTRITION EDUCATION WORKING TO IMPROVE AMERICANS' DIETS?

The Healthy Eating Index (HEI) is a measure developed in 1990 by the USDA to assess the overall health value of Americans' diets. It captures the type and quantity of foods people eat and the degree to which diets comply with specific recommendations in the USDA dietary guidelines. The HEI assigns points for eating consistently within USDA guidelines. It assesses 10 dietary components—grains, vegetables, fruits, milk, meat, total fat, total saturated fat, cholesterol, sodium, and a varied diet—on a scale of 0 to 10. Individuals who eat grains, vegetables, fruits, milk, meat (including chicken and fish), as well as a variety of foods at or above the USDA-recommended levels, receive a maximum score of 10. A score of 0 is assigned when the recommended amount of those components is not eaten. For fat, saturated fat, cholesterol, and sodium, a score of 10 is awarded for eating the recommended amount or less. The highest possible score is 100; a score of 80 or above is considered a healthy diet, scores between 51 and 80 show a need for dietary improvement, and scores below 50 indicate a poor diet.

Researchers use the HEI to evaluate Americans' diets. For example, Sibylle Kranz and George P. McCabe used the HEI to assess children's diet quality and reported their findings in "Examination of the Five Comparable Component Scores of the Diet Quality Indexes HEI-2005 and RC-DQI Using a Nationally Representative Sample of 2–18 Year Old Children: NHANES 2003–2006" (*Journal of Obesity*, September 2013). The researchers find that although most of the children scored between the ideal (25 points) and very low scores, 12% of the children had zero scores, meaning that they scored no points in any of the five components: dairy, total grains, whole grains, fruits, and vegetables.

The market research firm NPD Group reports in *28th Annual Report on Eating Patterns in America* (2013, https://www.npd.com/lps/pdf/28th-Eating-Patterns-in-America.pdf) that Americans have changed some, but not all, of their food purchasing and eating habits. The top-10 foods in the U.S. diet in 2013 were sandwiches, fruit, vegetables, carbonated soft drinks, milk, coffee, potatoes, salty snacks, fruit juice, and cold cereal, and they accounted for 50% of all food consumed. Adults surveyed in 2013 said they were:

- Eating more fresh fruit—fruit is the number-one snack and dessert and is present in 6% of foods Americans consume

- Drinking less fruit juice and more bottled water and eating more yogurt at home

- Purchasing more fresh foods at supermarkets and restaurants

- Spending an average of 70 minutes per day eating

- Continuing to favor easy meal preparation methods and one-dish meals when eating at home

- Cooking on the stove top—90% of dinners were cooked on the stove top

Although restaurant visits remained flat in 2013, the NPD Group reports that discounted or restaurant visits on a coupon or deal increased 2% in the year ending August 2013, compared with the year ending August 2012, when deal visits were down 1%. Despite the uptick of discounted and deal visits, the casual dining restaurant business decreased 1% in 2013 from the previous year, while quick service restaurant traffic increased 2%.

Americans' Make Some Healthier Choices at Restaurants

The NPD Group reports in the press release "Consumers Make Healthy Choices at Restaurants by Cutting Out or Down, Reports NPD" (June 11, 2013, https://www.npd .com/) that Americans are more likely to cut out a food item or cut down on an order rather than choose a more healthful menu item. More than one-third (38%) forgo dessert or sweets, 37% choose water over other beverages, 23% opt for smaller portions, and 22% forgo an appetizer. Other strategies include ordering a salad (39%) or an appetizer (10%) as a meal, sharing an entrée (12%), and choosing a more healthful protein or meat (28%).

Americans' Snack Food Choices

The NPD Group observes in "Snacking in America: The Changing Role of Snack Foods in America" (2012, http://www.siicex.gob.pe/siicex/documentosportal/alertas/ documento/doc/837721679radF98D9.pdf) that one out of every five eating occasions at home and away from home is a snack. Snacking at home during the morning and afternoon increased between 2002 and 2012. Interestingly, people with the healthiest eating habits snacked the most frequently, but they snacked on healthful foods such as fruit and yogurt.

Snacking remains popular among U.S. consumers. In "Consumers Munch Away in the U.S.A." (*Food Technology*, vol. 67, no. 8, August 2013), Lamine Lahouasnia reports that there is growing demand for sweet and savory snacks, a category that includes fruits and meat snacks as well as chips and trail mix. There is also increasing demand for more healthful, "guilt-free" snacks such as nuts and jerky, which are high in protein, and for single-serving, portion-controlled treats such as chocolate and popcorn, which are portable and can be consumed "on the go." According to Lahouasnia, Millennials (people born between the mid-1970s and the early 1990s, also known as Generation Y) want to snack on foods with exotic flavors, such as spicy potato chips, flavored nuts, and chocolate with sea salt.

Snacking May Help to Promote Weight Management

In the press release "The Right Snack May Aid Satiety, Weight Loss" (July 16, 2013, http://www.ift.org/news room/news-releases/2013/july/16/the-right-snack-may-aid-satiety.aspx), the Institute for Food Technologists observes that healthy snacks that promote satiety may reduce the quantity of food consumed at subsequent meals. In a presentation at the 2013 Institute of Food Technologists Annual Meeting & Food Expo, Roberta Re of Leatherhead Food Research in Surrey, England, explained that the food industry is trying to offer consumers snacks that improve satiety to help them reduce their total daily food intake. Re reports that midmorning snacks of cereal or nuts reduced food consumption at lunch and dinner, effectively decreasing the total daily food intake.

Portion-controlled snacks, such as Nabisco 100-Calorie Packs, aim to help dieters control their caloric intake while still enjoying their favorite snacks, which are often sweet, salty, or low-nutrient-value foods. Brian Wansink, Collin R. Payne, and Mitsuru Shimizu conducted research to determine whether the 100-calorie packages reduced the caloric intake of normal-weight and obese people and whether they enabled people to accurately track their caloric intake. The conduct and results of the study were published in "The 100-Calorie Semi-solution: Sub-packaging Most Reduces Intake among the Heaviest" (*Obesity*, vol. 19, no. 5, May 2011). The researchers asked 42 college students to eat snack crackers while watching television. Half of the study subjects were given a large 400-calorie package of crackers and the other half were given four 100-calorie packages. After the show, the subjects were asked to estimate how many crackers they had consumed, and then their actual consumption was calculated. Subjects ate an average 25% less when given four 100-calorie packages of crackers than when given one 400-calorie package, and overweight subjects' intake decreased 54%. Nonetheless, all of the subjects underestimated their consumption by 60% or more, which suggests that portion-controlled packaging does not improve the accuracy of estimated intake.

Interventions to Promote Healthy Weight

In "Obesity Prevention and Control: Interventions in Community Settings" (February 13, 2014, http://www.the communityguide.org/obesity/communitysettings.html), the CDC's Community Preventive Services Task Force reviews the effectiveness of interventions that prevent obesity and promote healthy eating and physical activity. The task force considers the effectiveness of population-based interventions that promote healthy growth and development of children and adolescents and that support healthy weights among adults. It also focuses on school-based strategies, work-site programs, health care system interventions, and community-wide initiatives.

The task force recommends interventions that reduce the time children and teens spend watching television, playing video or computer games, and surfing the Internet. It endorses work-site programs that combine nutrition and physical activity as effective strategies to reduce and control overweight and obesity. It also indicates that more research is needed to determine the extent to which school-based programs help control overweight and obesity. Table 10.3 is an overview of the interventions and task force ratings.

Proven Community-Based Prevention Programs

In October 2013 the Trust for America's Health and the New York Academy of Medicine published *A Compendium of Proven Community-Based Prevention Programs* (http://healthyamericans.org/assets/files/Compendium _Report_1016_1131.pdf), which details 79 community-based prevention programs that have demonstrated the ability to improve health and save lives. Examples of programs that have increased physical activity include the installation of a six-block walking path and school playground in a low-income African American neighborhood in New Orleans, Louisiana, and a comprehensive nutrition

TABLE 10.3

Obesity prevention interventions and task force ratings

	Ratings
Interventions to reduce screen time (e.g., time in front of a TV, computer monitor)	
Behavioral interventions to reduce screen time	Recommended
These interventions may include:	
• Skills building, tips, goal setting, and reinforcement techniques	
• Parent or family support through provision of information on environmental strategies to reduce access to television, video games, and computers	
• A "TV turnoff challenge" in which participants are encouraged not to watch TV for a specified number of days	
Mass media interventions to reduce screen time	Insufficient evidence
In these campaigns, one or more components is designed to:	
• Increase knowledge about screen time	
• Influence attitudes	
• Change behavior by transmitting messages through newspapers, radio, television, and billboards	
Technology-supported interventions (e.g., computer or web applications)	
Technology-supported components may include use of the following:	
• Computers (e.g., internet, CD-ROM, e-mail, kiosk, computer program)	
• Video conferencing	
• Personal digital assistants	
• Pagers	
• Pedometers with computer interaction	
• Computerized telephone system interventions that target physical activity, nutrition, or weight.	
Non-technological components may include use of the following:	
• In-person counseling	
• Manual tracking	
• Printed lessons	
• Written feedback	
Multicomponent coaching or counseling interventions:	
• To reduce weight	Recommended
• To maintain weight loss	Recommended
Interventions in specific settings	
Worksite programs	Recommended
• Informational and educational strategies aim to increase knowledge about a healthy diet and physical activity. Examples include:	
Lectures	
Written materials (provided in print or online)	
Educational software	
• Behavioral and social strategies target the thoughts (e.g. awareness, self-efficacy) and social factors that effect behavior changes. Examples include:	
Individual or group behavioral counseling	
Skill-building activities such as cue control	
Rewards or reinforcement	
Inclusion of co-workers or family members to build support systems	
• Policy and environmental approaches aim to make healthy choices easier and target the entire workforce by changing physical or organizational structures. Examples of this include:	
Improving access to healthy foods (e.g. changing cafeteria options, vending machine content)	
Providing more opportunities to be physically active (e.g. providing on-site facilities for exercise)	
• Policy strategies may also change rules and procedures for employees such as health insurance benefits or costs or money for health club membership.	
• Worksite weight control strategies may occur separately or as part of a comprehensive worksite wellness program that addresses several health issues (e.g., smoking cessation, stress management, cholesterol reduction).	
School-based programs	Insufficient evidence
These interventions are conducted in the classroom and may seek to increase physical activity and/or improve nutrition, both in school and at home. Classroom and physical education teachers may receive special training to carry out the programs.	

SOURCE: Adapted from "Summary of Task Force Recommendations," in *Obesity Prevention and Control: Interventions in Community Settings*, Guide to Community Preventive Services, September 27, 2013, http://www.thecommunityguide.org/obesity/communitysettings.html (accessed November 18 2013)

and health education program in Somerville, Massachusetts, that helps prevent overweight in elementary school students.

PREVENTION PROGRAMS AT THE WORK SITE

Along with school-based nutrition programs and education initiatives aimed at the public at large, several notable obesity prevention efforts involve developing and implementing strategies to integrate physical activity and healthful food choices into routine work-site activities. Examples of such activities include incorporating planned activity breaks with music into long meetings; offering healthful food choices during meetings and breaks and in employee cafeterias; and hosting walking meetings.

Because more than 100 million Americans (over one out of every three people in the United States, as of the end of 2013) spend a large number of their waking hours at work, the work site presents another opportunity for prevention programs. In "Obesity Prevention and Control: Interventions in Community Settings," the Community Preventive Services Task Force advises moving beyond traditional workplace health education programs. It recommends more intensive and comprehensive efforts, such as modifying physical and social environments, instituting policies consistent with the objective of preventing overweight and obesity, and extending work-site prevention efforts not only to employees but also to the families of employees and their communities.

Examples of work-site obesity prevention and weight-control strategies include:

- Educating workers using lectures, written materials provided in print or online, and educational software

- Ensuring that healthy food options are available in cafeterias and vending machines

- Establishing work-site exercise facilities or creating incentives for employees to join local fitness centers

- Developing incentives, rewards, and reinforcements for workers to achieve and maintain a healthy body weight

- Encouraging employers to require weight management and physical activity counseling as covered benefits in health insurance contracts

- Providing individual or group behavioral counseling

James A. Levine of the Mayo Clinic in Rochester, Minnesota, observes in "Poverty and Obesity in the U.S." (*Diabetes*, vol. 60, no. 11, November 2011) that there is evidence of a link between a sedentary lifestyle, obesity, diabetes, other metabolic diseases, and premature death. People who are sedentary, like many office workers, move an average of two hours less per day than active people and as a result expend less energy, increasing their risk for obesity, chronic metabolic disease, and cardiovascular death. Levine notes that "more than half of county-to-county variance in obesity can be accounted for by variance in sedentariness."

Offices and Work Sites Can Improve, Rather Than Imperil, Health and Fitness

Mary Murphy notes in "Obesity Expert Says Daily Workouts Can't Undo Damage Done from Sitting All Day" (NBCNews.com, January 9, 2013) that Levine, who studies nonexercise activity thermogenesis (NEAT; the calories people burn during everyday activities such as standing, walking, or even fidgeting), believes that sitting imperils health. Levine asserts that even a daily workout at the gym does not counteract the harmful effects of sitting all day long. He says it is crucial to break up the hours of sitting and suggests walking at lunchtime and moving more at work.

James A. Levine and Selene Yeager explain in *Move a Little, Lose a Lot: New NEAT Science Reveals How to Be Thinner, Happier, and Smarter* (2009) that Americans' reliance on electronics and especially the Internet has deprived them of the opportunity to be physically active and burn calories. They assert that changing office workers' routines to include more standing, turning, and bending throughout the course of the workday can burn 2,100 calories per week, boost metabolism, reduce blood pressure, and increase mental clarity.

In "Effects of a Worksite Physical Activity Intervention for Hospital Nurses Who Are Working Mothers" (*AAOHN Journal*, vol. 59, no. 9, September 2011), Sharon J. Tucker et al. report the results of a study that tested an innovative 10-week work-site physical activity intervention that was incorporated into the work flow of hospital-based nurses. The intervention involved redesigning and changing the physical environment and providing social reinforcements and strategies for engaging in physical activities while at work and away from work. The nurses were given an intervention toolkit that contained a water bottle, tote bag, research-grade pedometer, resistance band, relaxation ball, relaxation CD, exercise DVD, nutrition and physical activity tips brochure, nutritious snack, walking meeting tag, and wellness journal. After a 30- to 60-minute introductory session, the nurses were asked to increase their overall physical activity for 10 weeks by one hour each workday, 30 minutes of which were to be through walking. The study met its objective: increasing overall daily hours of physical activity by one hour per day over the study period. Tucker et al. conclude that "it is feasible to target the worksite of hospital-based registered nurses to improve body composition and physical activity."

DOES PARTICIPATION IN WORK-SITE HEALTH PROMOTION PROGRAMS INCREASE PHYSICAL ACTIVITY?
Work-site health promotion programs have demonstrated the ability to help workers improve their health, increase productivity, and manage health care costs. Lisa J. Leininger et al. compared the physical activity of state university workers on campuses with formal health promotion programs to the physical activity levels of workers on campuses without such programs to determine if the programs served to increase physical activity levels. The research and its results were described in "Differences in Physical Activity Participation between University Employees with and without a Worksite Health Promotion Program" (*Californian Journal of Health Promotion*, vol. 11, no. 1, March 2013). The researchers find that the presence of a health promotion program was only associated with more walking days per week and made no difference in the amount of vigorous physical activity workers engaged in. Leininger et al. conclude, "Overall findings of this study indicate that if health promotion programs are to carry out their mission of improved health behaviors and increased [physical activity] levels, best practices must be implemented and further research must be conducted."

INTENSIFYING THE PREVENTION AGENDA IN THE HEALTH CARE SYSTEM

Interactions with health care professionals are important opportunities to deliver powerful prevention messages. Physicians' and other health professionals' prescriptions and recurring advice to maintain a healthy weight to prevent disease or reduce symptoms of existing disease are often powerful inducements for behavioral change. Most Americans have at least annual contact with a health care professional, and if this contact includes information about the importance of weight management, then it may reinforce prevention messages received in other settings such as schools and work sites. Furthermore, health care professionals are instrumental in shaping public policy and can leverage their expertise and credibility to present accurate messages in the media and catalyze sweeping changes in the community at large.

Examples of strategies to expand on prevention efforts in the health care delivery system include:

- Training health care providers and health profession students to use effective techniques to prevent and treat overweight and obesity
- Cultivating partnerships between health care providers, schools, faith-based groups, and other community organizations to target social and environmental causes of overweight and obesity
- Classifying obesity as a disease to enable reimbursement for prevention efforts

- Partially or fully covering weight-management services including nutrition education and physical activity programs as health plan benefits

The Patient Protection and Affordable Care Act (ACA), the health reform legislation that expands health care coverage, was signed into law in March 2010. The bill effectively eliminates insurers' ability to deny or cancel coverage because of preexisting medical conditions. It also emphasizes community prevention as an important strategy for improving the nation's health and curbing the huge costs that are associated with untreated chronic disease. The act requires health plans to fully cover obesity screening and counseling for adults and children, appropriates funds for demonstration projects to develop model programs for reducing childhood obesity, and requires the disclosure of specified nutrient information for food sold in many chain restaurants and vending machines.

In "Improving Obesity Prevention at the Local Level—Emerging Opportunities" (*New England Journal of Medicine*, vol. 368, no. 19, May 9, 2013), Sara N. Bleich and Lainie Rutkow opine that the ACA requirement that chain restaurants with 20 or more locations provide calorie information on their menus and menu boards, along with recommended daily caloric intake, may help prevent obesity. The researchers note that for menu labeling to be optimally effective, it must be understandable, particularly to people with limited nutritional knowledge who may not, for example, appreciate the impact of consuming a 1,000-calorie lunch. Bleich and Rutkow suggest that displaying calorie information in the form of a physical-activity equivalent, such as minutes of walking required to burn the calories in a particular food, is more effective than presenting calorie counts alone.

USING THE MEDIA TO COMMUNICATE THE PREVENTION MESSAGE

The media play a pivotal role in prevention efforts. The media can communicate and educate the public about healthy behaviors and health risks that are associated with overweight and obesity, introduce and reinforce prevention messages from health care professionals, and assist to alter attitudes and perceptions by celebrating healthy eating and physical activity.

The International Food Information Council (IFIC) has tracked media coverage of diet, nutrition, and food safety since 1995. In its first report, *Food for Thought* (1995), the IFIC noted that the leading nutrition and food issues receiving newspaper, television, and other media coverage during the previous 12 months were reducing fat intake; the impact of diet on disease risks; and discussions of foodborne illnesses, vitamin and mineral intake, disease causation, caloric intake, antioxidants, cholesterol intake, sugar intake, and fiber intake.

As obesity became a more prominent issue during the late 1990s, the IFIC reports in "Executive Summary" (*Food for Thought VI* [December 2005, http://www.food insight.org/Content/3651/ExecSummaryFFTVI.pdf]) that the number of stories about diet, weight loss, nutrition, and obesity increased from 1,270 in 1995 to 2,412 in 2005. This increase reflected both a rising volume of coverage and an escalation in the number of media outlets reporting about diet, overweight, and obesity. In *Food for Thought VI*, the IFIC reports that obesity was the leading topic in food and nutrition media stories during 2004, followed by disease prevention, physical activity, weight management, disease causation, vitamin and mineral intake, fat intake, functional foods, mad cow disease, caloric intake, and biotechnology.

Eight years later, the IFIC published *2013 Food and Health Survey* (May 2013, http://www.foodinsight.org/Link Click.aspx?fileticket=spavtJtVkzM%3d&tabid=1482), which looks at trends in consumer attitudes toward food safety, nutrition, and health. The IFIC notes that although about two-thirds (65%) of Americans look to the media for information about food and nutrition, just 15% say information from the media is believable. By contrast, 4% are very willing to believe food and nutrition information obtained via social media and 41% say they are most likely to find food and nutrition information credible if they hear it from different sources.

The media have responded with advertising and public service campaigns intended to heighten awareness of the risks that are associated with obesity and help Americans make healthier choices. By early 2014, however, it was not yet known if these antiobesity advertising campaigns were effective. For example, Rebecca M. Puhl, Joerg Luedicke, and Jamie Lee Peterson report in "Public Reactions to Obesity-Related Health Campaigns: A Randomized Controlled Trial" (*American Journal of Preventive Medicine*, vol. 45, no. 1, July 2013) that public health campaigns that consumers perceive as stigmatizing obese people are considered less motivating for improving lifestyle behaviors and promoting healthy

behavior change than those that have neutral or less stigmatizing messages.

TARGETING CHILDHOOD OBESITY

Giving children the right kind of food is crucial to their well-being and success. The Healthy Schools Program proves that, with proper planning and support, there seems to be no reason why all districts can't meet nutritional standards and serve their students healthy, enjoyable meals.

—Former President Bill Clinton, cofounder of the Alliance for a Healthier Generation along with the American Heart Association, September 29, 2013

In 2005 the American Heart Association and the William J. Clinton Foundation launched a new initiative, the Alliance for a Healthier Generation (2013, https://www .healthiergeneration.org/about_us/), to combat childhood obesity. The alliance's mission is to "reduce the prevalence of childhood obesity and to empower kids to develop lifelong, healthy habits." Working with companies that influence children's lives—food, beverage, fitness, gaming, and technology—the alliance seeks to improve children's health and nutrition at home, in school, in physicians' offices, and in the community at large.

The alliance's Healthy Schools Program works with 28,000 schools and supports administrators, teachers, parents, and students to institute policies and programs that enable students to eat better and move more. It also involves insurers, employers, and health care provider associations to encourage reimbursement to physicians and registered dietitians for obesity prevention–related services. The alliance has helped forge voluntary agreements with the beverage, snack food, and dairy industries to significantly reduce the amount of high-calorie foods that are available to students in schools. According to the press release "President Bill Clinton to Recognize 267 U.S. Schools for Efforts to Prevent Childhood Obesity" (https://www.healthiergeneration.org/), in September 2013 Bill Clinton (1946–), the former president, honored 267 schools for meeting or exceeding federal standards for healthy school meals.

CHAPTER 11
PUBLIC OPINION AND ACTION ABOUT DIET, WEIGHT, NUTRITION, AND PHYSICAL ACTIVITY

At the end of the day, I don't see obesity as different from many other bad habits and behaviors that people have. We're not telling the people who don't wear motorcycle helmets to go home, and we're not telling people who have dangerous occupations or play tackle football that they better leave our shores because they are going to drive up our healthcare bill. In fact, the fastest way to lower our healthcare bill is to get rid of everybody who is a sinner because then the hospitals will be empty. The game of medicine is to try to figure out how to make people behave better, how to pursue their health, and not threaten them, penalize them, or make them pariahs.

—Arthur L. Caplan, "Kick Out Fat People to Lower Healthcare Costs?" (October 22, 2013)

Americans are growing heavier each year. According to Lindsey Sharpe of the Gallup Organization, in *U.S. Obesity Rate Climbing in 2013* (November 1, 2013, http://www.gallup.com/poll/165671/obesity-rate-climbing-2013.aspx), in 2013 the adult obesity rate was 27.2%, up from 26.2% in 2012. (See Figure 11.1.) This increase is not only the largest in a single year since 2009 but also reverses the trend of lower rates reported in 2011 and 2012.

In the United States obesity rates rose from 2012 to 2013 in nearly every age and socioeconomic group and among people of all races and ethnicities in every geographic region. The greatest increases between 2012 and 2013 were among people aged 45 to 64 years and workers earning between $30,000 and $74,999. (See Table 11.1.) African Americans continue to have the highest rates of obesity; young people aged 18 to 29 years and people with annual incomes in excess of $75,000 annually continue to be the least likely to be obese.

The highest rates of obesity are among people who have low incomes and low access to grocery stores—people living in so-called food deserts. In *Income, Not*

"Food Deserts," More to Blame for U.S. Obesity (September 20, 2013, http://www.gallup.com/poll/164513/income-not-food-deserts-blame-obesity.aspx), Kyley McGeeney and Elizabeth Mendes of the Gallup Organization report that low income is more strongly associated with obesity than is low access—28% compared with 25%—but people with low income and low access, such as those living in food deserts, have the highest rates of obesity (30%). (See Table 11.2.)

AMERICANS ARE WORRIED ABOUT THEIR WEIGHT

In *In U.S., Gender Gap in Personal Weight Worries Narrows* (July 1, 2012, http://www.gallup.com/poll/155903/Gender-Gap-Personal-Weight-Worries-Narrows.aspx), Alyssa Brown of the Gallup Organization observes that although the majority of Americans continue to describe their weight as "about right," 40% of men and 42% of women say that they are "somewhat" or "very" overweight. The percentages of people describing themselves as overweight, about right, or underweight have fluctuated but not changed dramatically since 2002. (See Figure 11.2.)

In 2012 about half (48%) of Americans were worried about their weight some of the time. (See Figure 11.3.) Although this percentage has not changed since 2005, it is considerably higher than the 34% who were worried about their weight in 1990. Women (55%) are much more likely to worry about their weight than are men (41%), but the percentage of men who said they worried about their weight all or some of the time nearly doubled from 1990 to 2012. (See Figure 11.4.) Not surprisingly, people who consider themselves overweight are much more likely to worry about their weight than those who feel that they are underweight or about right. (See Table 11.3.)

FIGURE 11.1

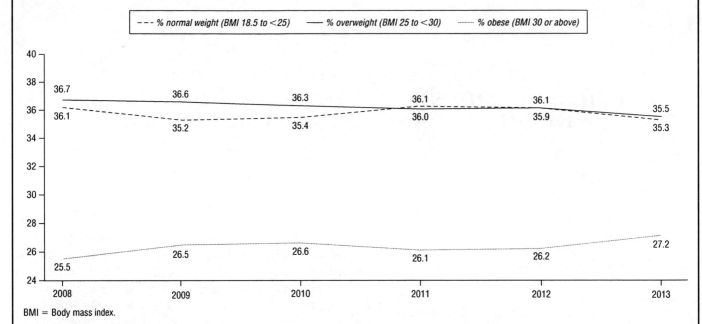

Adults by weight category, annual average, 2008–13

[Weight category as determined by BMI]

--- % normal weight (BMI 18.5 to <25) ⎯⎯ % overweight (BMI 25 to <30) ········ % obese (BMI 30 or above)

BMI = Body mass index.

SOURCE: Lindsey Sharpe, "American Adults, by Weight Category—Yearly Averages," in *U.S. Obesity Rate Climbing in 2013*, November 1, 2013, http://www.gallup.com/poll/165671/obesity-rate-climbing-2013.aspx (accessed November 16, 2013). Copyright © 2013 Gallup, Inc. All rights reserved. The content is used with permission; however, Gallup retains all rights of republication.

TABLE 11.1

Obesity rates by demographic characteristics, 2012 and 2013

[Sorted by difference between 2012 and 2013. Among adults aged 18 and older.]

	2012	2013	Difference
	%	%	(pct. pts.)
Aged 45–64	30.7	32.5	1.8
Annual income $30,000–$74,999	26.0	27.8	1.8
Aged 65+	25.2	26.6	1.4
South	28.1	29.4	1.3
Women	25.0	26.3	1.3
Annual income less than $30,000	30.4	31.6	1.2
West	23.2	24.4	1.2
Aged 30–44	28.1	29.1	1.0
Midwest	27.4	28.4	1.0
National adults	26.2	27.2	1.0
Whites	25.1	26.1	1.0
Annual income $75,000+	21.2	22.2	1.0
Men	27.3	28.2	0.9
Blacks	34.9	35.7	0.8
Hispanics	27.1	27.9	0.8
East	25.0	25.6	0.6
Aged 18–29	17.2	17.1	−0.1

SOURCE: Lindsey Sharpe, "Percentage Obese in U.S. among Various Demographic Groups," in *U.S. Obesity Rate Climbing in 2013*, November 1, 2013, http://www.gallup.com/poll/165671/obesity-rate-climbing-2013.aspx (accessed November 16, 2013). Copyright © 2013 Gallup, Inc. All rights reserved. The content is used with permission; however, Gallup retains all rights of republication.

TABLE 11.2

Percentage of Americans that are obese, low income versus low access, 2013

Food desert groups	% obese
Low-income and low-access	30
Low-income only	28
Low-access only	25
Neither low-income nor low-access	26

SOURCE: Kyley McGeeney and Elizabeth Mendes, "The Percentage of Americans Who Are Obese in Food Deserts Vs. Not in Food Deserts," in *Income, Not "Food Deserts," More to Blame for U.S. Obesity*, The Gallup Organization, September 20, 2013, http://www.gallup.com/poll/164513/income-not-food-deserts-blame-obesity.aspx (accessed November 16, 2013). Copyright © 2013 Gallup, Inc. All rights reserved. The content is used with permission; however, Gallup retains all rights of republication.

AMERICANS FAVOR LOW-FAT OVER LOW-CARB DIETS

According to a 2012 Gallup poll, twice as many Americans (63%) think that a low-fat diet is healthier than a low-carb diet (30%). In *Americans Still Say Low-Fat Diet Better Than Low-Carb* (August 17, 2012, http://www.gallup.com/poll/156710/Americans-Say-Low-Fat-Diet-Better-Low-Car.aspx), Andrew Dugan and Frank

FIGURE 11.2

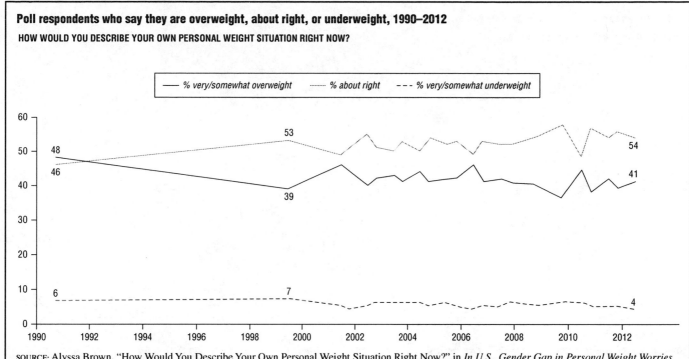

Poll respondents who say they are overweight, about right, or underweight, 1990–2012

HOW WOULD YOU DESCRIBE YOUR OWN PERSONAL WEIGHT SITUATION RIGHT NOW?

FIGURE 11.3

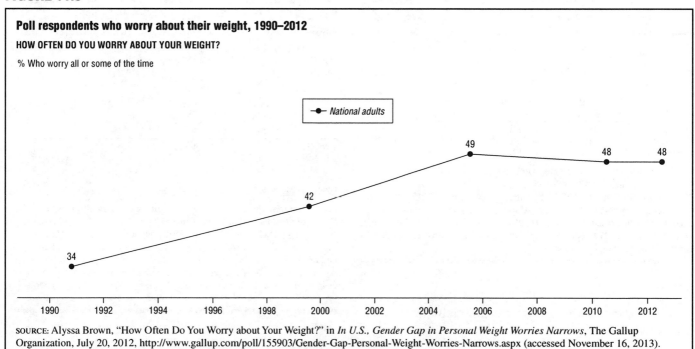

Poll respondents who worry about their weight, 1990–2012

HOW OFTEN DO YOU WORRY ABOUT YOUR WEIGHT?

% Who worry all or some of the time

Newport of the Gallup Organization note that the percentage of Americans who feel that a low-carbohydrate diet is more beneficial for the average American increased from 22% in 2002 to 30% in 2012. (See Table 11.4.)

More women (36%) than men (24%) think that a low-carb diet is healthier than a low-fat diet, and people aged 30 to 64 years are more likely to endorse the low-carb diet than are younger and older adults. (See Table 11.5.) Non-whites

FIGURE 11.4

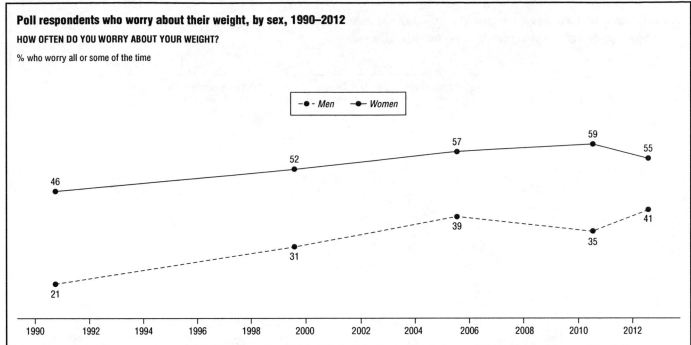

Poll respondents who worry about their weight, by sex, 1990–2012

HOW OFTEN DO YOU WORRY ABOUT YOUR WEIGHT?

% who worry all or some of the time

SOURCE: Alyssa Brown, "How Often Do You Worry about Your Weight?" in *In U.S., Gender Gap in Personal Weight Worries Narrows*, The Gallup Organization, July 20, 2012, http://www.gallup.com/poll/155903/Gender-Gap-Personal-Weight-Worries-Narrows.aspx (accessed November 16, 2013). Copyright © 2012 Gallup, Inc. All rights reserved. The content is used with permission; however, Gallup retains all rights of republication.

TABLE 11.3

Poll respondents who worry about their weight, by self-reported weight, 2012

HOW OFTEN DO YOU WORRY ABOUT YOUR WEIGHT?

By self-reported current weight situation

	All of the time	Some of the time	Not too often	Never
Overweight	24%	48%	22%	6%
About right	9%	23%	38%	29%
Underweight	11%	5%	19%	61%

SOURCE: Alyssa Brown, "How Often Do You Worry about Your Weight? By Self-Reported Current Weight Situation," in *In U.S., Gender Gap in Personal Weight Worries Narrows*, The Gallup Organization, July 20, 2012, http://www.gallup.com/poll/155903/Gender-Gap-Personal-Weight-Worries-Narrows.aspx (accessed November 16, 2013). Copyright © 2012 Gallup, Inc. All rights reserved. The content is used with permission; however, Gallup retains all rights of republication.

TABLE 11.4

Public opinion on low-fat versus low-carb diets, 2002, 2004, and 2012

FROM A HEALTH PERSPECTIVE, WHICH OF THE FOLLOWING DO YOU THINK IS MORE BENEFICIAL FOR THE AVERAGE AMERICAN—A DIET LOW IN FAT, OR A DIET LOW IN CARBOHYDRATES?

	Low in fat	Low in carbohydrates	Both/ equally (vol.)	Neither/no opinion (vol.)
	%	%	%	%
July 2012	63	30	2	4
July 2004	67	23	5	5
July 2002	68	22	5	5

(vol.) = Volunteered response

SOURCE: Andrew Dugan and Frank Newport, "From a Health Perspective, Which of the Following Do You Think is More Beneficial for the Average American—a Diet Low in Fat, or a Diet Low in Carbohydrates?" in *Americans Still Say Low-Fat Diet Better Than Low-Carb*, The Gallup Organization, August 17, 2012, http://www.gallup.com/poll/156710/Americans-Say-Low-Fat-Diet-Better-Low-Car.aspx (accessed November 16, 2013). Copyright © 2012 Gallup, Inc. All rights reserved. The content is used with permission; however, Gallup retains all rights of republication.

(37%) are more likely to favor the low-carb diet than are whites (28%).

Americans who describe themselves as overweight are more likely to favor the low-carb diet (34%) than people who assessed their weight as about right (28%). (See Table 11.6.) Dugan and Newport observe that despite mounting scientific evidence of the health benefits of low-carbohydrate diets, Americans still feel that a low-fat diet is the healthier choice.

CONSUMER ATTITUDES AND BEHAVIORS TOWARD DIET AND HEALTH

According to the International Food Information Council Foundation, in *2013 Food & Health Survey* (May 2013, http://www.foodinsight.org/LinkClick.aspx?fileticket=spavtJtVkzM%3d&tabid=1482), the majority of Americans say that they are giving "a lot" (56%) or "a little"

TABLE 11.5

Public opinion on low-fat versus low-carb diets, by selected characteristics, 2012

FROM A HEALTH PERSPECTIVE, WHICH OF THE FOLLOWING DO YOU THINK IS MORE BENEFICIAL FOR THE AVERAGE AMERICAN—A DIET LOW IN FAT, OR A DIET LOW IN CARBOHYDRATES?

	Low in fat	Low in carbohydrates
	%	%
Men	69	24
Women	58	36
Aged 18 to 29	70	27
Aged 30 to 49	63	34
Aged 50 to 64	59	31
Aged 65+	64	28
White	65	28
Non-white	57	37

SOURCE: Andrew Dugan and Frank Newport, "From a Health Perspective, Which of the Following Do You Think Is More Beneficial for the Average American—a Diet Low in Fat, or a Diet Low in Carbohydrates?" in *Americans Still Say Low-Fat Diet Better Than Low-Carb*, The Gallup Organization, August 17, 2012, http://www.gallup.com/poll/156710/Americans-Say-Low-Fat-Diet-Better-Low-Car.aspx (accessed November 16, 2013). Copyright © 2012 Gallup, Inc. All rights reserved. The content is used with permission; however, Gallup retains all rights of republication.

TABLE 11.6

Public opinion on low-fat versus low-carb diets, by self-reported weight, 2012

FROM A HEALTH PERSPECTIVE, WHICH OF THE FOLLOWING DO YOU THINK IS MORE BENEFICIAL FOR THE AVERAGE AMERICAN—A DIET LOW IN FAT, OR A DIET LOW IN CARBOHYDRATES?

	Low in fat	Low in carbohydrates	Both/equally/neither/ no opinion (vol.)
	%	%	%
Overweight	59	34	7
About right	66	28	7
Underweight	62	30	8

SOURCE: Andrew Dugan and Frank Newport, "From a Health Perspective, Which of the Following Do You Think Is More Beneficial for the Average American—a Diet Low in Fat, or a Diet Low in Carbohydrates?" in *Americans Still Say Low-Fat Diet Better Than Low-Carb*, The Gallup Organization, August 17, 2012, http://www.gallup.com/poll/156710/Americans-Say-Low-Fat-Diet-Better-Low-Car.aspx (accessed November 16, 2013). Copyright © 2012 Gallup, Inc. All rights reserved. The content is used with permission; however, Gallup retains all rights of republication.

(40%) thought to the healthfulness of their foods and beverages, and 38% often or always think about the number of calories they consume. When respondents were asked how they could improve their diet, the top three responses they gave, garnering 17% each, were to eat healthier or have a more balanced diet, eat more fruits or vegetables, and cut back on sweets and junk food.

The survey reveals that the changes Americans made to improve their diets include eating more fruits and vegetables (88%), reducing calorie consumption by drinking water or low- and no-calorie beverages (82%), eating more whole grains (78%), limiting foods with added sugars (75%), consuming smaller portions (73%), and cutting back on foods high in salt (70%).

The majority (81%) of Americans say that they eat more healthfully at home than at restaurants. The majority (89%) agree that displaying calorie counts on menus is helpful. Roughly same percentage favor listing calories on the nutrition facts panel on foods and beverages or on the front of packaging and showing the number of calories contained in recipes. About two-thirds, especially women and individuals under the age of 65 years, would like to use websites with tools that estimate calorie consumption and measure calories consumed each day, and 58% think that smartphone apps that count and track calorie consumption would be useful. More than half (56%) of those surveyed said that they were trying to lose weight, and an additional 27% indicated that they were trying to maintain their weight.

Americans are thinking about physical activity—60% think about it a lot, and 37% think about it a little. More Americans (90%) believe that they have control over their physical activity level than believe that they can control the healthfulness of their diet (88%) or their weight (81%). Although 60% believe that a great amount of control over physical activity levels is possible, just 31% try to exert control their level of activity. There is a similar gap in terms of perceived control over the healthfulness of the diet: about half of Americans (49%) feel that it is possible to control their diet, but just 29% attempt to do so. The gap is smaller in terms of control over weight: 40% feel that complete control is possible, and 30% attempt to exert this control. Those with higher incomes feel that they can exert more control over their physical activity, diet, and weight.

Americans cite lack of willpower (23%), dislike of exercise (21%), and the cost of healthful foods (19%) as major reasons that they do not assume more control over their weight. Among those trying to lose weight, 72% say that lack of willpower is an obstacle, 65% dislike exercise, and 56% cite the expense of healthful foods as a barrier to weight loss. More than half of Americans admit that they eat when they are under emotional stress (58%), and nearly half (48%) indicate that they have other, more important concerns.

Are Americans Getting Enough Exercise to Help Them Manage Their Weight?

In *Americans Exercising Less in 2013* (July 29, 2013, http://www.gallup.com/poll/163718/americans-exercising-less-2013.aspx), Mendes reports that about half (53.8%) of Americans were exercising at least 30 minutes on three or more days per week in mid-2013. According to Mendes,

FIGURE 11.5

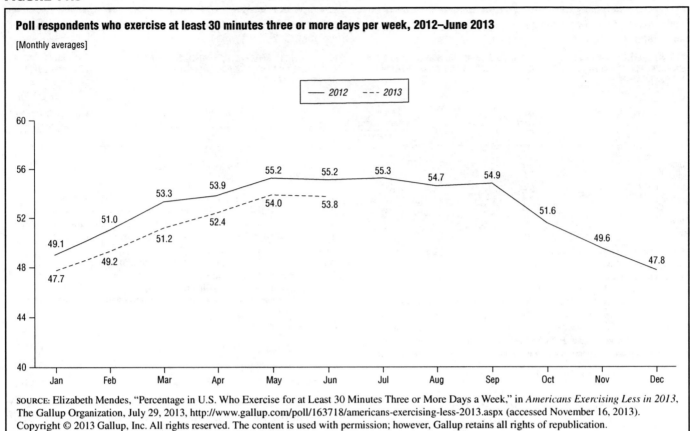

Poll respondents who exercise at least 30 minutes three or more days per week, 2012–June 2013

[Monthly averages]

— 2012   --- 2013

the rate of exercise declined from 2012, when the percentage of Americans exercising reached a high of 55.2%. (See Figure 11.5.)

Americans Feel That Obesity Is a Serious Public Health Problem

According to a November 2013 Pew Research Center survey, the majority of Americans (69%) think that obesity poses a very serious threat to public health, and 63% of Americans feel that obesity has consequences for society beyond its personal impact. In "Public Agrees on Obesity's Impact, Not Government's Role" (November 12, 2013, http://www.people-press.org/2013/11/12/public-agrees-on-obesitys-impact-not-governments-role/), the Pew Research Center indicates that concern about obesity outpaces concern about mental illness, prescription drug and alcohol abuse, cigarette smoking, and acquired immune deficiency syndrome.

Only 28% of Americans feel that the country is making progress in reducing obesity, and 34% believe that the nation is losing ground. By contrast, more than half (54%) of survey respondents said that the country is making progress in dealing with cancer, and 48% see gains in addressing acquired immune deficiency syndrome.

Although Americans generally believe that obesity poses a serious problem, more than one-half (54%) feel that the government should not play a significant role in addressing it. Just 42% favor government action to reduce obesity, and support for specific anti-obesity measures varies. Around two-thirds (67%) favor requiring chain restaurants to list calorie counts on their menus, and 55% support banning television advertisements for unhealthful foods during children's programs. Only 35%, however, support raising taxes on unhealthful food and sugary drinks, and just 31% favor size limits on sugary drinks in restaurants and convenience stores.

The former New York City mayor Michael Bloomberg (1942–) has had a long-standing interest in public health measures and was among the first to ban the use of trans fats and to require calorie counts on chain restaurant menus. In 2013, as mayor, Bloomberg moved to ban the sale of sodas and other sugary beverages larger than 16 ounces (473 ml) in restaurants, movie theaters, stadium concession stands, and other venues in New York City. Convenience stores, vending machines, and some newsstands were unaffected by the ban. In "Health Panel Approves Restriction on Sale of Large Sugary Drinks" (NYTimes.com, September 13, 2012), Michael M. Grynbaum reports that despite protests from some city council members, the former city comptroller, and groups funded by the soft-drink industry, the New York City Board of Health approved the measure.

In "Bloomberg's Ban on Big Sodas Is Unconstitutional: Appeals Court" (Reuters.com, July 30, 2013), Joseph Ax reports that in July 2013 the New York Supreme Court's Appellate Division deemed the mayor's proposed ban unconstitutional, declaring that it "violated the state principle of separation of powers." The appeals court explained that the ruling did not reflect disapproval of the effort to restrict the sale of large sodas; rather it asked that only "the government body with the authority to do so" enact the laws.

In November 2013 Bloomberg's successor, Mayor-Elect Bill de Blasio (1961–), vowed to appeal the court rejection of the soda ban. In "Bill de Blasio Must Fight New York City's Legal Battles Left by Mike Bloomberg" (NYDailyNews.com, November 18, 2013), Dareh Gregorian and Daniel Beekman report that de Blasio agrees with Bloomberg about the ban on supersized sodas and will take on the appeal when he assumes office in 2014.

Should Public Policy Stigmatize and Penalize People Who Are Obese?

In 2013 Albert Buitenhuis, a South African chef living in New Zealand—the third-most obese developed country (after the United States and Mexico)—faced deportation because the government of New Zealand determined that he did not have an "acceptable standard of health." When Buitenhuis moved to Christchurch, New Zealand, six years earlier, he weighed 350 pounds but had lost 60 pounds by the time he was to be deported. He worked as a chef, his wife worked as a waitress, and they paid taxes, yet the government argued that the demands Buitenhuis's obesity might place on New Zealand's health care system, which provides free medical care to all permanent residents, could be excessive.

Some observers opined that the country had a right to protect its economy from the ravages of the obesity epidemic. Others, however, decried New Zealand's actions as unfair, observing that the country does not seek to deport smokers, who also may be costly for the health care system. Arthur L. Caplan declares in "New Zealand's Solution for Rising Health Costs? Deport Fat People" (NBCNews.com, August 11, 2013) that "deporting Albert, especially while he is losing weight, looks for all the world like a sudden attack of unbridled prejudice." In "Kick Out Fat People to Lower Health-Care Costs?" (Medscape.com, October 22, 2013), Caplan states, "There are many ways to wage war on obesity. Deporting people is not one of them. I think we have to take a lesson here. It's important to say that there are all kinds of weaknesses and temptations that

have led to our obesity epidemic. We took a long time to eat ourselves into the problem. It will take a long time to work our way out of the problem. But I don't think citizens should have to worry that they are not going to get benefits, that they are going to be penalized or, at the far extreme, thrown out of the country because they have a medical problem."

Buitenhuis appealed the deportation and in September 2013 was granted a 23-month reprieve. In "'Too Fat' South African Wins Reprieve from New Zealand Deportation" (News24.com, September 9, 2013), New Zealand's associate immigration minister Nikki Kaye explains that although Buitenhuis has been granted a work visa, "under this arrangement he is not entitled to publicly-funded health care and he will have to meet any health costs himself."

Americans Are Concerned about Childhood Obesity

In "Overweight in Children" (November 7, 2013, http://www.heart.org/HEARTORG/GettingHealthy/WeightManagement/Obesity/Overweight-in-Children_UCM_304054_Article.jsp), the American Heart Association reports that childhood obesity is number one on parents' lists of health concerns, outpacing smoking and drug abuse. According to the University of Michigan C. S. Mott Children's Hospital National Poll on Children's Health, in "Top Child Health Concerns: Obesity, Drug Abuse & Smoking" (August 2013, http://mottnpch.org/sites/default/files/documents/081913Top10.pdf), childhood obesity is the leading concern of American adults, with 38% naming it as a "big problem." Concern is greatest among Hispanic and white adults—both groups named childhood obesity as their leading health concern, 47% and 39%, respectively. Fewer African American adults (29%) view childhood obesity as a serious problem, behind smoking and tobacco use (40%), drug abuse (34%), school violence (33%), sexually transmitted infections (32%), and teen pregnancy (30%).

Americans Want Schools to Provide Healthful Food

According to Lydia Saad and Brandon Busteed of the Gallup Organization, Americans support legislation that would sharply limit the kinds of foods schools can include in meals or sell on their campuses. In *Americans Favor Limiting Sale of Unhealthy Food in Schools* (March 12, 2013, http://www.gallup.com/poll/161318/americans-favor-limiting-sale-unhealthy-food-schools.aspx), Saad and Busteed report that 67% of adults and 75% of parents of public school students want schools to provide food that is high in nutritional value and would vote for a federal law that would strictly limit the kinds of foods schools could serve or sell. (See Table 11.7.)

Half of public school parents and 57% of American adults favor federal legislation to improve the nutritional

TABLE 11.7

Poll respondents who favor legislation limiting the sale of unhealthy food in schools, 2013

NEXT, I'M GOING TO READ SOME PROPOSALS THAT HAVE BEEN MADE TO IMPROVE THE NUTRITIONAL VALUE OF FOODS STUDENTS EAT WHILE AT SCHOOL. PLEASE SAY WHETHER YOU WOULD VOTE FOR OR AGAINST EACH OF THE FOLLOWING—A NEW FEDERAL LAW THAT WOULD STRICTLY LIMIT THE KINDS OF FOOD THAT CAN BE SERVED IN SCHOOL MEALS OR SOLD ELSEWHERE IN PUBLIC SCHOOLS TO FOOD THAT MEETS CERTAIN STANDARDS FOR HIGH NUTRITIONAL VALUE.

	National adults	Public school parents	Nonpublic school parents
	%	%	%
For	67	75	64
Against	31	22	34
No opinion	2	3	2

SOURCE: Lydia Saad and Brandon Busteed, "Americans' Support for New Nutritional Restrictions on School-Based Food," in *Americans Favor Limiting Sale of Unhealthy Food in Schools*, The Gallup Organization, March 12, 2013, http://www.gallup.com/poll/161318/americans-favor-limiting-sale-unhealthy-food-schools.aspx (accessed November 16, 2013). Copyright © 2013 Gallup, Inc. All rights reserved. The content is used with permission; however, Gallup retains all rights of republication.

TABLE 11.8

Poll respondents who favor legislation limiting the sale of unhealthy competitive food in school snack bars and vending machines, 2013

NEXT, I'M GOING TO READ SOME PROPOSALS THAT HAVE BEEN MADE TO IMPROVE THE NUTRITIONAL VALUE OF FOODS STUDENTS EAT WHILE AT SCHOOL. PLEASE SAY WHETHER YOU WOULD VOTE FOR OR AGAINST EACH OF THE FOLLOWING—A NEW FEDERAL LAW THAT WOULD STRICTLY LIMIT THE KINDS OF FOODS THAT CAN BE SERVED IN SCHOOL MEALS OR SOLD IN VENDING MACHINES, AT SNACK BARS AND BAKE SALES IN PUBLIC SCHOOLS TO FOOD THAT MEETS CERTAIN STANDARDS FOR HIGH NUTRITIONAL VALUE.

	National adults	Public school parents	Nonpublic school parents
	%	%	%
For	57	50	59
Against	41	49	38
No opinion	3	1	3

SOURCE: Lydia Saad and Brandon Busteed, "Americans' Support for New Nutritional Restrictions on School-Based Food, Specifically Including Snack Bars, Vending Machines, and Bake Sales," in *Americans Favor Limiting Sale of Unhealthy Food in Schools*, The Gallup Organization, March 12, 2013, http://www.gallup.com/poll/161318/americans-favor-limiting-sale-unhealthy-food-schools.aspx (accessed November 16, 2013). Copyright © 2013 Gallup, Inc. All rights reserved. The content is used with permission; however, Gallup retains all rights of republication.

TABLE 11.9

Poll respondents who feel strict nutritional standards in schools will effectively reduce childhood obesity and improve students' academic performance, 2013

STILL THINKING ABOUT A FEDERAL LAW REGULATING WHAT SCHOOL DISTRICTS COULD SERVE FOR MEALS AND SNACKS ON SCHOOL GROUNDS, HOW EFFECTIVE DO YOU THINK SUCH A LAW WOULD BE IN TERMS OF [ROTATE: REDUCING OBESITY IN CHILDREN/IMPROVING STUDENTS' ACADEMIC PERFORMANCE]? WOULD IT BE VERY EFFECTIVE, SOMEWHAT EFFECTIVE, NOT TOO EFFECTIVE, OR NOT EFFECTIVE AT ALL?

	National adults	Public school parents	Nonpublic school parents
Reducing obesity	%	%	%
Very effective	19	19	18
Somewhat effective	40	36	42
Not too effective	20	24	19
Not effective at all	19	17	20
No opinion	2	4	2
Improving academic performance			
Very effective	13	18	12
Somewhat effective	38	31	40
Not too effective	21	22	20
Not effective at all	25	24	25
No opinion	3	5	3

SOURCE: Lydia Saad and Brandon Busteed, "Perceived Effectiveness of School-Wide Nutritional Standards at Reducing Childhood Obesity, Improving Academic Performance," in *Americans Favor Limiting Sale of Unhealthy Food in Schools*, The Gallup Organization, March 12, 2013, http://www.gallup.com/poll/161318/americans-favor-limiting-sale-unhealthy-food-schools.aspx (accessed November 16, 2013). Copyright © 2013 Gallup, Inc. All rights reserved. The content is used with permission; however, Gallup retains all rights of republication.

value of competitive foods—items sold in school snack bars, in vending machines, and at bake sales and other school events. (See Table 11.8.) Not only do Americans want legislation to improve school nutrition but they are also confident that policies regulating the nutritional value of foods served in schools would effectively reduce obesity in children and improve their academic performance. More than half (59%) of adults feel that strict standards would effectively reduce obesity, and one in five (19%) thinks that such policies would be "very effective." (See Table 11.9.) Around half (51%) believe that higher nutritional standards would improve students' academic performance.

Are Parents to Blame for Children's Obesity?

There is no question that parents play a pivotal role in terms of preventing childhood obesity by shaping their children's early eating and physical activity habits. However, should overweight children be taken away from their parents?

In "State Intervention in Life-Threatening Childhood Obesity" (*JAMA*, vol. 306, no. 2, July 13, 2011), Lindsey Murtagh and David S. Ludwig support the use of state intervention in cases of life-threatening obesity. Murtagh and Ludwig point out that "improper feeding practices, causing undernourishment and failure to thrive, have long been addressed through the child abuse and neglect framework." Murtagh and Ludwig assert that physicians are or should be obligated to inform child protective services in "cases of children for whom chronic parental neglect has resulted in severe weight-related health complications." In contrast, Susan Z. Yanovski, Jack A. Yanovski, and Mary Horlick note in "Life-Threatening Childhood Obesity and Legal Intervention" (*JAMA*, vol. 306, no. 16, October 26, 2011) that obesity is highly heritable and that genetic factors play a key role in risk for obesity.

The article "200 Pound Child Removed from Home Because of Weight" (UPI.com, November 28, 2011) reports that in November 2011 an eight-year-old boy who weighed more than 200 pounds (91 kg) was removed from his home in Ohio and placed in foster care. This action was the first recorded instance of a government agency intervening to remove a child from his or her home because of concern about the child's physical health. According to a spokesperson for the Cuyahoga County Department of Children and Family Services, the third grader was removed because his mother had not done enough to help him lose weight and had failed to comply with his physician's orders. As a result, "case workers considered his mother's failure to reduce his weight a form of medical neglect." A lawyer representing the boy's mother argued that the boy's weight did not pose an imminent danger to his health and that removing him from his family, school, and friends could result in emotional distress.

According to Tara Dodrill, in "Ohio Boy Removed from Home Because of Obesity Concerns" (Yahoo-News.com, November 28, 2011), the case created a firestorm of commentary in the blogosphere via e-mail, Twitter, and other social media. Many people spoke out in favor of protecting the boy's health and preventing increasingly dire consequences of obesity, whereas others decried removing the child from his home because they feared that the trauma would only compound his problems. Still others called for support services and counseling to help parents and children who are overweight or obese.

In March 2012, after having lived in a foster care home and later with an uncle, the boy had lost 50 pounds and was returned to his mother. The article "200-lbs. Ohio Boy Returned to Mother's Custody after Losing 50 Pounds" (Associated Press, May 11, 2012) notes that despite having moved several times and having changed schools, the boy appeared to be doing well and was continuing to exercise to control his weight.

Parents Misjudge Children's Weight

Several studies find that parents often misperceive their children's weight and underestimate their risk for obesity in adulthood. For example, one study examined the relationship between parents' underestimation of their child's weight and concerns about their child's weight and health. Jillian M. Tschamler et al. interviewed parents in a pediatric clinic, measured the height and weight of the children, and reported their findings in "Underestimation of Children's Weight Status: Views of Parents in an Urban Community" (*Clinical Pediatrics*, vol. 49, no. 5, May 2010). The researchers found that many parents—nearly half of parents of overweight children and about one-fourth of parents of normal-weight children—underestimated their children's weight. Parents of normal-weight children who underestimated their children's weight were more likely to be concerned about their children's weight than those who did not underestimate. Parents of overweight children who underestimated were less likely to be concerned about their children's weight than those who recognized their children as being overweight. Tschamler et al. conclude that parents who underestimate their children's weight status are not likely to be receptive to initiatives aimed at preventing childhood obesity.

Schools Send Parents Letters about Children's Weight

Some school districts have begun to issue letters to parents of students who are considered overweight. In "California Sends 'Fat Letters' Informing Parents Their Children Are Overweight" (NYDailyNews.com, September 6, 2013), David Knowles describes one such initiative in Los Angeles County, California. A registered dietician weighs preschoolers in this community and then contacts their families if the children are overweight. In 2013, of the 900 children aged two to five years who were screened by the dietician, 200 were considered obese, and their families received letters, dubbed "fat letters," informing them of the issue. They also received educational materials about the relationship between nutrition, weight, and health.

Other school districts are considering ending the practice of sending fat letters. For example, Massachusetts schools have been sending letters to parents since 2010, identifying children who, based on body mass index, were determined to be normal weight, underweight, overweight, or obese. In "Massachusetts Mulls Doing Away with 'Fat Letters' That Report Schoolkids' BMI to Parents" (NYDailyNews.com, February 26, 2013), Tracy Miller reports that a group of state representatives is seeking to halt the practice, arguing that it creates unnecessary administrative costs, that it is not always an accurate assessment of a student's health because many athletes have higher-than-average body mass indexes, and that it has the potential to harm children's self-esteem.

IMPORTANT NAMES
AND ADDRESSES

Academy for Eating Disorders
111 Deer Lake Rd., Ste. 100
Deerfield, IL 60015
(847) 498-4274
FAX: (847) 480-9282
E-mail: info@aedweb.org
URL: http://www.aedweb.org/

Academy of Nutrition and Dietetics
120 S. Riverside Plaza, Ste. 2000
Chicago, IL 60606-6995
(312) 899-0040
1-800-877-1600
URL: http://www.eatright.org/

American Academy of Sleep Medicine
2510 N. Frontage Rd.
Darien, IL 60561
(630) 737-9700
FAX: (630) 737-9790
URL: http://www.aasmnet.org/

American Cancer Society
250 Williams St. NW
Atlanta, GA 30303
1-800-227-2345
URL: http://www.cancer.org/

American Diabetes Association
1701 N. Beauregard St.
Alexandria, VA 22311
1-800-342-2383
URL: http://www.diabetes.org/

American Heart Association
7272 Greenville Ave.
Dallas, TX 75231
(214) 570-5978
1-800-242-8721
URL: http://www.americanheart.org/

American Society of Bariatric Physicians
2821 S. Parker Rd., Ste. 625
Aurora, CO 80014-2735
(303) 770-2526

FAX: (303) 779-4834
URL: http://www.asbp.org/

American Society for Metabolic and Bariatric Surgery
100 SW 75th St., Ste. 201
Gainesville, FL 32607
(352) 331-4900
FAX: (352) 331-4975
E-mail: info@asmbs.org
URL: http://www.asmbs.org/

Arthritis Foundation
1330 W. Peachtree St., Ste. 100
Atlanta, GA 30309
(404) 872-7100
1-800-283-7800
URL: http://www.arthritis.org/

Atkins Nutritionals, Inc.
1050 17th St., Ste. 1500
Denver, CO 80265
1-800-628-5467
URL: http://www.atkins.com/

Center for Science in the Public Interest
1220 L St. NW
Washington, DC 20005
(202) 332-9110
FAX: (202) 265-4954
E-mail: cspi@cspinet.org
URL: http://www.cspinet.org/

Centers for Disease Control and Prevention
1600 Clifton Rd.
Atlanta, GA 30333
1-800-232-4636
URL: http://www.cdc.gov/

Council on Size and Weight Discrimination
PO Box 305
Mt. Marion, NY 12456
(845) 679-1209
FAX: (845) 679-1206
E-mail: info@cswd.org
URL: http://www.cswd.org/

Eating Disorders Coalition
720 Seventh St. NW, Ste. 300
Washington, DC 20001
(202) 543-9570
E-mail: manager@eatingdisorder
scoalition.org
URL: http://www.eatingdisorder
scoalition.org/

Federal Trade Commission
600 Pennsylvania Ave. NW
Washington, DC 20580
(202) 326-2222
1-877-382-4357
URL: http://www.ftc.gov/

**International Food
Information Council**
1100 Connecticut Ave. NW, Ste. 430
Washington, DC 20036
(202) 296-6540
E-mail: info@foodinsight.org
URL: http://www.foodinsight.org/

National Association of Anorexia Nervosa and Associated Disorders
750 E. Diehl Rd., Ste. 127
Naperville, IL 60563
(630) 577-1330
E-mail: anadhelp@anad.org
URL: http://www.anad.org/

**National Association of
Cognitive-Behavioral Therapists**
102 Gilson Ave.
Weirton, WV 26062
(304) 224-2534
1-800-253-0167
URL: http://www.nacbt.org/

**National Association to Advance
Fat Acceptance**
PO Box 4662
Foster City, CA 94404-0662
(916) 558-6880
URL: http://www.naafa.org/

National Center for Health Statistics
3311 Toledo Rd.
Hyattsville, MD 20782
1-800-232-4636
URL: http://www.cdc.gov/nchs/

**National Center on Sleep Disorders
Research**
National Heart, Lung, and Blood Institute
National Institutes of Health
6701 Rockledge Dr.
Bethesda, MD 20892
(301) 435-0199
FAX: (301) 480-3451
URL: http://www.nhlbi.nih.gov/about/ncsdr/

**National Diabetes Information
Clearinghouse**
One Information Way
Bethesda, MD 20892-3560
1-800-860-8747
FAX: (703) 738-4929
E-mail: ndic@info.niddk.nih.gov
URL: http://diabetes.niddk.nih.gov/

**National Digestive Diseases Information
Clearinghouse**
Two Information Way
Bethesda, MD 20892-3570
1-800-891-5389
FAX: (703) 738-4929
E-mail: nddic@info.niddk.nih.gov
URL: http://digestive.niddk.nih.gov/

**National Eating
Disorders Association**
165 W. 46th St.
New York, NY 10036
(212) 575-6200
1-800-931-2237
FAX: (212) 575-1650

E-mail: info@NationalEatingDisorders.org
URL: http://
www.nationaleatingdisorders.org/

National Heart, Lung, and Blood Institute
PO Box 30105
Bethesda, MD 20824-0105
(301) 592-8573
FAX: (301) 592-8563
E-mail: nhlbiinfo@nhlbi.nih.gov
URL: http://www.nhlbi.nih.gov/

**National Institute of Diabetes and
Digestive and Kidney Diseases**
Bldg. 31, Rm. 9A06
31 Center Dr., MSC 2560
Bethesda, MD 20892-2560
(301) 496-3583
E-mail: niddkinquiries@nih.gov
URL: http://www.niddk.nih.gov/

National Mental Health Association
2000 N. Beauregard St., Sixth Floor
Alexandria, VA 22311
(703) 684-7722
1-800-969-6642
FAX: (703) 684-5968
URL: http://www.nmha.org/

**National Women's Health
Information Center**
157 Broad St., Ste. 200
Red Bank, NJ 07701
1-877-986-9472
FAX: (732) 530-3347
E-mail: info@healthywomen.org
URL: http://www.healthywomen.org/

Obesity Society
8757 Georgia Ave., Ste. 1320
Silver Spring, MD 20910

(301) 563-6526
FAX: (301) 563-6595
URL: http://www.obesity.org/

Office on Women's Health
**U.S. Department of Health and
Human Services**
200 Independence Ave. SW, Rm. 712E
Washington, DC 20201
(202) 690-7650
1-800-994-9662
FAX: (202) 205-2631
URL: http://www.womenshealth.gov/

Rudd Center for Food Policy and Obesity
Yale University
309 Edwards St.
New Haven, CT 06511
(203) 432-6700
FAX: (203) 432-9674
URL: http://www.yaleruddcenter.org/

TOPS Club Inc.
4575 S. Fifth St.
Milwaukee, WI 53207
(414) 482-4620
URL: http://www.tops.org/

Weight Watchers International Inc.
175 Crossways Park West
Woodbury, NY 11797
(516) 390-1400
1-800-651-6000
URL: http://www.weightwatchers.com/

Weight-Control Information Network
One WIN Way
Bethesda, MD 20892-3665
1-877-946-4627
E-mail: win@info.niddk.nih.gov
URL: http://win.niddk.nih.gov/index.htm

RESOURCES

The Centers for Disease Control and Prevention (CDC) tracks nationwide health trends, including overweight and obesity, and reports its findings in several periodicals, especially its *Health, United States* and *Morbidity and Mortality Weekly Reports*. The *National Vital Statistics Reports*, which is issued by the CDC's National Center for Health Statistics (NCHS), gives detailed information on U.S. births, birth weights, and death data and trends. The NCHS also compiles and analyzes demographic data—the heights and weights of a representative sample of the U.S. population—to develop standards for desirable weights. The National Health Interview Surveys, the National Health Examination Surveys, the National Health and Nutrition Examination Surveys, and the Behavioral Risk Factor Surveillance System offer ongoing information about the lifestyles, health behaviors, and health risks of Americans. Working with other agencies and professional organizations, the CDC produced *Healthy People 2020*, which serves as a blueprint for improving the health status of Americans.

The U.S. Department of Agriculture provides nutrition guidelines for Americans, and the Federal Trade Commission (FTC) has launched initiatives to educate consumers and the media about false and deceptive weight-loss advertising. The FTC is one of about 50 members of the Partnership for Healthy Weight Management, a coalition of scientific, academic, health care, government, commercial, and public-interest representatives, that aims to increase public awareness of the obesity epidemic and to promote responsible marketing of weight-loss products and programs.

The relationship between birth weight and future health risks has been examined by many researchers, and the studies cited in this text were reported in *American Journal of Epidemiology, American Journal of Obstetrics and Gynecology, Circulation, International Journal of Cancer, Journal of Clinical Endocrinology and Metabolism, Journal of Women's Health, Obesity,* and *Pediatrics*. Data from the CDC Pregnancy Nutrition Surveillance System show that very overweight women benefit from reduced weight gain during pregnancy to help reduce the risk for high-birth-weight infants.

The World Health Organization and the National Institutes of Health provide definitions, epidemiological data, and research findings about a comprehensive range of public health issues, including diet, nutrition, overweight, and obesity. The Central Intelligence Agency's *World Factbook* provides longevity estimates. The National Heart, Lung, and Blood Institute conducts research about obesity and overweight. Weight-control information and updated weight-for-height tables that incorporate height, weight, and body mass index are published by the National Institute of Diabetes and Digestive and Kidney Diseases (the part of the National Institutes of Health that is primarily responsible for obesity- and nutrition-related research). The National Institute of Mental Health offers information about eating disorders as well as the mental health issues that are related to obesity.

The origins, causes, and consequences of the obesity epidemic have been described in numerous professional and consumer publications, including *American Journal of Clinical Nutrition, American Journal of Epidemiology, American Journal of Nutrition, American Journal of Preventive Medicine, American Journal of Public Health, Appetite, Archives of General Psychiatry, Bariatric Nursing and Surgical Patient Care, Diabetes, Obesity, and Metabolism, Eating Disorders, Endocrinology Nutrition, European Eating Disorders Review, Global Health, Health Affairs, International Journal of Eating Disorders, International Journal of Obesity, Journal of Obesity, New England Journal of Medicine, Nutrition in Clinical Practice, Obesity, Obesity Surgery, Preventing Chronic Diseases,* and *Proceedings of the Nutrition Society*.

Many excellent books and publications provided valuable insight into the obesity epidemic. Peter N. Stearns, in *Fat History: Bodies and Beauty in the Modern West* (1997), and Laura Fraser, in *Losing It: False Hopes and Fat Profits in the Diet Industry* (1998), offer detailed histories of magical cures and weight-loss fads. In *Diabesity: The Obesity-Diabetes Epidemic That Threatens America—And What We Must Do to Stop It* (2005), Francine Ratner Kaufman, the former president of the American Diabetes Association, contends that the diabesity epidemic "imperils human existence as we now know it." David A. Kessler, the former commissioner of the U.S. Food and Drug Administration, explains in *The End of Overeating: Taking Control of the Insatiable American Appetite* (2009) how the desire to eat and overeat originates in the brain and is triggered by a variety of combinations of salt, fat, and sugar in the American diet.

Medical and public health societies, along with advocacy organizations, professional associations, and foundations, offer a wealth of information about the relationship between weight, health, and disease. Sources cited in this edition include the Academy of Nutrition and Dietetics, the American Heart Association, the American Medical Association, the American Obesity Association, the Center for Consumer Freedom, the Center for Science in the Public Interest, the International Size Acceptance Association, the National Academy of Sciences, the National Association to Advance Fat Acceptance, the National Eating Disorders Association, the Pharmacy Benefit Management Institute, the Public Health Advocacy Institute, and the Trust for America's Health.

The Trust for America's Health/Robert Wood Johnson Foundation publication, *F as in Fat: How Obesity Threatens America's Future 2013*, provided data and insight into the obesity epidemic. The Gallup Organization makes available valuable poll and survey data about Americans' attitudes about overweight, obesity, physical activity, diet, and nutrition. Finally, many professional associations, voluntary medical organizations, and foundations dedicated to research, education, and advocacy about eating disorders, overweight, and obesity provided up-to-date information that was included in this edition.

INDEX

from sugar consumption, 131–132

very-low-calorie diets, 158

See also Reduced calorie menus

Calories Don't Count (Herman), 87

"Campaign for Real Beauty" (Dove), 57

Camuto, Vince, 127

Cancer

birth weight and, 4

obesity and, 42

Cancer Prevention and Early Detection: Facts and Figures, 2013 (American Cancer Society), 42

Caplan, Arthur L., 173, 179

Carbohydrates

low-carbohydrate diets, 94–96

low-carbohydrate foods, myths about, 149

low-fat *vs.* low-carbohydrate diets, 97–99

recommended proportions of by age group, 91*t*

See also Low-carbohydrate diets

Cardiovascular disease, 7

Carlsson, A. C., 7

Carroll, Margaret D., 9

Casazza, Krista, 147–148

Castellini, Giovanni, 55

"The Causal Link between Financial Incentives and Weight Loss: An Evidence-Based Survey of the Literature" (Paloyo et al.), 152

Cawley, John, 153

CBT. *See* Cognitive-behavioral therapy

CCAs (Commonsense Consumption Acts), 138

CDC. *See* Centers for Disease Control and Prevention

CDC Division of Nutrition, Physical Activity, and Obesity, 166

Center for Consumer Freedom, 134–135

Center for Science in the Public Interest (CSPI), 134–135

Centers for Disease Control and Prevention (CDC)

"Adult Obesity Facts," 1

"Announcements: Arthritis Awareness Month—May 2013," 39

"Basics about Childhood Obesity," 61

on community strategies to prevent obesity, 160–162

"Frequently Asked Questions about Calculating Obesity-Related Risk," 33

on funding for obesity prevention efforts, 166

"Genomics and Health: Genes and Obesity," 31

"How Much Physical Activity Do Adults Need?," 103

"Identifying Effective Strategies to Help Combat Childhood Obesity," 137

"Obesity Prevention and Control: Interventions in Community Settings," 167–168

"Obesity Trends in Adults with Arthritis," 39

Pregnancy Nutrition Surveillance System, 44

"Progress on Childhood Obesity," 59

State Indicator Report on Fruits and Vegetables, 2013, 15

weight-loss program of, 126

Centers for Medicare and Medicaid Services (CMS), 119

Cereal products, 15

Cesa, Gian Luca, 54

"Challenges and Opportunities for Change in Food Marketing to Children and Youth—Workshop Summary" (IOM), 76

Chamber of Fashion (Milan), 57

Chang, Maria, 42

Chang, Virginia W., 33

"Changes in Eating, Physical Activity, and Related Behaviors in a Primary-Care-Based Weight-loss Intervention" (Volger et al.), 112–113

"The Changing American Diet" (Liebman), 90

"Changing Definitions of Metabolic Syndrome" (Parikh & Mohan), 45

Cheese, 14

Child and Adult Care Food Program, 135

"Childhood Anxiety Associated with Low BMI in Women with Anorexia Nervosa" (Dellava), 52

Childhood obesity

Alliance for a Healthier Generation, work of, 171

cost of treating, 118–119

Healthy Weight Commitment Foundation and, 139–140

public opinion on, 179

public opinion on parents' role in, 180–181

Childhood Obesity Demonstration Project, 137

Children

BMI age variation, 63*f*

BMI percentiles for boys, 62*f*

calorie consumption, decrease of among, 70

diet/nutrition/weight issues among, 59–61

eating disorders among, 83–84

health risks/consequences of obesity for, 76–78

Healthy, Hunger-Free Kids Act, 135–136

high school students engaging in dangerous dieting behaviors, 50(*t*3.2)

high school students who vomited/took laxatives to lose/maintain weight, 50(*t*3.3)

intervention/treatment of overweight/obesity for, 81–83

low-income preschoolers, changes in obesity prevalence among, 64*f*

marketing of food to, WHO strategy to limit, 129, 131

media, nutrition/health education provided by, 75–76

media, role in obesity epidemic among, 70–73

MyPlate, praise/criticism for, 164–165

MyPlate dietary guidelines for children, 163–164

MyPlate guidelines, knowledge/use of, 165

obesity among, 60*t*–61*t*

overweight, reasons for, 64–67

parents underestimation of children's weight, 181

poll respondents who favor legislation limiting sale of unhealthy competitive food in school snack bars, vending machines, 180(*t*11.8)

poll respondents who favor legislation limiting sale of unhealthy food in schools, 180(*t*11.7)

poll respondents who feel strict nutritional standards in schools will effectively reduce childhood obesity/improve students' academic performance, 180(*t*11.9)

prevention efforts at schools, 160

prevention initiatives to promote healthy eating/physical activity, 160

public opinion on parents' role in children's obesity, 180–181

public opinion on schools providing healthful food, 179–180

school letters to parents about children's weight, 181

schools, innovative programs supporting healthy meals at, 75

schools, role in obesity epidemic, 73

schools, unhealthy food choices offered by, 73, 75

screening/assessment of overweight, 78, 81

unborn, effects of caloric intake of mother on, 33

war on obesity in U.S. and, 132–133

weight status categories by BMI-for-age percentiles, 64*t*

weight-based discrimination in, 140

See also Birth weight

"Children in U.S. Are Eating Fewer Calories, Study Finds" (Tavernise), 70

Children's Health Insurance Program Reauthorization Act, 137

Cholesterol levels

among adults, 35*t*

Gofman, John, on, 86

ChooseMyPlate.gov, 163

Food labels
  added sugars that appear on food labels, names for, 131, 132(*t*8.3)
  nutritional labeling, effect on consumer choices, 134
Food Marketing and the Diets of Children and Youth (IOM Committee on Progress in Preventing Childhood Obesity), 76
Food Marketing to Children and Youth: Threat or Opportunity? (IOM), 76
Food Rules: An Eater's Manual (Pollan), 89
Food service industry, lawsuits against, 137
"Food Spending Adjustments during Recessionary Times" (Kumcu & Kaufman), 15
"For a Healthier Country, Overhaul Farm Subsidies" (ScientificAmerican.com), 131
Formula, baby, 5
Forney, K. Jean, 52, 84
44 Healthy Teaching Kitchens (VA), 160
Fox, Renee Ellen, 13
Fox, Steven, 113
Franck, Caroline, 137
Fraser, Laura, 152
Freeman, Gulnur, 9
Frenk, Julio, 83
"Frequently Asked Questions about Calculating Obesity-Related Risk" (CDC), 33
"The Freshman 15: A Critical Time for Obesity Intervention or Media Myth?" (Zagorsky & Smith), 151
Froguel, Philippe, 31–32
"Front-of-Package Food and Beverage Labeling: New Directions for Research and Regulation" (Pomeranz), 134
Front-of-package labels, 134
Front-of-Package Nutrition Rating Systems and Symbols: Promoting Healthier Choices (Institute of Medicine), 134
Fructose, 20–21
Fruits
  Americans' consumption of, 15
  community strategies to prevent obesity, 160–161
  consumption by adults/adolescents, by state, 16*t*
  Fruits & Veggies: More Matters initiative, 165–166
  increasing availability of at school/workplace, 159
  prevention initiatives to promote healthy eating, 160
  servings of fruit/vegetables with 100 calories or less, 166*t*
  teenagers' consumption of, 67
Fruits & Veggies: More Matters initiative, 165–166
Fryar, Cheryl D., 9
FTC. *See* Federal Trade Commission

"FTC Charges HCG Marketer with Deceptive Advertising" (FTC), 157
"FTC Mails Refund Checks to Consumers Who Bought Skechers' Shape-Ups and Other 'Toning' Shoes" (FTC), 157
FTO (fat mass and obesity associated) gene variant, 32, 108
Funding, for prevention efforts, 166
"The Future Direction of Personalised Nutrition: My Diet, My Phenotype, My Genes" (Gibney & Walsh), 152

G

Gagne, Danielle, 150
Galbraith, John Kenneth, 1
Gallbladder disease, 40–41
Gallop, Rick, 89
Gallstones, 77
Gallup Organization
  public opinion on low-fat vs. low-carb diets, 174–176
  public opinion on schools providing healthful food, 179–180
  on U.S. obesity rate, 173
Games, video, 76
Garrison, Jordan M., Jr., 111–112
Gastric bypass surgery, 111
Gastric restriction surgery, 111
"Gastrointestinal System and Obesity" (Ashburn & Reed), 41
Geithner, Timothy, 145
Gender
  BMI for children/teens and, 59
  calorie needs, estimated, by age, sex, physical activity, 164*t*
  deaths, leading causes/numbers of, by sex/race, 28*t*–29*t*
  life expectancy at birth/65/75 years of age, by race/sex, 26*t*–27*t*
  obesity among adults aged 20+ by age/sex, 13*f*
  obesity among adults aged 20+ by sex/race/ethnicity, 14*f*
  worry about weight by, 173
Gene variants, 108
"Genes and Obesity: A Cause and Effect Relationship" (González Jiménez), 13
"Genetic Association of Recovery from Eating Disorders: The Role of GABA Receptor SNPs" (Bloss et al.), 54–55
Genetic density, myths regarding, 149–150
Genetics
  eating disorders, influence of, 48
  eating disorders, statistics on influence of on, 51
  environmental influences on obesity *vs.*, 33
  as factor in obesity, 30–31
  genes variants associated with obesity, 32*t*
  multiple gene variants, effects on body weight/obesity, 32–33

obesity and, 31*t*
obesity-related genes, exercise countering of, 108
reduction of weight bias and, 143
role in childhood obesity, 181
role in obesity, 13
single mutant genes, 31–32
thinness, genetic cause of, 33
"The Genetics of Eating Disorders" (Trace et al.), 48
"The Genetics of Human Obesity" (Xia & Grant), 13–14
"Genome-Wide Linkage Scan for the Metabolic Syndrome in the HERITAGE Family Study" (Loos et al.), 45
Genomics, 30
"Genomics and Health: Genes and Obesity" (CDC), 31
Gertner, Jon, 158
"Getting Paid for Treating Obesity, Now That It's a 'Disease'" (Page), 30
GI. *See* Glycemic index
The G.I. Diet: The Easy, Healthy Way to Permanent Weight Loss (Gallop), 89
Gibney, Michael J., 152
Gibson, Sigrid, 148
Gierut, Kristen, 119
Gilboa, Suzanne M., 44
Girls (TV show), 144
Global politics of obesity, 129–131
Global Strategy on Diet, Physical Activity, and Health (World Health Organization), 129–131
Glucose
  effects on brain/body, 20–21
  intolerance among children, 77
Glycemic index (GI)
  diets focusing on, 89
  overview of, 94–96
"Glycemic Status, Metabolic Syndrome, and Cardiovascular Risk in Children" (Berenson et al.), 77
Godfrey, Keith M., 4
Gofman, John W., 86
Goldhaber-Fiebert, Jeremy D., 61
Goldstein, Andrea N., 43
Gonadal steroids, 54
González Jiménez, Emilio, 13
Government
  coverage for treatment of obesity, 119–120
  food marketing restrictions by, 72
  in global strategy to combat overweight/obesity, 129
Graff, Samantha K., 72
Grains
  Americans' consumption of, 15
  dietary guidelines on, 163
  ways to make half of total grain intake whole grains, 91*f*

IFIC. *See* International Food Information Council

Iliadou, Anastasia, 4

"Impact of Bariatric Surgery on Health Care Costs of Obese Patients" (Weiner et al.), 126

"The Impact of Sleep Deprivation on Food Desire in the Human Brain" (Greer, Goldstein, & Walker), 43

"Implicit and Explicit Anti-fat Bias among a Large Sample of Medical Doctors by BMI, Race/Ethnicity and Gender" (Sabin, Marini, & Nosek), 140–141

Implicit Associations Test (IAT), 140–141

"Impossible Weight-Loss Claims: Summary of an FTC Report" (Barrett), 153

"Improving Obesity Prevention at the Local Level—Emerging Opportunities" (Bleich & Rutkow), 170

"Improving School Lunch by Design" (Martin), 75

Impulsive behavior, 53

In the Groove (video game), 76

In U.S., Gender Gap in Personal Weight Worries Narrows (Brown), 173

Income
    effects of obesity on, 117
    obese, percentage of Americans that are, low income *vs.* low access, 174(*t*11.2)
    obesity rates by, 173

Income, Not "Food Deserts," More to Blame for U.S. Obesity (McGeeney & Mendes), 173

"Inflammation, a Link between Obesity and Cardiovascular Disease" (Wang & Nakayama), 34

Ingall, Marjorie, 57

Insel, Thomas, 48

Inskip, Hazel M., 4

Institute for Food Technologies, 167

Institute of Medicine (IOM), 76, 134

Insulin
    metabolic syndrome and, 45
    resistance in type 2 diabetes, 37
    role of in high-protein diet, 88

Insurance
    coverage for treatment of obesity, 30
    for treatment of obesity, 120

Integrated threat theory, 142

Interagency Working Group (IWG), 71–72

Internal Revenue Service (IRS), 30

International Diabetes Federation, 45

International Food Information Council (IFIC)
    tracking of media coverage of diet/ nutrition/food issues, 170–171
    2013 Food & Health Survey, 176–177

International Size Acceptance Association (ISAA), 144

International Sugar Organization, 129

Internet
    behavioral therapy program delivered via, cost of, 126
    online counseling on, 113–114

"Internet Programs Targeting Multiple Lifestyle Interventions in Primary and Secondary Care Are Not Superior to Usual Care Alone in Improving Cardiovascular Risk Profile: A Systematic Review" (Vegting), 126

Interpersonal factors, of eating disorders, 48

Interpersonal psychotherapy (IPT), 53

Intervention, for adolescents, 81–83

"Introducing the New Torrid" (Hot Topic), 127

"An Investigation of Goodman's Addictive Disorder Criteria in Eating Disorders" (Speranza et al.), 50–51

"Investigation of Mendelian Forms of Obesity Holds out the Prospect of Personalized Medicine" (Blakemore & Froguel), 31–32

IOM. *See* Institute of Medicine

IPT (interpersonal psychotherapy), 53

IRS (Internal Revenue Service), 30

"Is Obesity in Women Protective against Osteoporosis?" (Migliaccio et al.), 30

"Is the Association between Low Birth Weight and Asthma Independent of Genetic and Shared Environmental Factors?" (Villamor, Iliadou, & Cnattingius), 4

ISAA (International Size Acceptance Association), 144

IWG (Interagency Working Group), 71–72

J

Jackvony, Elizabeth H., 113–114

Jacquemont, Sébastien, 33

Jameson, Gardner, 87

Jamie Oliver's Food Revolution, 76

Jansen, Pauline W., 78

Jazzercise Inc., 142

Jebb, Susan A., 113

Jefferson, Thomas, 85

Jenny Craig
    market share increase of, 125
    overview of, 88–89

Jeukendrup, Asker E., 115

John, Leslie K., 152

Johnson, Mark S., 111–112

Johnson, Rebecca J., 111

Joints
    injury from overweight/obesity, 39–40
    pain reported by adults, 40*t*

Jones, Peter B., 52

Joy of Cooking (Rombauer & Becker), 19

Juice fasts, 90

Junk food
    addiction to, food industry and, 133–136
    taxes on, 137

Just Dance 3/4 (video game), 76

K

Karhunen, Leila, 151

Kaufman, Phil, 15

Kaye, Nikki, 179

Kaye, Walter, 53

Keel, Pamela K.
    on eating disorders treatment/outcome, 54
    "Psychosocial Risk Factors for Eating Disorders," 52, 84

Keep Off Pounds Sensibly (KOPS), 86

Kessler, David A., 20

Ketosis, 88

KFC, lawsuit against, 137

Khan, Muhammad Asad, 111

"Kick Out Fat People to Lower Healthcare Costs?" (Caplan), 173, 179

The Kids' Safe and Healthful Foods Project, 73

Kilpeläinen, Tuomas O., 108

Kinetic (video game), 76

King, Kyla, 42

King, Nancy, 144

Kirschenbaum, Daniel S., 119

Klein, Calvin, 127

Klein, Olivier, 15

Klein, Samuel, 157

Knowles, David, 181

KOPS (Keep Off Pounds Sensibly), 86

Kors, Michael, 127

Kraft, Lunchables, 134

Kranz, Sibylle, 166

Kratina, Karin, 144

Krook, Anna, 107–108

Kuk, Jennifer L., 115

Kumcu, Aylin, 15

L

Lahouasnia, Lamine, 167

Lancet (medical journal), 7

Landaverde, Carmen, 41–42

Land-use policies, to increase physical activity, 161

Lanzalotta, Stephen, 89

Larson-Meyer, D. Enette, 150

Lasater, Gentry, 69–70

The Last Chance Diet—When Everything Else Has Failed (Linn), 88

Laws
    legislation protects food industry interests, 138
    regarding overweight/obesity, 137–138
    use of legal system to change Americans' diets, 134–135
    against weight discrimination, 142

Lawsuits
    Commonsense Consumption Acts and, 138
    against food service industry, 137

Laxatives, 51

Prescription drugs. *See* Medication

"Prescription Medications for the Treatment of Obesity" (Weight-Control Information Network), 110

"President Bill Clinton to Recognize 267 U.S. Schools for Efforts to Prevent Childhood Obesity" (Alliance for a Healthier Generation), 171

Presidential Youth Fitness Program (HHS), 160

President's Council on Fitness, Sports, and Nutrition (PCFSN), 160

"Prevalence and Correlates of Eating Disorders in Adolescents: Results from the National Comorbidity Survey Replication Adolescent Supplement" (Swanson et al.), 52

"Prevalence of Obesity, in the United States, 2009–2010" (Ogden et al.), 1

"Prevalence of Obesity and Trends in the Distribution of Body Mass Index Among US Adults, 1999–2010" (Flegal et al.), 1

"Prevalence of Overweight, Obesity, and Extreme Obesity among Adults: United States, Trends 1960–1962 through 2009–2010" (Fryar, Carroll, & Ogden), 9

Prevention, eating disorders, 55–58, 55*t*

Prevention of overweight/obesity
  calorie needs, estimated, by age, sex, physical activity, 164*f*
  childhood obesity, targeting, 171
  community strategies, 160–162
  Fruits & Veggies: More Matters initiative, 165–166
  health care system, prevention agenda in, 170
  media for communication of prevention message, 170–171
  MyPlate, praise/criticism for, 164–165
  MyPlate dietary guidelines for children, 163–164
  MyPlate guidelines, knowledge/use of, 165
  national nutrition education, 162–163
  nutrient density, comparison of calorie content between foods that are not nutrient dense/foods that are nutrient dense, 163*f*
  nutrition education, effect on improving Americans' diets, 166–169
  nutrition/physical activity decisions, factors shaping, 161*f*
  obesity prevention interventions/task force ratings, 168*t*
  servings of fruit/vegetables with 100 calories or less, 166*t*
  solid fats/oils, differences between commonly used, 162*f*
  state/community funding for prevention efforts, 166
  U.S. surgeon general's recommendations for, 159–160

work site, prevention programs at, 169–170

"Preventive Care and Health Behaviors among Overweight/Obese Men in HMOs" (Quinn et al.), 141

Preventive health services, 141

"Primary Care Referral to a Commercial Provider for Weight Loss Treatment versus Standard Care: A Randomised Controlled Trial" (Jebb et al.), 113

"Primary Prevention of Cardiovascular Disease with a Mediterranean Diet" (Estruch et al.), 149

Print media. *See* Media

Pritikin, Nathan, 88

Pritikin diet, 88

Pritikin Longevity Center, 88

The Pritikin Program for Diet and Exercise (Pritikin), 88

Private sector, 139

Processed foods
  names for added sugars that appear on food labels, 132(*t*8.3)
  names of added sugars in, 131
  See also Junk food

Produce for Better Health Foundation (PBH), 165–166

Products, weight-loss
  checklist for evaluating, 154*t*
  creams/patches, 156
  fat blockers, 155–156
  natural, myths regarding, 148–149
  over-the-counter, 153
  permanent weight-loss schemes, 155
  phony, campaign targeting, 156–157
  product claims, assessing, 153
  quick weight-loss schemes, 156
  targeted weight-loss products, 156

"Profits and Pandemics: Prevention of Harmful Effects of Tobacco, Alcohol, and Ultra-processed Food and Drink Industries" (Moodie et al.), 138–139

Progress in Preventing Childhood Obesity, 76

"Progress on Childhood Obesity" (CDC), 59

"Promoting Healthy Food Consumption: A Review of State-Level Policies to Improve Access to Fruits and Vegetables" (Hood, Martinez-Donate, & Meinen), 165

"Protecting Children from Harmful Food Marketing: Options for Local Government to Make a Difference" (Harris & Graff), 72

Proteins
  MyPlate on, 164, 165
  recommended proportions of by age group, 91*t*

Pryor, Laura E., 59

"PS3–20: Prevalence of Obesity and Extreme Obesity in Children Aged Three to Five Years" (Lo et al.), 59

"Psychobehavioural Factors Are More Strongly Associated with Successful Weight Management Than Predetermined Satiety Effect or Other Characteristics of Diet" (Karhunen et al.), 151

Psychological health
  bulimia and, 52
  diet/appetite, influence on, 47
  eating disorders, factors predisposing people towards, 48
  psychological problems, weight-related, 2
  See also Mental health

"Psychosocial Origins of Obesity Stigma: Toward Changing a Powerful and Pervasive Bias" (Puhl & Brownell), 142

"Psychosocial Risk Factors for Eating Disorders" (Keel & Forney), 52, 84

"Public Agrees on Obesity's Impact, Not Government's Role" (Pew Research Center), 178

Public opinion
  adults by weight category, annual average, 174*f*
  consumer attitudes/behaviors toward diet/health, 176–181
  on low-fat *vs.* low-carb diets, 174–176, 176(*t*11.4)
  on low-fat *vs.* low-carb diets, by selected characteristics, 177(*t*11.5)
  on low-fat *vs.* low-carb diets, by self-reported weight, 177(*t*11.6)
  obese, percentage of Americans that are, low income *vs.* low access, 174(*t*11.2)
  obesity rates, 173
  obesity rates by demographic characteristics, 174(*t*11.1)
  poll respondents who exercise at least 30 minutes three or more days per week, 178*f*
  poll respondents who favor legislation limiting sale of unhealthy competitive food in school snack bars, vending machines, 180(*t*11.8)
  poll respondents who favor legislation limiting sale of unhealthy food in schools, 180(*t*11.7)
  poll respondents who feel strict nutritional standards in schools will effectively reduce childhood obesity/improve students' academic performance, 180(*t*11.9)
  poll respondents who say they are overweight, about right, or underweight, 175(*f*11.2)
  poll respondents who worry about their weight, 175(*f*11.3)
  poll respondents who worry about their weight, by self-reported weight, 176(*t*11.3)
  poll respondents who worry about their weight, by sex, 176*f*
  worry about weight, 173

poll respondents who feel strict nutritional standards in schools will effectively reduce childhood obesity/improve students' academic performance, 180(t11.9)

prevention efforts at, 160

public opinion on schools providing healthful food, 179–180

unhealthful food choices offered by, 73, 75

Schreffler, Laura, 57

Schroeder, Robin, 111–112

ScientificAmerican.com, 131

Screening, overweight children, 78, 81

Sealey, Geraldine, 137

Sears, Barry, 89

Sebelius, Kathleen

on childhood obesity reduction, 129

NAAFA letter to, 145

"Self-Reported Clothing Size as a Proxy Measure for Body Size" (Hughes et al.), 8

"Separate and Combined Associations of Body-Mass Index and Abdominal Adiposity with Cardiovascular Disease: Collaborative Analysis of 58 Prospective Studies" (*Lancet*), 7

"Serving Healthy School Meals: Despite Challenges, Schools Meet USDA Nutrition Requirements" (Kids' Safe and Healthful Foods Project), 73

Sesame Street (television show), 75–76

Sex hormones, 54

Sexual activity, 148

Sharpe, Lindsey, 173

Sherwood, Thomas A., 125

Shimizu, Mitsuru, 167

Shinall, Jennifer Bennett, 142

Simple carbohydrates, 94

Sin taxes, 137

Singhal, Atul, 5

Single mutant genes, 31–32

Single nucleotide polymorphisms (SNPs), 32

Single sugars, 94

Size acceptance movement, 144–145

Skin care advertising, 57

Skinfold measurement, 7

Sleep disorders

resulting from overweight, 42–43

sleep apnea among children, 77

Slusser, Wendy, 118–119

Smart Snacks in Schools

nutrition standards for, 135–136

snack choices before/after Smart Snacks in School nutrition standards, 136f

"Smart Snacks in Schools" (USDA), 73

"Smart Snacks in School: USDA's 'All Foods Sold in Schools' Standards" (USDA), 135

Smartphones, 114

Smith, Daniel L., Jr., 158

Smith, Patricia K., 151

"Snacking in America: The Changing Role of Snack Foods in America" (NPD Group), 167

Snacks

Americans' snack food choices, 167

calories obtained from, 20

snack choices before/after Smart Snacks in School nutrition standards, 136f

SNPs (single nucleotide polymorphisms), 32

Social consensus theory, 143–144

Social identity theory, 142

Social-ecological model

factors shaping nutrition/physical activity decisions, 161f

for food/physical activity decisions, 160

Society

adolescents, eating disorders and, 83

eating disorders, influence of, 48

norms of, effects on behavior, 33

overweight children, challenges for in, 78

prevention of overweight/obesity and, 159

social support interventions in community settings, 161

weight-related social problems, 2

Sodas

ban on sale of large sugary drinks in New York City, 178–179

students who drank/did not drink soda, 71t

taxes on, 137

See also Beverages

Sodium, 162

Solovay, Sondra, 142

Solving the Problem of Childhood Obesity within a Generation: White House Task Force on Childhood Obesity Report to the President (White House Task Force on Childhood Obesity), 119

Sonnenberg, Lillian, 134

The South Beach Diet: The Delicious, Doctor-Designed, Foolproof Plan for Fast and Healthy Weight Loss (Agatston), 89

South Beach/Glycemic Index, 89

Southwest Airlines, 141

Spain, 57

SparkPeople, 114

Speranza, Mario, 50–51

Sprehe, Michael R., 4

Spurlock, Morgan, 134

SSBs (sugar-sweetened beverages), 69–70

Stanley, Alessandra, 144

Starchy foods, 149

"State- and Payer-Specific Estimates of Annual Medical Expenditures Attributable to Obesity" (Trogdon et al.), 118

State Indicator Report on Fruits and Vegetables, 2013 (CDC), 15

"State Intervention in Life-Threatening Childhood Obesity" (Murtagh & Ludwig), 180

"State Survey of Coverage of Obesity Interventions Finds Coverage of Treatment Options Limited for Overweight and Obese Populations across the United States" (Ferguson), 119

States

fruit/vegetable consumption by adults/adolescents, by state, 16t

Medicaid coverage for obesity treatment, 119–120

obesity epidemic, cost of to, 118

state attorneys call to action for war on obesity, 133

state/community funding for prevention efforts, 166

Statistical information

adult BMI chart, 10t

adults age 18+ who engaged in regular physical activity, by race/ethnicity, 107f

adults age 18+ who engaged in regular physical activity, percentage of, 106f

adults by weight category, annual average, 174f

arthritis, obesity among adults with/without, 40f

binge eating, prevalence of, 48f

bulimia prevalence/demographics/treatment, 51f

caloric sweeteners for domestic food/beverage use, total estimated deliveries of, by calendar year, 130t

calorie needs, estimated, by age, sex, physical activity, 164f

cholesterol levels among persons, 35t

diagnosed diabetes among adults aged 18+ years, 39f

food away from home, total expenditures for, 18t–19t

food expenditures as share of disposable personal income, 23t–24t

food marketed to children via "advergames," 73t

fruit/vegetable consumption by adults/adolescents, by state, 16t

funding for various research/conditions/disease categories, 121t–124t

high school students engaging in dangerous dieting behaviors, 50(t3.2)

high school students who ate fruit/drank fruit juice 2+ times/day, 68(t4.6)

high school students who met recommended levels of physical activity, 77t

high school students who used computers/played video games/watched television for 3+ hours/day, 68(t4.5)